Depression in Late Life

SECOND EDITION

Depression in Late Life

Dan G. Blazer, II, M.D., Ph.D.
J.P. Gibbons Professor of Psychiatry
Dean of Medical Education
Duke University School of Medicine
Durham, North Carolina

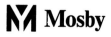 Mosby

St. Louis Baltimore Boston Chicago London Philadelphia Sydney Toronto

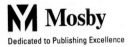
Mosby

Dedicated to Publishing Excellence

Editor: Robert Farrell
Editorial Assistant: Andrea Whitson
Project Manager: Carol Sullivan Wiseman
Senior Production Editor: Diana Lyn Laulainen
Senior Designer: Jeanne Wolfgeher

Second Edition
Copyright © 1993 by Mosby–Year Book, Inc.

Previous edition copyrighted 1982

Printed in the United States of America

Mosby–Year Book, Inc.
11830 Westline Industrial Drive
St. Louis, Missouri 63146

Library of Congress Cataloging in Publication Data

Blazer, Dan G. (Dan German)
    Depression in late life / Dan G. Blazer II. — 2nd ed.
        p.   cm.
    Includes bibliographical references and index.
    ISBN 0-8016-7434-4
    1. Depression in old age.   I. Title.
    [DNLM: 1. Depression—in old age.   WM 171 B645d 1993]
    RC537.5.B58   1993
    618.97'68527—dc20
    DNLM/DLC   93-513
    for Library of Congress   CIP

93 94 95 96 97 CL/DC 9 8 7 6 5 4 3 2 1

To
Sherrill,
Tasha,
and
Trey.

Preface to the First Edition

This book is intended for professionals providing care and treatment for depressed elderly persons. It is aimed at those clinicians who are most likely to encounter such patients, including primary care physicians, geriatricians, psychiatrists, geriatric psychiatrists, psychologists, psychiatric nurses, and social workers. Students of the phenomenon of late life depression may also find the material of value. I wrote this book from my own experience as a clinician who has found depression to be the most prevalent psychiatric symptom in the inpatient wards of Duke Hospital and in the outpatient medical and psychiatric clinics. The orientation of the material presented is eclectic, reflecting my own view of the understanding and management of this problem. Multiple factors must be considered in the etiology, and multiple targets are available to the clinician for intervention. I realize that this orientation may appear cumbersome to some, but my clinician experience suggests that it simplifies rather than complicates management. Readers must judge for themselves, for the measure of this approach is its usefulness.

A major purpose for writing this monograph is to demarcate the body of knowledge regarding late life depression. What do we know, and what do we speculate? A comprehensive approach to patient care must be grounded in our knowledge of the condition that we are treating. Basic biologic, psychologic, social, and epidemiologic data provide a framework upon which diagnosis and treatment can be effected. No attempt has been made to cite every study relevant to the subject, but many studies are drawn upon that are representative of both the present and past literature. Material presented on diagnosis and treatment has been made to conform to the third edition of the *Diagnostic and Statistical Manual of Mental Disorders* (Washington, D.C., 1980, American Psychiatric Association) whenever possible. This recent approach to diagnosis represents a revolution in psychiatric nomenclature.

The organization of the book reflects its purpose. First, an overview of late life depression in its historic context helps clarify the present discrepancy in orientation and subsequent debates about the phenomenon of depression in late life. In Part Two depression in late life is described in terms of its symptoms, signs, and outcomes. In Part Three the psychobiology, psychology, sociology, and epidemiology of depression are interlaced with our knowledge of the normal aging process. The diagnostic workup and differential diagnosis are presented in Part Four. Unipolar and bipolar affective disorders, bereavement and depressive neuroses, and depression secondary to physical illness and alcohol use are among the more common subtypes of late life depression. Each of these is reviewed in Part Five with case presentations to illustrate diagnostic and treatment techniques. Finally, in Part Six the common therapeutic techniques of psychotherapy, family therapy, pharmacologic therapy, electroconvulsive therapy, physical therapies, and nutritional therapies are reviewed. The unique applications in the long-term care facility of treatment that requires careful attention to milieu are also presented in Part Six.

Styles of learning are different. Some students prefer to obtain a firm grasp of the clinical picture of a disorder prior to acquiring basic science information. Others prefer to build their clinical knowledge on a foundation of basic data. To accommodate these various styles of learning, some persons may want to read Part Five before Part Three. Others may prefer to go back and forth from one section to another. Still others may wish to read the entire monograph in sequence.

No preface could do justice to the many individuals who have contributed either directly or indirectly to this book. A few deserve special mention, however. First, I wish to thank my fellow faculty members who helped review chapters of this book. They include Jim Moore, M.D., Assistant Professor of Psychiatry; Ron Taska, M.D., Assistant Professor of Psychiatry; John Rhoads, M.D., Professor of Psychiatry; Jeffrey Houpt, M.D., Associate Professor of Psychiatry; Berton Kaplan, Ph.D., Professor of Epidemiology, School of Public Health, University of North Carolina; Linda George, Ph.D., Associate Professor of Medical Sociology; Ralph Cooper, Ph.D., Assistant Professor of Psychiatry; Ilene Siegler, Ph.D., Associate of Medical Psychology; and William P. Wilson, M.D., Professor of Psychiatry.

My colleagues and mentors in the Department of Psychiatry and in the Center for the Study of Aging at Duke University Medical Center are a major part of the social network that facilitates the scholarly pursuit and clinical application of knowledge relevant to the care of the elderly. First, I wish to express my gratitude for their continued support and constant availability to my mentors, Ewald W. Busse, M.D.; J.P. Gibbons, Professor of Psychiatry and Dean of the Medical School; George Maddox, Ph.D., Professor of Medical Sociology and Director of the Center for the Study of Aging; and Keith H. Brodie, M.D., Professor and Chairman of the Department of Psychiatry. To my colleagues, Alan Whanger, M.D., Professor of Psychiatry; Adrian Verwoerdt, M.D., Professor of Psychiatry; James Moore, M.D., Assistant Professor of Psychiatry; Shan Wang, M.D., Professor of Psychiatry; and Dan Gianturco, M.D., Professor of Psychiatry, I express my thanks for being included in a group of clinicians and scholars who have devoted themselves to the study and care of the elderly.

Joanne Steuer, Ph.D., and Lee Hyer, Ph.D., were most gracious to provide their own orientations in two areas in which they are especially qualified. Dr. Steuer has been my colleague and associate for the past 2 years, and I have been impressed with her knowledge and dedication to the psychotherapeutic treatment of the depressed elderly. Dr. Hyer has been a postdoctoral student with me and has taught me much about the measurement of and intervention in the long-term care facility. He adds a unique perspective to this book.

Finally, I wish to thank Mrs. Thelma Jernigan, my secretary, who has labored through many manuscripts in the past 3 years, and especially Ms. Karen Berger, Editor at Mosby. Ms. Berger has been vigilant and supportive throughout this process and has made my association with Mosby a pleasure.

Dan G. Blazer II

Preface to the Second Edition

The pupose for writing a second edition of *Depression in Late Life* is the same as the original purpose for writing this monograph (i.e., to demarcate the current body of knowledge relevant to the clinical care of elders experiencing depression). There has been an explosion of knowledge regarding late life depression since I wrote the first edition, and therefore the second edition cannot be properly entitled a "revision" but is, more properly, a new book. The structure of the monograph, however, remains unchanged. I have eliminated the introductory chapter (combining it with the chapter on epidemiology) and the chapter on depression in long-term care facilities (since the basic knowledge for managing depressed elders in long-term care facilities fits well into the other chapters). A chapter has been added on depression and cognitive impairment, and the original chapter on unipolar and bipolar mood disorders has been split into two separate chapters. The chapter on bereavement has been separated from the chapter on depressive neuroses and minor depressive disorders. In addition,I have added a chapter on existential depression, a topic about which sparse hard data are available, yet a chapter that is essential to understanding late life depression in its broader context.

In contrast to the first edition, I have personally written this entire book. In this era of increased specialization, I believe it even more important for someone to research a broader topic, such as late life depression, comprehensively. By adopting a biopsychosocial perspective derived from my investigative efforts and applying this perspective to my clinical experience, I have attempted to be both thorough and consistent in my review.

Many persons from Duke University Medical Center have contributed directly by reviewing the chapters of this edition. They include the following: Stephen Ford, M.D., Associate in Psychiatry; Linda George, Ph.D., Professor of Medical Sociology in Psychiatry; Dana Hughes, Ph.D., Assistant Professor, School of Nursing; William McDonald, M.D., Assistant Professor of Psychiatry; Ranga Krishnan, M.D., Associate Professor of Psychiatry; Bernard J. Carroll, M.D., Ph.D., Professor of Psychiatry; Richard Weiner, M.D., Ph.D., Associate Professor of Psychiatry; Carolyn Haynes, M.D., Ph.D., Associate in Psychiatry; John C.S. Breitner, M.D., M.P.H., Associate Professor of Psychiatry; Harold Koenig, M.D., M.H.S., Assistant Professor of Psychiatry; Karen Wells, Ph.D., Assistant Professor of Medical Psychology; and Eugene Broadhead, M.D., Ph.D., Associate Professor of Community and Family Medicine.

The Department of Psychiatry, the Center for the Study of Aging and Human Development, and the Clinical Research Center for the Study of Depression in Late Life, supported by the National Institute of Mental Health (MH-40159) were major supports of this endeavor. I wish to express my special gratitude for the continued support and constant availability of my mentors, Ewald W. Busse, M.D., J.P. Gibbons Professor of Psychiatry, Emeritus, and Associate Provost, Emeritus; George Maddox, Ph.D., Professor of Medical Sociology and Emeritus Director of the Center for the Study of Aging and Human Development; Bernard J. Carroll, M.D. Ph.D., Professor and Chair Emeritus of the Department of Psychiatry; and Harvey J. Cohen, M.D., Professor of Medicine and Director of the Center for Aging and Human Development.

Finally, I wish to thank Denise Smith, my Staff Assistant, who has labored through the many manuscripts and coordinated this activity in my office. Mosby Publishing has been exemplary in their work with me and, therefore, are major contributors to the quality of this text.

Dan G. Blazer, II, M.D., Ph.D.
Durham, North Carolina

Contents

Description and Distribution of Late Life Depression

P A R T O N E

Description and
Definition of
Late-Life
Depression

1

The Epidemiology of Depression in Late Life

"I'm old and getting older. There is nothing I can do about it." "I am lonely." "I forget what day it is because each day is just like another. The days are gray and run together." "I am so disgusted with my life. Some people always did everything exactly right. I did everything wrong." Older adults are thought to frequently make such statements. Depressive, hopeless, and helpless expressions are considered ubiquitous with the aging process. We view late life as a time of sadness and bitterness. Simone de DeBeauvoir (1970) tells of the young Buddah, Prince Siddartha, who would often leave his beautiful palace and ride into the countryside. Once on such a journey, he saw a tottering, wrinkled, white-haired, decrepit old man who was bent over, trembling, and mumbling something incomprehensible while he tottered along, balanced by a stick he used for a cane. The young prince was astonished and told the charioteer that "it's the world's pity, that weak and ignorant beings, drunk with the vanity of youth, do not behold old age. Let us hurry back to the palace. What is the use of pleasures in life, since I myself am the future dwelling-place of old age?"

Yet this perception of old age as depressing is not confirmed in scientific studies of the elderly. One of the best places to implement science is to study the nature and extent of sadness and depression among older adults. Epidemiology is the science that clinicians and clinical investigators implement to determine the burden of a health problem in a population, such as the problem of depression among older adults. Therefore epidemiology serves as a useful organizing theme to introduce the study of depression in late life.

Both art and science are necessary, however, to practice clinical medicine, psychiatry, and counseling. Although clinicians vary in the degree to which science influences their practices, more often than not the clinical practitioner in the community tends to degrade the science of clinical practice (while at the same time taking advantages of scientific breakthroughs). Science to the clinician is not always intelligible and frequently is not relevant to clinical practice. Therefore the clinicion may revert to a case history approach to clinical psychiatry and devalue the results of systematic studies.

Platt (1952) further commented on the use of science in clinical practice. "Wherein then lies the need for training physicians in science . . . first . . . the training is needed because scientific discipline is the anecdote to a surfeit of the art of medicine, which, carried too far, degenerates into medical lifemanship. . . All power corrupts . . . power which a physician has to influence the lives of his patients is formidable. . . . The clinician who knows only the art (of medicine) may end by deceiving not only his patients but himself . . . self-deception is the sin against which scientific discipline protects."

Epidemiology places late life depression in its larger context and therefore is a useful place to begin the study of late life depression. Science cannot be limited to the clinician's office nor to the laboratory. Hippocrates recognized that "who ever wishes to investigate medicine properly should proceed thus: in the first place to consider the seasons of the year, and what effect each then produces. Then the winds . . . in the same manner, when one comes into a city to which he is a stranger, he should consider his situation, how it lies as to the wind and the rising of the sun . . . one should consider most attentively the water . . . and the mode in which the inhabitants live, and what are their pursuits, whether they are fond of drinking to excess, and given to indolence, or are fond of exercising and labor" (Hippocrates, 400 BC/1938).

Psychiatric epidemiology is the study of the distribution of psychiatric disorders or symptoms in human populations and the study of factors that influence those distributions, thus the goals of psychiatric epidemiology provide a framework for the humane scientific study of late life depression (Lilienfeld, 1980).

■ THE GOALS OF THE EPIDEMIOLOGIC STUDY OF LATE LIFE DEPRESSION

Morris (1975) described the domain of epidemiology as a set of tasks (or goals) to be accomplished before the clinical picture of a disease is completed. These tasks are especially applicable to chronic disorders such as late life depression. A modification of the tasks proposed by Morris and examples of questions relevant to the individual tasks include the following:

1. Identification of cases—can the symptom pattern of late life depressive disorders across populations be easily recognized and defined consistently across settings, such as the community versus a nursing home?
2. Distribution of late life depressive disorders in the population (prevalence and incidence)—what is the frequency of depressive disorders in older adults in long-term care facilities versus the community?
3. Historical trends of depressive disorders and suicide—have the rates of depressive disorders among the elderly decreased over the past 25 years?
4. Identification of causes of depressive disorders—does impaired social support contribute to the chronicity of depressive disorders in late life?

5. Prognosis—what is the likelihood of recovery from an episode of major depression in the elderly 1 year after diagnosis of the episode?
6. Need, demand, supply, and use of psychiatric services for depressed older adults—do older adults with depressive disorders seek psychiatric care?
7. Effectiveness of psychiatric treatment for late life depression—does long-term maintenance therapy with tricyclic antidepressants decrease the likelihood of relapse in an older adult who recovers from a major depressive episode?

These goals and the results of studies devoted to accomplishing them are reviewed in this chapter, with the following exceptions. The fifth task, making a prognosis, is discussed in detail in the chapter on the outcome from major depression. The fourth task, identification of causes, is reviewed in overview, with specific etiologic studies described in chapters devoted to the biologic, psychologic, social, and existential contributions to late life depression. The seventh goal, effectiveness of psychiatric treatment, is discussed in more detail in chapters devoted to specific treatment modalities, such as psychotherapy, pharmacotherapy, and electroconvulsive therapy. The evaluation of the effectiveness of treatment, however, is addressed at the end of this chapter.

■ IDENTIFICATION OF CASES

Grouping of individuals into classes for comparison is essential to the scientific method. Manifestational criteria are used to group persons according to similarity of symptoms, signs, or physiologic changes. These groupings can be made a priori or a posteri. The DSM diagnostic system is an example of an a priori grouping of symptoms, a consensus of clinical opinion about the core criteria of psychiatric disorders. A committee was convened by the National Institute of Mental Health and the American Psychiatric Association to explore the possibilities for modifying DSM-III (and DSM-III-R) to better accommodate psychiatric disorders in the elderly. Regarding the mood disorders, three a priori modifications to DSM-III-R were recommended by clinicians. The first was to simultaneously evaluate cognitive status and depressive symptoms. This could be accomplished by including symptoms of cognitive dysfunction in the Axis I diagnostic criteria or by adding an additional axis to permit evaluation of cognitive functioning. A second recommendation was to include a category of *minor depression* in DSM-IV to accommodate older adults who do not meet criteria for major depression or dysthymia but nevertheless suffer clinically significant depressive symptoms not explained by environmental stressors. The third recommendation was a diagnostic category that recognized the frequent coexistence of depression and anxiety. These recommendations, in general, were not derived from nor substantiated by empirical studies of clusters of symptoms and signs in the elderly. Instead, they were developed on the basis of clinical experience. A posteri case identification has also been applied to the study of depressive symptoms in older adults. We (Blazer et al, 1987) reviewed 37 subjects (18 middle-aged and 19 elderly) who were hospitalized with the diagnosis of major depression with melancholia. Neither depressive symptoms in general nor symptoms specifically associated with melancholic or endogenous depression differed across age groups, except for a higher prevalence of weight loss and a lower prevalence of suicidal thoughts in the elderly.

Using a new statistical procedure, grade-of-membership analysis, to classify adults suffering depressive symptoms in both the clinical and community populations, we found that older adults cluster on two "pure types": one that is similar to major depression with melancholia and another that can be described as mild-to-moderate depressive symptoms associated with significant cognitive difficulties (Blazer et al, 1989). Therefore the a posteri approach to case identification confirms the usefulness of the a priori defined major depression with melancholia (as per DSM-III) in diagnosing depressed older adults. Nevertheless, other depressive syndromes appear to be present among older persons, especially a mixed depressive and cognitive impairment syndrome (which supports the recommendation to include cognitive dysfunction in the diagnostic criteria for depression in late life).

Causal criteria, in contrast to manifestational criteria, are used to group individuals according to a specified experience believed to be the cause of the disorder (MacMahon and Pugh, 1970). An example of causal criteria is the cluster of symptoms that, as Lindemann (1944) suggested, follow a catastrophe and constitute bereavement.

Persons classified by one set of criteria may be distributed differently if other criteria are used, yet clinical groupings often correspond closely. For example, bereaved individuals, as described by Lindemann, usually qualify for a diagnosis of bereavement according to DSM-III. In studies of etiology using epidemiologic methods, clinicians and clinical investigators must take care not to include causal criteria in the diagnostic classification. In clinical practice, however, use of one scheme of classification does not exclude the concurrent use of the other. Axis IV of DSM-III (and DSM-III-R) in contrast to Axis I (which codes diagnosis) provides a coding of the overall severity of the stressor judged to have been a contributor to the development or exacerbation of the disorder classified according to the symptoms in Axis I (DSM-III, 1980; DSM-III-R, 1987).

Copeland (1981), when posing the question: "What is a case?" asked a second question "A case for what?" He noted that the concept of *case* is a chimera that exists only in the mind of the investigator and is not a "reality." Case identification can therefore be accomplished by methods other than diagnosis. In reality, diagnosed "cases" of major depression are not isolated from cognitive impairment, anxiety, and disruptions in the support networks of the depressed individual. Two approaches to case identification, other than specific diagnoses, have been used in psychiatric epidemiologic studies, depending on the goals of the investigator.

The most frequently used approach in epidemiologic studies is not diagnoses (because diagnoses are difficult to assign, especially in community populations) but rather the frequency of depressive symptoms (Murrell et al, 1983; Berkman et al, 1986). Yet another approach to case identification, frequently used in the study of psychiatric disorders in late life, is *mental health functioning*. Blazer (1978) reported the prevalence of mental health impairment in a community population of 997 adults 65 years of age and older, disregarding diagnoses. Over 13% of the sample suffered "moderate to complete mental impairment," defined as having "definite psychiatric symptoms and/or intellectual impairment which interfered at least in part with the ability of subjects to handle major problems of life."

The potential of biologic markers, and laboratory diagnostic tests, such as the dexamethasone suppression test (Carroll et al, 1981) and polysomnography (Kupfer et al,

1978), for identifying cases of depressive disorders in the elderly must be evaluated on the basis of the ability of the clinician to identify a case reliably. Validity tests of these diagnostic procedures depend on a reliable classification of subjects clinically into categories of either experiencing a disorder or not experiencing a disorder. In other words the gold standard for evaluating biologic markers is case identification.

Currently, reliability refers to the repeatability of diagnostic classification across clinicians and through time. Two clinicians evaluating a subject simultaneously should classify that individual into the same diagnostic category. Clinicians evaluating a subject at two points in time should be able to classify the individual as meeting criteria for the same diagnosis at two different points in time. These tests of reliability are designated respectively *interrater reliability* and *test-retest reliability*. A change in status of older adults experiencing mood disorders (their symptoms do not remain static) complicates test-retest reliability.

For a diagnosis to be valid, according to Goodwin and Guze (1979) the diagnostic criteria that define a category should do the following:

1. Permit the category to be distinguished on the basis of patterns of symptomatology;
2. Predict the outcome of the disorder;
3. Reflect underlying biologic reality, confirmed by family history in genetic studies;
4. Correspond with laboratory studies that are markers for the pathophysiology of the disease process;
5. Identify persons who will respond to specific therapeutic interventions, such as a particular psychotherapy or a specific group of medications (Weissman and Klerman, 1978; Blazer, 1989).

The scientific study of late life depression depends on reliable and valid case identification. Prevalence and incidence studies, discussed next, are especially dependent on accurate case identification.

■ DISTRIBUTION OF DEPRESSIVE DISORDERS IN LATE LIFE

Sources of Data

Three sources of data have been used to study the distribution of depressive disorders in late life: psychiatric case registries, surveys of institutional and clinical populations, and general population surveys. Each of these sources has advantages and limitations for determining the distribution of depressive disorders in the population. The best means for estimating the prevalence and distribution of the late life depressive disorders is to use these methods complementarily, especially if the sources use similar diagnostic criteria.

Psychiatric case registries are the least effective of the approaches to case identification and are reviewed briefly. A psychiatric case registry is a central file that includes information about all persons with the diagnosis of a mental disorder, such as depressive disorder, and contact with a group of psychiatric care facilities over time. Demographic variables, such as age, gender, race, and socioeconomic status, are usually available in case registries. Inpatient facilities, outpatient clinics, private psychiatric practitioners, and social service agencies are contacted periodically to obtain information about use. Case registries are most useful in the investigation of the use of psychiatric treatments by the chronically ill, especially those with long-term disability resulting from a particular disorder. The recurrent nature of depressive disorders across the life cycle leads to multiple contacts with several service providers over time. For example, the reports by Angst (1986) on the course of mood disorders were derived from case registry studies in Switzerland. From these studies, Angst determined that the usual course of mood disorders over the life span is of recurrent, solitary depressive episodes separated by intervals of many symptom-free years. Previous number of episodes is the best predictor of recurrence of depressive episodes in the future and rate of recurrence does not vary by age.

The psychiatric case registry is a poor source of data for estimating the prevalence and incidence of depressive disorders in the elderly, especially in the United States. Many elderly individuals who suffer depressive symptoms do not contact mental health professionals (or any professionals for that matter). If they are seen by a primary care physician or social agencies, the depressive symptoms may be overlooked or may not be diagnosed as a depressive disorder and therefore are not counted. Depression in late life is usually not so severe as to require inevitable psychiatric care, especially hospitalization in a psychiatric facility. In countries, such as in Scandinavia, where the delivery of psychiatric care is more centralized, case registries may useful for estimating prevalence. For example, Sorensen and Stromgren (1961), from a case registry of Samso, Denmark (n = 1412), estimated that 3% of the population had active or inactive depression. Rates were higher for women and persons 60 to 70 years of age.

Surveys of institutions and outpatient facilities are a second source of epidemiologic data about the distribution of late life depression. These surveys have traditionally fallen into two groups, based on methods of case identification: those using symptoms screens and those using structured clinical interviews. The latter have predominated in recent years (Koenig et al, 1988; O'Riordan et al, 1989; Parmelee et al, 1989; Ames, 1990). These surveys have an advantage over psychiatric case registries in that uniform methods of case identification are used, thus avoiding the potential classification bias of the psychiatric case registry. When all treatment sites within the same geographic area are surveyed simultaneously, however, individuals receiving treatment from multiple facilities may be counted more than once, which overestimates the number of cases. Surveys of treatment facilities, however, are likely to underestimate the prevalence of mood disorders in the elderly because most elderly do not seek help for their depressive symptoms.

The third source of data for determining the frequency and distribution of mood disorders is a population survey. Most psychiatric epidemiology surveys have used symptom screens to evaluate the burden of symptoms of community residents rather than using diagnostic criteria for specific psychiatric disorders. Symptom screens, usually in the form of checklists, are easily administered by nonprofessionals to community residents and are nonthreatening to persons being interviewed. Unfortunately, they cannot identify cases of specific psychiatric disorders. The Epidemiologic Catchment Area study, the results of which are reviewed later, therefore used the Diagnostic Interview Schedule (DIS). The DIS was designed for use by lay interviewers, but, unlike its predecessors, it reliably identifies cases of specific psychiatric disorders as defined by the DSM-III nomenclature.

Some population surveys have used clinicians for case identification. The cost of fielding a survey with trained mental health personnel to screen enough persons within the community for reliable prevalence estimates of major psychiatric disorders, such as depression, is usually economically unfeasible. Even when such surveys are feasible, the reliability of psychiatric diagnosis may be poor. To facilitate improved reliability of clinical interviews in the community, Wing, Cooper, and Satorious (1974) designed the Present State Examination (PSE), a semistructured interview in which the clinician determines the presence or absence of a series of symptoms and signs, such as depressed mood, delusions, and ideas of reference. The diagnosis is then generated by a computerized program that identifies clusters of symptoms. The Schedule for Affective Disorders and Schizophrenia (SCADS) and Structured Clinical Interview for DSM-III Diagnoses (SCID) are more structured than the PSE but less than the DIS. Both require clinicians to administer the instruments.

Community surveys are the only direct means for estimating prevalence, assuming that it is possible to accurately identify cases. However, most community surveys fail to accurately sample persons with psychiatric disorders who intermittently reside in institutions and the more impaired elders in the community who may refuse to participate in the community survey. Accurate assessment of prevalence is possible only when community and institutional residents have been surveyed simultaneously. Care must be taken to avoid double counting. The impact of the increasing rates of institutionalization on overall rates of depressive symptoms among the elderly is presented in Figure 1-1.

Measures of the Frequency of Depressive Disorders

Measures of disease frequency, stated in terms permitting comparison across populations or subgroups within a population, are the foundation of epidemiology (MacMahon and Pugh, 1970). To allow for differences in population size or for comparisons within populations, disease frequency is expressed as the number of cases of a disease or char-

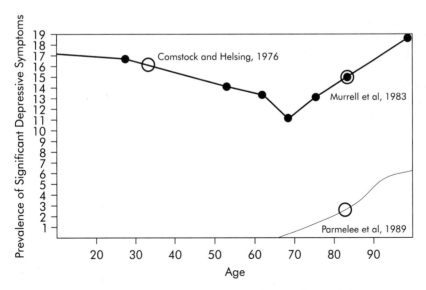

Figure 1-1. The association of institutionalization and the prevalence of depressive symptoms by age.

acteristic per unit of the population or group in which it is observed per unit of time. The most commonly used measure in psychiatric epidemiology is point prevalence— the number of persons with current symptoms of a psychiatric disorder, such as depression, in a sample of the population studied at a particular point in time. Point prevalence provides an estimate of the current burden of a disease but does not provide information about either disease course or changing patterns in disease frequency through time.

Estimating point-prevalent cases of late life depression in a sample can be used in retrospective or prospective studies. For example, incidence (discussed next) can only be determined once point prevalence is determined.

Since point prevalence can rarely be measured directly (i.e., a community survey cannot be completed in a single day), most prevalence studies actually estimate period prevalence (the number of cases coming into existence during a given period— usually the period of the survey). Lifetime prevalence of depressive disorders is the percentage of individuals at a given point in time with a history, past or present, of a depressive disorder. A past history of a depressive disorder is a major predictor for future depressive episodes (Angst, 1980). The problem of recall affects lifetime prevalence estimates in most community surveys, especially among the elderly.

Incidence complements prevalence estimates. Cumulative incidence is the probability of developing a disorder during a specified period of time, usually 1 year. In other words, incidence is the number of new cases of depression in a sample not suffering from depression at the time of the onset of the period of surveillance (which can only be determined if prevalent cases of depression are identified at the beginning of the study).

Incident measures, however, present a problem to the psychiatric epidemiologist. Dysthymic disorder (chronic depression) is a chronic condition and therefore equivalent to chronic physical illnesses, such as arteriosclerotic heart disease and diabetes mellitus. Therefore those who suffer dysthymic disorder would not be included in an incidence study, although they may not be suffering clinically significant symptoms currently. Other depressive disorders, however, are isolated events that more closely parallel the infectious disease model (an adjustment disorder with depressed mood). In such cases, exposure to a stressor, such as an illness, can cause depressive symptoms that spontaneously remit when the stressor is removed or adaption occurs. Unipolar depressive disorders of predominantly biologic etiology tend to be episodic and thus fall between the chronic disease model and the infectious disease model. These disorders are chronic in that they have a propensity to recur. They are acute in that each episode may be strongly influenced by environmental factors at the time of onset and may remit completely. The types of mood disorders differentiated by symptom presentation through time are illustrated in Figure 1-2. Individuals with a history of symptoms of a depression should be excluded from studies that estimate new cases of depression. However, these same individuals could be included in studies of recurrent depressive episodes.

The lifetime expectancy for developing a specific psychiatric disorder, such as depression, although of great interest to researchers and clinicians, can rarely be estimated directly but must be calculated from measures including predictions of the life span and prevalence rates for different age groups. Lifetime expectancy must not be confused with incidence, the likelihood of people at risk (but who do not presently experience the illness) developing the illness over a specified period of time (usually 1 year).

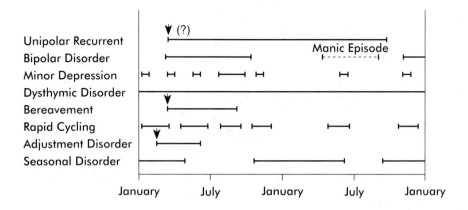

Figure 1-2. Examples of mood disorders as they are differentiated by symptom presentation through time.

If an etiologic factor is periodically operational, a population may be at risk for the de-velopment of a psychiatric disorder for only a circumscribed period of time (MacMahon and Pugh, 1970). An unpredictable catastrophic event (e.g., a nursing home fire) or a predictable but stressful event (e.g., movement from a house to a different living arrange-ment) can lead to the onset of depressive symptoms during and for a time after the event. The usual measure of the likelihood of developing a disorder such as depression in these circumstances is the *attack rate*, which represents the number of persons developing an ill-ness divided by the number of individuals effected by the event under study.

The duration of a depressive episode interacts with both incidence and prevalence. In studies of late life depression the point at which a case is identified rarely corresponds to the onset of the disorder (i.e., the individual does not seek medical care at the onset of a depressive episode). Most surveys do not assess people at enough points in time to identify the exact point at which the depressive episode began, and the time of onset usually cannot be attributed to a given day or even month. In most cases of depression in older adults a series of events lead to the overt syndrome. Environmental etiologic factors may influence a vulnerable individual, causing subclinical biologic changes (e.g., changes in circadian rhythms or hormone levels). These changes are later manifested as symptoms and subsequently a diagnosis is made. Recall of the day or week of symptom onset not only can be biased by poor memory but usually does not represent the point at which the biologic and psychologic changes characteristic of the depressive disorder began. As descriptions of depressive symptoms become more reliable with the use of operational diagnostic criteria, such as DSM-III, III-R, and IV, the points of onset and termination will be more accurately measured. Yet symptoms alone will never provide an accurate determination of the onset of depression.

Duration of an illness episode is also a criterion for many diagnoses. Cross-sectional symptom measures that do not include a measure of duration are less useful in identifying cases of psychiatric disorder. Examples of illness episodes from the major categories of mood disorders are presented in Figure 1-2. At a given point in time, the prevalence incidence of depressive symptoms in a population are determined by both the frequency and duration of the mood disorders in the population. Prevalence studies usually include dysthymic disorders, episodes of bereavement and adjustment disorders with depressive features, major depression, and less well-defined syndromes (e.g., minor depression).

A subject in a population study may suffer from more than one syndrome at a given point in time. Diagnosis also may predict the probability of depressive symptoms being present at the time of assessment in some cases. For example, individuals with seasonal affective disorders are more likely to experience depressive symptoms in the fall and winter than in the spring and summer. Persons with melancholic depression are more likely to experience depressive symptoms in the morning and than the afternoon, in contrast to more psychogenic depressive syndromes. A 1-year period prevalence study of depressive symptoms could identify cases of many different disorders (see Figure 1-2). Without differential diagnosis, the relative contribution of each diagnostic category to overall depressive morbidity would be unknown.

The interrelation of prevalence, incidence, and duration of depressive episodes is diagramed in Figure 1-3. When duration does not vary according to age (such as the studies by Keller et al [1981] and Murphy [1983] suggest), prevalence and incidence present as almost overlapping lines. In the incidence study by Hagnell et al (1990), previous history of a depressive episode does not rule out an individual from developing an incident case of depression. Incidence, therefore, almost parallels prevalence across the life cycle. Similar data are not available for minor depression, but a hypothetical case is presented based on the clinical observation that minor depressive episodes are of shorter durations as individuals age. In such a circumstance, even if the incidence of minor depression were to increase with age, prevalence would remain constant or perhaps even decrease (because duration of episodes would decrease).

An understanding of the interaction of prevalence, incidence, and duration, as well as the mix of depressive syndromes that may contribute to the burden of depression in a population, is necessary if the prevalence and distribution of depressive symptoms in a population study are to be understood.

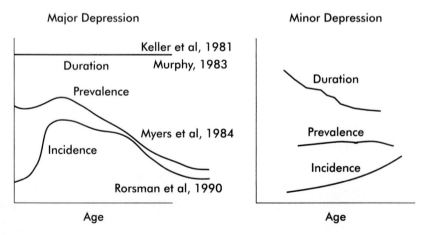

Figure 1-3. The interrelation of prevalence and duration of depressive episodes with incidence. Major and minor depression are used as examples.

■ RESULTS FROM EPIDEMIOLOGIC STUDIES

Estimates of the prevalence and incidence of depression in late life are presented below from a variety of community and clinical samples. The cited studies do not exhaust the literature but demonstrate the consistency of results found using different methods of case identification. Lack of a standard method of case identification makes comparisons across studies difficult. Most investigators report only prevalence rates and do not report the duration of those prevalent cases identified. In such cases, exploration of the interaction of prevalence, incidence, and duration is impossible.

A variety of symptom checklists have been used to evaluate the burden of clinically significant depressive symptoms in community samples (Table 1-1). The results of these studies are remarkably consistent, with the vast majority of reports estimating a prevalence of approximately 15%, with a range from 10% to 25%. Results vary geographically, even when the same case identification instrument is used. For example, Kennedy

TABLE 1-1. Prevalence of Depression Symptoms in Community Samples of Older Adults

Author	Sample	n	Screening Method	Findings
Blazer and Williams, 1980	Community sample of Durham, N.C. (65+)	997	OARS Depression Scale	14.7% significant dysphoric symptoms. No significant age, gender, or racial differences in prevalence.
Murrell et al, 1983	Community sample of Kentucky (55+)	2517	CES-D	16% significant depressive symptoms. Symptoms more prevalent in the oldest old and females.
Kivela et al, 1986	Community sample in Finland	1529	Zung SDS	29.7% of females and 22.4% of males with significant depressive symptoms.
Ben-Arie et al, 1987	Community sample of the elderly "coloured persons" in Cape Town, South Africa	139	PSE symptoms	13% with significant depressive symptoms.
Berkman et al, 1986	Community sample in New Haven	2806	CES-D	16% with significant depressive symptoms. Symptoms more prevalent in females and the oldest old.
Kennedy et al, 1989	Community sample in the Bronx	2137	CES-D	16.9% with significant depressive symptoms. Symptoms more prevalent in females and the oldest old.
O'Hara et al, 1985	Community sample in Iowa	3159	CES-D	9% with significant depressive symptoms. Symptoms more common in females.

found almost double the prevalence of significant depressive symptoms in the elderly in an intercity population (Bronx, New York) as that reported by O'Hara et al (1985) in rural Iowa using the CES-D.

Estimates of the prevalence of dysthymia and major depression from various community surveys are presented in Table 1-2. Estimates from the ECA studies by age and gender are presented in Figure 1-4. The prevalence of major depression is much lower in community samples than is the prevalence of depressive symptoms, approximating 1% to 5%. Again, samples that are geographically separated reveal different estimates. The period prevalence of major depression in a mixed urban and rural sample in North Carolina (Blazer et al, 1987) was less than 1% compared with 5.4% in northeastern, urban New Haven (Weissman and Myers, 1978). If the prevalence of dysthymic disorder and depression are added (which will overestimate the prevalence of subjects suffering both disorders, because they often occur simultaneously), the majority of subjects suffering significant depressive symptoms in the community do not meet the criteria for either disorder. One of the major tasks facing psychiatric epidemiologists studying depression in the elderly is to explain the residue of depressive symptoms in community samples. Minor depression, one potential explanation, is discussed in Chapter 11.

The prevalence of depression in acute medical facilities as reported in a number of studies, is presented in Table 1-3. Estimates range from around 5% to 10% for major depression. More significantly, approximately 25% suffer clinically significant symptoms not captured by the diagnosis of major depression. The same is true for estimates of prevalence in long-term care facilities (Table 1-4). Estimates again range between 5%

TABLE 1-2. Prevalence of Dysthymic and Major Depression in Community Samples of Older Adults

Author	Sample	n	Screening Method	Findings
Bollerup, 1975	Community sample of nine Copenhagen suburbs	626	Psychiatric evaluation	1% with bipolar or unipolar depression; 12 with depressive neurosis.
Weissman and Myers, 1978	Community sample of New Haven	111	SADS	5.4% with major depression; 2.7% with minor depression.
Copeland et al, 1987	Community sample of Liverpool	1070	Geriatric Mental State Schedule	2.9% with depressive psychosis; 8.3% with depressive neurosis.
Kua, 1990	Community sample of Chinese in Singapore	612	Geriatric Mental State Schedule	4.6% with depressive disorder (both psychosis and neurosis).
O'Hara et al, 1985	Community sample in Iowa	3159	RDC criteria	2.9% with major depression.
Blazer et al, 1987	Community sample in North Carolina	1304	DIS	0.8% with major depression; 2% with dysthymia.
Weissman et al, 1988	Samples of the US community	18,000	DIS	1.8% to 0.6% with major depression; 3.0% to 1.5% with dysthymia.

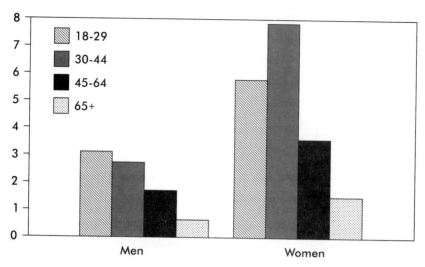

Figure 1-4. Current (1 year) prevalence of mood disorders by age and gender. Estimates derived from the epidemiologic catchment area study.

TABLE 1-3. Prevalence of Depression in Acute Care Medical Facilities

Author	Sample	n	Diagnostic Method	Findings
Koenig et al, 1988	VA inpatient service of men (70+)	171	Screening and modified DIS	11.5% major depression; 23% other depressive syndromes.
O'Riordan et al, 1989	Acute medical geriatric assessment unit (66+)	111	Geriatric Depression Scale and clinical interview	4.5% major depression; 3.6% dysthymic disorder; 10.8% depressive symptoms with dementia.
Rapp et al, 1988	VA medical and surgical patients (65+) (not cognitively impaired)	150	Screening Scales and SADS/RDC	6% major depression; 3.3% minor depression; 6% with intermittent depression.
Cheah and Beard, 1980	Medical geriatric evaluation clinic	262	Psychiatric evaluation	31.3% dysphoria and depression; 7% moderate-to-severe cases.

and 15% for major depression, yet approximately 30% of the remaining subjects suffered clinically significant depressive symptoms. Prevalence studies of depression in outpatient facilities are relatively rare (Table 1-5). In general the estimates are lower than those reported for acute care settings and long-term care facilities, yet higher than found in community surveys.

Incidence studies are extremely rare, although two recent studies are reported. Rorsman et al (1990) provided data from the Lundby Cohort in Sweden of 2612 individuals evaluated in 1957 and 1972 (15-year incidence figures). Until 70 years of age, the cumulative probability over 15 years of developing a first episode of depression was 27% in

TABLE 1-4. Prevalence of Depression in Longer Term Facilities

Author	Sample	n	Diagnostic Method	Findings
Parmelee et al, 1989	Nursing home and congregate apartment resident	708	DSM-III-R checklist	12.4% major depression; 30.5% less severe but marked depressive symptoms.
Burns et al, 1988	National nursing home survey	526	Chart review and interview with nurse	23% "depressed."
Bond et al, 1989	Three British NHS nursing homes	568	Crichton Royal Behavioral Scale and the Survey Psychiatric Assessment Schedule	Between 31% and 43% with some affective disorder or psycho neurosis.
Ames, 1990	Twelve homes for the elderly	390	Geriatric Mental State Schedule	6% major depression; 11% other DSM-III diagnosis of affective disorder; 12.3% depressive symptoms with organic disorder.
Jensen, 1966	Residents of four homes for the aged	126	Psychiatric Evaluation	4% endogenous depression; 1% reactive.

TABLE 1-5. Prevalence of Depression in Outpatient Facilities among the Elderly

Author	Sample	n	Diagnostic Method	Findings
Boorson et al, 1986	Medical clinic at VA Hospital	406	Self-rating Depression Scale (SDS)	24% clinically significant depressive symptoms; 10% major depression.
Barrett et al, 1988	Primary care clinic	349	Screening instrument and SADS	5.6% major depression and episodic minor depression; 2.1% characterologic depression; 7.9% masked/suspected depression.

men and 45% in women (very high incidence estimates). The annual age-standardized first incidence for depression, all degrees of impairment included, was 0.43 for men and 0.76 for women. Incidence appeared to decrease in this study as individuals aged, especially for men. Foster et al (1990) reported the incidence of depression in medical long-term care facilities. In a cohort of 104 new admissions followed for 1 year, they estimated an incidence of approximately 14%. Approximately one third of these cases were diagnosed as major depression and two thirds as minor depression.

■ HISTORICAL TRENDS OF DEPRESSIVE DISORDERS AND SUICIDE

Historical investigations in epidemiology are directed to the frequency of events among populations at different points in time. Some diseases, such as tuberculosis, wax and wain in incidence and prevalence. Other diseases, such as AIDS dementia, appear, and still others, such as small pox, are eradicated (or disappear naturally) (Morris, 1975). Historical studies in psychiatric epidemiology are rare and therefore temporal changes in mental illness are difficult to determine. The reasons for the scarcity of such studies are threefold. First, temporal changes in psychiatric disorders usually evolve over years rather than months (e.g., the gradual disappearance of the dementia secondary to tertiary syphilis). Therefore longitudinal studies lasting the decades necessary to detect historical trends are rare. Second, concepts of case identification change through time, as most recently evidenced by the change in the approach to psychiatric diagnosis in the United States with the emergence of DSM-III. Finally, historical studies are plagued by methodologic difficulties, primarily the loss of subjects in longitudinal studies to follow-up.

Despite these difficulties, some interesting although infrequent reports of historical trends have emerged. The most consistent theme in recent reports is that psychiatric disorders have become more frequent in young adults and less frequent in older adults. Although this trend has been suggested for a variety of disorders, data are most plentiful for depression.

Klerman (1978) notes that in contrast to the "age of anxiety" that followed World War II, western society has entered an "age of melancholy," precipitated in large part by social factors such as the threat of nuclear warfare, the population explosion, and environmental pollution. Cross-sectional estimates by age from the Epidemiologic Catchment Area studies (Myers et al, 1984; Robins et al, 1984) show a significant decrease in both current and lifetime prevalence of major depression with increasing age. Klerman et al (1985), analyzing family history data from the Psychobiology of Depression Study, found a progressive increase in rates of depression in successively younger birth cohorts through the twentieth century and earlier age of onset of depression in each birth cohort. These trends, however, were not present in an underdeveloped county using similar methodology (Canino et al, 1987).

These cross-sectional data, however, must be considered within the context of historical trends. This context can be best exemplified by reviewing data on suicide by age, age of death, and birth cohort. Although suicide frequency is known to increase with increasing age, significant fluctuations in the association between age and suicide occur through time.

Suicide frequency, at a given point in historical time, is determined by three factors: age, generational or cohort effects, and unique stressors impacting on a particular age group at a particular point and time (i.e., period effects). Table 1-6 illustrates the impact of both age and birth cohort on suicide rates. If one attends to the rows (i.e., evaluates the suicide rates as age increases for a given birth cohort over a 20-year period), suicide rates for each birth cohort increase with age (at least after age 70) for white males. The older birth cohorts, however, experienced higher suicide rates at specific ages than the younger cohorts. This can be best appreciated by examining the diagonal of the table. For example, the suicide rate for 70 year olds declined from 43.5 per 100,000 population to 30.7 per 100,000 population among 70 year olds over the 20 years.

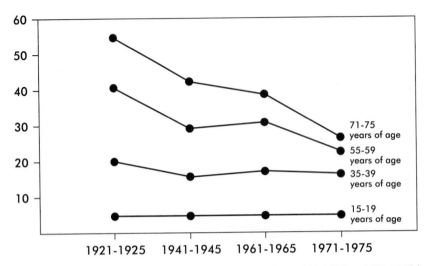

Figure 1-5. Suicide rate for males in the United Kingdom from 1921-1925 to 1971-1975 by age group. (From Murphy et al, 1986.)

TABLE 1-6. Suicide Rates for Males in the United States for Selected Birth Cohorts Over a 20-Year Period

Birth Cohort	1962	1972	1981
1922	23.7	28.4	26.7
	(40)	(50)	(50)
1912	34.6	33.9	30.7
	(50)	(60)	(70)
1902	38.5	39.0	43.5
	(60)	(70)	(80)
1892	43.5	45.8	54.2
	(70)	(80)	(90)

From Vital Statistics of the United States.
Figures in parentheses are ages of cohorts.

The impact of period effects can be observed in Figure 1-5 derived from a study by Murphy et al in the United Kingdom (1986). In this study, suicide among older males declined dramatically from 1961-1965 to 1971-1975, yet suicide for younger males remains relatively constant. Why did they find such a dramatic change in rates, especially for one age group in contrast to another? Murphy (and other investigators) has speculated that a change in the cooking gas used in the British Isles from a toxic (and therefore lethal) to a nontoxic gas may have eliminated one of the more common means of committing suicide by older males (i.e., by placing one's head in an oven and turning on the gas).

To interpret historical trends, one must consider age, period, and cohort effects. In relationship to the rates of depression (especially major depression) and suicide (which may be a marker of the more severe depressions), four consistent trends have emerged as the twentieth century nears its end. First, there is a trend for the prevalence of depression to be relatively constant across the life cycle for a given birth cohort (Srole and Fischer, 1980). Second, younger birth cohorts in the latter decades of the twentieth century appear to suffer much higher prevalences of depression than the older birth cohorts (Myers et al, 1984; Robins et al, 1984). Third, suicide rates increase with age for white males, regardless of birth cohort, therefore driving the overall suicide rate to increase with age, regardless of birth cohort (Blazer et al, 1986). Fourth, changes in the rates of suicide and depression by age group over the past 50 years have been of such magnitude that the varying rates are best explained by psychosocial rather than biologic or hereditary factors.

What factors contribute to the relative protection of older birth cohorts from depression and suicide in the 1990s compared with younger cohorts? What factors contribute to the relative increase in depression and suicide among younger cohorts in the 1990s? Definitive answers to these questions are not available, but informed speculation is possible. While speculating about these trends, investigators and clinicians must recognize the significant methodologic problems in historical studies. Reported suicide rates across the life cycle can be misleading, since suicide rates are obtained from review of death certificates and death certificates are subject to bias. For example, it is probably more likely that younger persons who commit suicide will be reported as suicide victims compared with older persons. For example, an older adult may take a fatal overdose of medication. Because the person is older it may be assumed, unless evidence suggests otherwise, that the elder died of natural causes and therefore late life suicide is probably underreported. Similar concerns exist for the estimates of prevalence by age (Tweed, in press). The reported trends are of such magnitude, however, that reporting bias alone cannot explain them.

One explanation for the increased prevalence of depression and suicide in younger compared with older birth cohorts is the relative protection of older cohorts (especially those between ages 70 and 90 during the early 1990s). After World War II, these cohorts fared well economically. They took advantage of the economic growth in Western society during the late 1940s and early 1950s. They became the first cohort of elders who consistently set aside retirement funds other than Social Security. They have full advantage of Medicare (often supplemented by private insurance).

From a review of mortality data, these older birth cohorts also appear to be significantly healthier than the cohorts that preceded them. Mortality rates among the elderly has decreased remarkably since 1970, especially among the oldest old, whereas rates of institutionalization have remained relatively constant. Therefore older people are living longer independently in the community. Given the well-recognized associations among depression, physical illness, and functional disability, current cohorts of elders may be less depressed because they are healthier.

Population statistics do not apply to all older adults, however. Many elders suffer significant depressive symptoms and these symptoms are often associated with economic impairment and/or functional disability (Kennedy et al, 1990). Suicide rates appear to increase among the young old, and suicide remains a major public health problem for older adults, regardless of birth cohort. The phenomena of relatively decreased rates of elderly depression compared with younger persons and the decline in suicide rates among the elderly from World War II until the 1980s may well be an historical phenomenon that is reversing in the 1990s. Perhaps the well-being of older adults is on the decline.

■ IDENTIFYING THE ETIOLOGY OF LATE LIFE DEPRESSION

Many theories attempt to explain the onset, manifestations, and durations of late life depression. These theories are explored in more detail in the chapters on biologic, psychologic, and social causes of depression (Chapters 4, 5, and 6). In most research the variables included in the study and interpretations drawn from the data reflect on hypothesized causal theory (Cassel and Leighton, 1969). In most of medicine, theories of causation are derived directly from discoveries of the association of an infectious agent, a genetic abnormality, or some type of external toxic agent. In the current era of biopathology, unitary causes are often sought. A unitary model, however, is inadequate for the study of late life depression. Psychopathologic disorders in general and late life depression in particular are not simply the result of some extraneous stress on normal aging but rather a "character of danger" that both normal and abnormal processes can acquire under given circumstances (Leighton et al, 1963). Multiple internal and external factors contribute to the onset of depression, including external physicochemical agents (e.g., food stuffs or pharmacologic agents), cognitive processes, physiologic substrates to emotions, and the social and cultural environment. From this large network of causes the clinical investigator searches for those few factors that are most important. To investigate causal factors, a representative model of the etiology of depression is necessary.

Even the concept of a network of causation, although useful, is oversimplified (MacMahon and Pugh, 1970). Some of the factors that enter into the etiology of late life depression are shown in Figure 1-6. Even in this complex diagram, not all causative factors are listed. Factors listed represent broad classes of factors rather than the specific factors that form the classes. Therefore the network of causative factors of late life depression may be thought of as a web, which, in its complexity and origins, is beyond total comprehension (MacMahon and Pugh, 1970). The factors represented within this web of causation lead to those behaviors and manifestations that are labelled *depression.* Yet depression is not a unitary construct. The relative contribution of the factors to the range of mood disorders will vary across those disorders. Therefore considerable emphasis has and will be directed in this monograph to the importance and difficulty in defining a *case* of late life depression and the importance of depressive subtypes.

Cassel and Leighton (1969) outlined a series of guidelines by which investigators can develop hypotheses regarding the causation of a disorder and then test these hypotheses. These guidelines, modified to determine the etiology of late life depression, include the following:

1. Genetic and biologic factors provide a substrate for the onset of depressive symptoms in late life, yet these biologic factors are neither necessary nor sufficient for the onset of late life depressions, except in rare circumstances.
2. Events during the entire course of an individual's life have the potential to precipitate the onset and course of depression in late life.
3. Depression, once it has emerged, merges with the older person's personality and perception of life satisfaction. Residual symptoms therefore frequently persist after the remission of the depressive disorder.
4. Sociocultural processes and situations concurrent with the mood disorder can contribute to a high level of disability or, conversely, can significantly reduce the level of disability secondary to late life depressions.

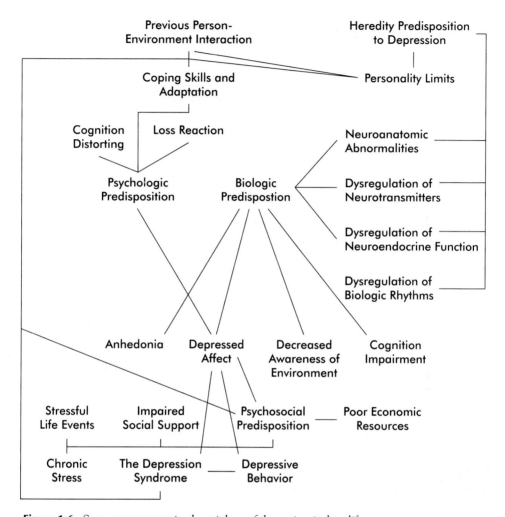

Figure 1-6. Some components in the etiology of depression in late life.

5. Depressive symptom complexes and clusters in late life may have their origins in combinations of innate factors, such as hereditary, biology, and psychology, and in social and cultural processes that mold these innate factors.

6. The degree of disability from late life depression is in part influenced by factors responsible for its origin but is, to a major degree, also influenced by psychologic stress resulting from social processes, such as conflict, rapid cultural change, migration, low socioeconomic status, and the disintegration and malfunction of social systems.

The clinician should not be discouraged when confronted with this complex etiologic web of causation. Exhaustive comprehension of the literature related to the etiology of late life depression is not necessary for effective treatment of patients. Instead, a general understanding of the interactive factors is essential. Therapeutic interventions may occur at various points in the web, each intervention having the potential to reverse or alleviate symptoms. Multiple interventions, if orchestrated effectively, are even more likely to be successful. Late life depression, however, is a complex disorder and, when simple treatments fail, a broader perspective may be necessary for effective intervention.

■ NEED, DEMAND, SUPPLY, AND USE OF PSYCHIATRIC SERVICES

The interaction of the depressed older adult with medical and psychiatric health care personnel is of particular interest to the clinical investigator, the clinician, and persons responsible for developing health care policy. Morris (1975) distinguishes the need for psychiatric or medical services from the demand for them. How does the clinician determine the need for such services? Most clinicians and health care planners would opt for the use of clinically trained personnel to evaluate all individuals within a community and/or a health care system to determine who can benefit from such services. In the United States, however, few medical examinations and no psychiatric evaluations are required of the general population. Individuals within the community are free to determine whether they suffer from a malady that can be alleviated by health care providers and to choose the type of provider to minister to their needs. When the health care system works properly, older adults suffering mood disorders are referred to the proper resource when they enter the system when the system is working properly.

A model of factors leading to effective use of medical and psychiatric care by depressed older adults is presented in Figure 1-7. As can be seen, assignment of a diagnosis is only one factor among many that determine use, recovery, and ultimate adaptation. Data from epidemiologic surveys can play a major role in planning for mental health services available to the elderly, yet service providers must consider the complicated pathway from a community-based diagnosis, such as that generated by a structured interview using DSM-III-R or DSM-IV criteria to the use of these services. This model is further complicated when service providers consider the many factors that intervene between use of medical and psychiatric services and recovery or adaptation of the mood disordered patient. These factors include the relationship between the patient and the clinician, the effectiveness of the therapeutic modality, and the integration of therapy into the patient's life-style.

Little information is available regarding the use of psychiatric and medical services by depressed older adults. A review of the literature suggests that older persons tend to use inpatient psychiatric facilities more often than do the remainder of the population, but they greatly underuse outpatient facilities. In a survey performed in Durham, North Carolina, only 1% of a randomly selected community sample of older persons were receiving some type of counseling or psychotherapy (Blazer, 1978). Approximately 20% of the subjects were taking some type of tranquilizer or "nerve medicine," usually prescribed by the primary care physician. On systematic questioning, 9.6% of the subjects perceived a need for some type of trained counseling or other mental health service. German et al (1986) found older persons with all mental disorders less likely to be seen and treated for these disorders than younger individuals. Of those under age 65, 8.7% had made a visit to a specialty or primary care provider for mental health care in the year before the survey compared with 4.2% of persons between ages 65 and 74 and only 1.4% of persons 75 and greater. The most likely source of care for older persons for emotional or psychiatric problems was their primary care provider. Most surveys reveal

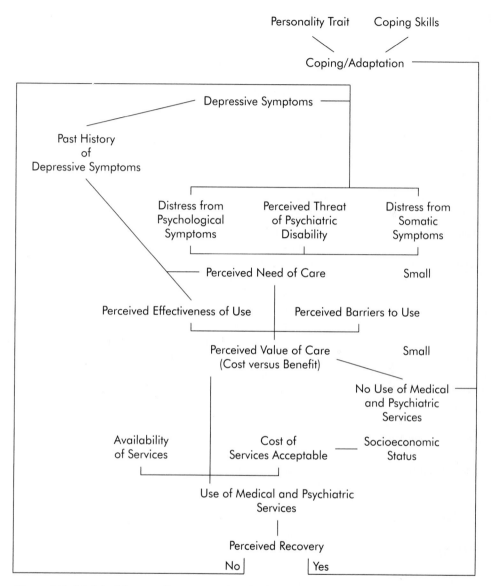

Figure 1-7. Model of factors affecting use of medical and psychiatric services by depressed older adults. (Adapted from Kalimo, 1969.)

that the use of psychiatric services for the mood disorders parallels the use for psychiatric disorders in general.

One aspect of the study of health services use is the evaluation of individual clinical performance. Every clinician working with depressed older adults should systematically evaluate his or her performance. This monograph provides background data and perspective for the clinician to develop a self-evaluation program. For example, in the next chapter, detailed data are presented regarding the outcome of depressive disorders across the life cycle.

Sackett et al (1985) suggests the following five determinates of clinical outcome:

1. The illness itself (e.g., is the elder suffering from a bipolar affective disorder with intermittent and unpredictable episodes of mania and depression or is the elder suffering a chronic dysthymic disorder with little change in symptomatology through time?).

2. The diagnostic tests that might be used to identify the cause of the illness (e.g., the laboratory tests suggest a significant contribution of physical illness, such as thyroid abnormalities, as contributors to the depressive disorder).

3. The potential treatments that might be prescribed for the illness (e.g., a medication, cognitive psychotherapy, intermittent family counseling, or simply waiting for the patient to recover spontaneously should be reviewed).

4. The performance of the clinician (e.g., how competent is the clinician to diagnose and prescribe effectively for the treatment of major depression in the older adults? How motivated is the clinician to treat an older person? Do external factors, such as insurance, preclude effective clinical performance?).

5. The degree of patient compliance (e.g., the willingness is the patient to take a medication or to join a group for therapy?).

Clinicians do not have the luxury of individually performing extensive and large clinical trials to quantify these predictors of clinical performance. Therefore the clinician must informally monitor performance based on existing data that clarify current concepts of the illness (including prognosis), available diagnostic tests, available therapies, and extent outcome studies in the literature. For this reason, the literature on late life depression is reviewed at depth in the subsequent chapters of this monograph. In the latter twentieth century the informed clinician working with depressed older adults can abstract not only clinical "pearls" from the literature but also can begin to develop a living textbook of data that assists in diagnosis, selection of appropriate therapy, and prediction of outcome.

REFERENCES

Ames D: Depression among elderly residents of local-authority residential homes: its nature and efficacy of intervention, *British Journal of Psychiatry* 156:667-675, 1990.

Angst J: The course of major depression, a typical bipolar disorder, and bipolar disorder. In Hippius H (ed): *New Results in Depression Research*. Berlin, Springer-Verlag, 1986, pp. 26-35.

Barrett JE, Barrett JA, Oxman TE, Gerber PD: The prevalence of psychiatric disorders in a primary care practice, *Archives of General Psychiatry* 45:1100-1106, 1988.

Ben-Arie Swartz L, Bickman BJ: Depression in the elderly living in the community: its presentation and features, *British Journal of Psychiatry* 150:169-174, 1987.

Berkman LF, Berkman CS, Kasl S, Freeman DH, Leo L, et al: Depressive symptoms in relation to physical health and functioning in the elderly, *American Journal of Epidemiology* 124:372-388, 1986.

Blazer DG: The Oars Durham surveys: description and application. In *Multidimensional Functional Assessment: The Oars Methodology/A Manual* (ed 2). Durham, North Carolina, The Center for the Study of Aging and Human Development, 1978.

Blazer DG, Bahar JR, Hughes DC: Major depression with melancholia: A comparison of middle-aged and elderly adults, *Journal of the American Geriatric Society* 35:927-932, 1987.

Blazer DG, Busse EW, Craighead WE, Evans D: Use of the laboratory in the diagnostic workup of the older adult. In Busse EW, Blazer DG (eds): *Geriatric Psychiatry*. Washington, DC, American Psychiatric Press, 1989, pp. 285-312.

Blazer DG, Hughes DC, George LK: The epidemiology of depression in an elderly community population, *The Gerontologist* 27:281-287, 1987.

Blazer DG, Williams CD: The epidemiology of dysphoria and depression in an elderly population, *American Journal of Psychiatry* 137:439-444, 1980.

Blazer DG, Woodbury M, Hughes DC, George LK, Manten KG, et al: A statistical analysis of the classification of depression in a mixed community and clinical sample, *Journal of Affective Disorders* 16:11-20, 1989.

Bollerup TR: Prevalence of mental illness among 70-year-olds domiciled in nine Copenhagen suburbs, *Acta Psychiatrica Scandinavica* 51:327-339, 1975.

Bond J, Atkinson A, Gregson BA: The prevalence of psychiatric illness among continuing-care patients under the care of departments of geriatric medicine, *International Journal of Geriatric Psychiatry* 4:227-233, 1989.

Boorson S, Barnes RA, Kukull WA, Okimoto JT, Vieth RC, et al: Symptomatic depression in elderly medical outpatients. I. Prevalence, demography, and health services utilization, *Journal of the American Geriatric Society* 34:341-347, 1986.

Burns DJ, Larson DB, Goldstrom ID, Johnson WE, Toube CA, et al: Mental disorder among nursing home patients: preliminary findings from the national nursing home survey pretest, *International Journal of Geriatric Psychiatry* 3:27-35, 1988.

Canino GJ, Bird HR, Shrout PE, Rubio-Stipec M, Brown M, et al: Prevalence of specific psychiatric disorders in Puerto Rico, *Archives of General Psychiatry* 44:727-730, 1987.

Carroll BJ, Feinberg M, Graden JF, Terika J, Albala AA: Specific laboratory tests for the diagnosis of melancholia, *Archives of General Psychiatry* 38:15-22, 1981.

Cassel JC, Leighton AH: Epidemiology in mental health. In Goldston SE (ed): *Mental Health Considerations in Public Health*. National Institute of Mental Health, PHS publication no. 1898, May 1969, pp. 69-85.

Cheah KC, Beard OH: Psychiatric findings in the population of a geriatric evaluation unit: implications, *Journal of the American Geriatric Society* 28:153-156, 1980.

Comstock GW, Helsing KJ: Symptoms of depression in two communities, *Psychological Medicine* 6:551-563, 1976.

Copeland J: What is a "case"? A case for what? In Wing JK, Bebbington P, Robins LN (eds): *What is a Case? The Problem of Definition in Psychiatric Community Surveys*. London, Grant McIntyre, 1981, pp. 9-11.

Copeland JMR, Dewey ME, Wood N, Searle R, Davidson IA, McWilliam C: Range of mental illness among the elderly in the community: prevalence in the Liverpool using in the GMS-AGECAT package, *British Journal of Psychiatry* 150:815-823, 1987.

de Beauvoir S: *The Coming of Age*. Paris, Editions Gallimard, 1970.

Diagnostic and Statistical Manual of Mental Disorders (ed 3—revised) (DSM-III-R). Washington, DC, American Psychiatric Association, 1987.

Diagnostic and Statistical Manual of Mental Disorders (ed 3) (DSM-III). Washington, DC, American Psychiatric Association, 1980.

Foster JR, Cataldo JK, Baksay JE: Incidence of depression in a medical long-term care facility: findings for a restricted sample of new admission, *International Journal of Geriatric Psychiatry* 5:1-8, 1990.

German PS, Shapiro S, Skinner EA: Mental health of the elderly: use of health and mental health services, *Journal of the American Geriatric Society* 33:246-252, 1985.

Goodwin DW, Guze B: *Psychiatric Diagnosis* (ed 2). New York, Oxford University Press, 1979.

Hippocrates on airs, waters and places, Circa 400 BC In *Medical Classics* III:19, 1938.

Jensen K: Psychiatric problems in four Danish old age homes, *Acta Psychiatrica Scandinavica* (supp) 169:411-418, 1966.

Kalimo E: *Determinates of Medical Care Utilization*. Helsinki, Institute for Social Security, 1969.

Keller MD, Lavori PW, Endicott J, Coryell W, Klerman GL: "Double depression:" two-year follow-up, *American Journal of Psychiatry* 140:689-694, 1983.

Kennedy GJ, Kelman HR, Thomas C: The emergency of depressive symptoms in late life: the importance of declining health and increasing disability, *Journal of Community Health* 15:93-104, 1990.

Kennedy GJ, Kelman HR, Thomas C, Wisniewski W, Metz H, et al: Hierarchy of characteristics associated with depressive symptoms in an urban elderly sample, *American Journal of Psychiatry* 146:220-225, 1989.

Kivela SL, Pahkela K, Laippala P: Prevalence of depression in an elderly population in Finland, *Acta Psychiatrica Scandinavica* 78:401-413, 1988.

Klerman GL: Affective disorders. In Nicholi A (ed): *The Harvard Guide to Modern Psychiatry.* Cambridge, Massachusetts, Belknap Press, 1978, pp. 253-281.

Klerman GL, Lavori PW, Rice J, Reich T, Endicott J, et al: Birth-cohort trends and rates of major depressive disorders among relatives of patients with affective disorder, *Archives of General Psychiatry* 42:689-695, 1985.

Koenig HG, Meador KG, Cohen HJ, Blazer DG: Depression in elderly hospitalized patients with medical illness, *Archives of Internal Medicine* 148:1929-1936, 1988.

Kua EH: Depressive disorder in elderly Chinese people, *Acta Psychiatrica Scandinavica* 81:386-388, 1990.

Kupfer DJ, Foster FG, Coble P, McPartland RJ, Ulrich RF: The application of EEG sleep for the differential diagnosis of affective disorders, *American Journal of Psychiatry* 135:69-74, 1978.

Leighton DC, Harding JS, Macklin DB, McMillan AM, Leighton AH: *The Character of Danger.* New York, Basic Books, 1963.

Lilienfeld AM, Lilienfeld DE: *Foundations of Epidemiology* (ed 2). New York, Oxford University Press, 1980, p. 3.

Lindemann E: Symptomology and management of acute grief, *American Journal of Psychiatry* 101:141-149, 1944.

MacMahon B, Pugh TF: *Epidemiology: Principles and Methods.* Boston, Little, Brown and Company, 1970.

Morris JN: *Uses of Epidemiology* (ed 3). London, Churchill Livingstone, 1975.

Murphy E: The prognosis of depression in old age, *British Journal of Psychiatry* 142:111-119, 1983.

Murphy E, Lindesay J, Grundy E: Sixty years of suicide in England and Wales, *Archives of General Psychiatry* 43:969-977, 1986.

Murrell SA, Himmelfarb S, Wright K: Prevalence of depression and its correlates in older adults, *American Journal of Epidemiology* 117:173-185, 1983.

Myers JK, Weisman MM, Tischler GL, Holzer CE, Leaf PJ, et al: Six-month prevalence of psychiatric disorders in three communities, *Archives of General Psychiatry* 41:959-970, 1984.

National Center for Health Statistics: *Final Statistics of the United States,* 1980. Vol 2—Mortality (Part B). DHHS Publication (PHS) 85-1102, 1985.

O'Hara MW, Cohout FJ, Wallace RB: Depression among the rural elderly: a study of prevalence and correlates, *Journal of Nervous and Mental Diseases* 173:582-589, 1985.

O'Riordan TG, Hayes JP, Shelley R, O'Neill D, Walsh JB, et al: The prevalence of depression in an acute geriatric medical assessment unit, *International Journal of Geriatric Psychiatry* 4:17-21, 1989.

Parmelee PA, Katz IR, Lawton MP: Depression among institutionalized aging: assessment in prevalence estimation, *Journal of Gerontology* 44:M22-29, 1989.

Platt R: Wisdom is not enough, reflections on art and science in medicine, *Lancet* ii:977, 1952.

Rapp SR, Walsh DA, Parisi SA, Wallace CE: Detecting depression in elderly medical inpatients, *Journal of Counselling in Clinical Psychology* 36:509-513, 1988.

Regier DA, Myers JK, Kramer M, Robins LN, Blazer DG, et al: NIMH epidemiologic catchment area program, *Archives of General Psychiatry* 41:934-941, 1984.

Roberts CJ: *Epidemiology for Clinicians.* London, Pitman Medical Publishing, 1977, p. 3.

Robins LN, Helzer JE, Croughan J: National Institute of Mental Health Diagnostic Interview Schedule: history, characteristics, validity, *Archives of General Psychiatry* 38:381-389, 1981.

Robins LN, Helzer JE, Weissman MM, Orvaschel H, Grunberg E, et al: Life time prevalence of specific psychiatric disorders in three sites, *Archives of General Psychiatry* 41:949-958, 1984.

Rorsman B, Grasbeck A, Hagnell O, Lanke J, Ohman R, et al: A prospective study of first-incidence depression: the Lundby study, 1957-1972, *British Journal of Psychiatry* 156:336-342, 1990.

Sackett DL, Haynes RB, Tugwell P: *Clinical Epidemiology: The Basic Science for Clinical Medicine.* Boston, Little, Browning, 1985, p. 255, 256.

Sorensen A, Stromgren E: Frequency of depressive states within geographically delimited population groups. II. Prevalence (the Samso investigation), *Acta Psychiatrica Scandinavica,* (supp) 162:62, 1961.

Srole L, Fischer AK: The midtown Manhatten longitudinal study versus "the mental paradise lost" doctrine, *Archives of General Psychiatry* 37:209-221, 1980.

Tweed DL: Identification of illness for case-finding studies. In Copeland J, Abou-Saleh M, Blazer D (eds): *The Psychiatry of Old Age: An International Textbook.* New York, John Wiley and Sons, in press.

Weissman MM, Klerman GL: Epidemiology of mental disorders, *Archives of General Psychiatry* 25:705-715, 1978.

Weissman MM, Leaf PJ, Tischler GL, Blazer DG, Kerno M, et al: Affective disorders in five United States communities, *Psychological Medicine* 18:141-153, 1988.

Weissman MM, Myers JK: Affective disorders in a US urban community, *Archives of General Psychiatry* 35:1304-1311, 1978.

Wing JK, Cooper JE, Satorius N: *Measurement and Classification of Psychiatric Symptoms: an Instruction Manual for the PSE and Catego Program.* Cambridge, Cambridge University Press, 1974.

2

Symptoms and Signs

In contrast with the diagnosis of most physical illnesses, clinicians who work with the psychiatrically ill must focus their diagnostic skills on the thoughts, feelings, and actions of the persons being examined (Linn, 1974). Symptoms of psychiatric disorder are changes in physical, psychologic, or social functioning subjectively reported by the patient that might be indicative of disease or maladaptation. Signs of psychiatric disorders, on the other hand, are objective indications that disease or maladaptation is present. Symptoms and signs of depression in late life are determined not only by reports and observable evidence of distress within the individual but also by observations that the personal environment interactions are disturbed. In fact, one of the most reliable measures of impaired mental health functioning is a disturbance in the quality of relationship with other persons.

Investigators and clinicians generally agree about the core symptoms and signs of depressions at all stages of the life cycle. Beck (1967) found a remarkable consistency in the descriptions of depressive disorders since ancient time. Core symptoms and signs of depression include sadness, low mood, pessimism about the future, self-criticism and self-blame, retardation or agitation, slow thinking, and difficulty concentrating. Core "vegetative" signs include appetite and sleep disturbances.

Unfortunately, few investigators objectively consider the symptoms and signs of depressive disorders without assuming that the symptoms and signs delineate preestablished syndromes or diseases. These assumptions cloud the ability to distinguish objectively the characteristics of the mood disorders and the variations of emotions throughout the life cycle. In this chapter the symptoms and signs that have been classically associated with depressed disorders that occur in later life are reviewed. First, attention is directed to categorizations of these symptoms and signs. Next, the patterns of symptoms present in late life are discussed. Finally, attention is directed to one symptom complex that can easily be confused with depressive symptoms in late life (i.e., demoralization).

Chief Complaint

The chief complaint made by the depressed older person may not immediately signal depression to the clinician. This complaint may reflect concern about physical health, difficulty in family and social relationships, dissatisfaction with economic circumstances, and so on. Skillful questioning, however, can usually uncover and cluster the symptoms that underlie the chief complaint. Older persons do not usually mask depressive symptoms more than younger persons when the clinician probes for presence of a depressed mood.

Point of entry into the health care system may determine the nature of the chief complaint. Watts (1957) found depressed persons treated in medical clinics by a primary care physician frequently presented symptoms suggestive of physical illness. Bradley (1963) noted that severe general pain may be the focus of depressed patients in a pain clinic. Because many older persons present depressive problems initially to a primary care physician, the recognition of physical complaints accompanying symptoms of mood disorders by clinicians is imperative.

■ SYMPTOMS

Beck (1967) categorized depressive symptoms into emotional, cognitive, physical, and volitional symptoms. The signs of depressive disorders include those observable behaviors that suggest depressive disorder. A modification of Beck's approach to the classification of depressive symptoms is presented in Table 2-1.

Emotional Symptoms

Emotional symptoms of depression are those changes in the person's feelings that accompany depression. When evaluating the emotional symptoms of depression, one must take into account the mood state before the onset of the symptoms. Changes in emotional symptoms within the context of a person's age, gender, race, and prior personality are more important than the absolute presence or absence of particular emotional symptoms.

The most common characteristic symptom described by depressed persons is dysphoria or sadness. Dysphoria is not thought to be as common in the elderly as in younger persons (Salzman and Shader, 1978; Goldfarb, 1974). Blazer et al (1984, 1987), however, found depressed older adults in both clinical and community samples with equivalent severity of depression and no complicating comorbidity (e.g., dementia or physical illness) were no less likely to respond that they were sad, blue, or down in the dumps during a depressive episode than persons in mid-life.

The recognition of psychologic discomfort as depression is characteristic of our psychologic society (Gross, 1978). Many older persons, however, have not been influenced by our psychologically oriented society. They may be less likely, therefore, to report psychic discomfort as depression. A parallel to this phenomenon can be seen in other cultures (e.g., African). Many western African languages do not contain a word that can be translated as depression. Because of this lack of a cultural construct for depression, the subjective report of a depressive mood may occur rarely in that society. On the other hand, the symptoms and signs (including physical symptoms) of depression are common in these cultures (Leighton et al, 1963). The

Symptoms and Signs of Depression in Late Life

Symptoms	Observable Signs

Emotional

Dejected mood or sadness
Decreased life satisfaction
Loss of interest
Impulse to cry
Irritability
Emptiness
Fearfulness and anxiety
Negative feelings toward self
Worry
Helplessness
Hopelessness
Sense of failure
Loneliness
Uselessness

Cognitive

Low self-esteem
Pessimism
Self-blame and criticism
Rumination about problems
Suicidal thoughts
Delusions
 Of uselessness
 Of unforgivable behavior
 Nihilistic
 Somatic
Hallucinations
 Auditory
 Visual
 Kinesthetic
Doubt of values and beliefs
Difficulty concentrating
Poor memory

Physical

Loss of appetite
Fatigability
Sleep disturbance
 Initial insomnia
 Terminal insomnia
 Frequent awakenings
Constipation
Loss of libido
Pain
Restlessness

Volitional

Loss of motivation or "paralysis of will"
Suicidal impulses
Desire to withdraw socially

Appearance

Stooped posture
Sad face
Uncooperativeness
Social withdrawal
Hostility
Suspiciousness
Confusion and clouding of consciousness
Diurnal variations of mood
Drooling (in severe cases)
Unkempt appearance (in severe cases)
Occasional ulcerations of skin secondary to
 picking
Crying or whining
Occasional ulcerations of cornea secondary to
 decreased blinking
Weight loss
Bowel impaction

Psychomotor retardation

Slowed speech
Slowed movements
Gestures minimized
Shuffling slow gait
Mutism (in severe cases)
Cessation of mastication and swallowing (in se-
 vere cases)
Decreased or inhibited blinking (in severe cases)

Psychomotor agitation

Continued motor activity
Wringing of hands
Picking at skin
Pacing
Restless sleep
Grasping others

Bizarre or inappropriate behavior

Suicidal gestures or attempts
Negativism, such as refusal to eat or drink and
 stiffness of the body
Outbursts of aggression
Falling backward

current cohort of older adults have lived within a somewhat different culture than younger adults.

Decreased life satisfaction is a pervasive emotional symptom among the depressed. Beck (1967) found that 92% of severely depressed patients reported loss of life satisfaction. Many assume that a decline in life satisfaction is a normal correlate. The symptom is not pervasive in late life, but it is common and is usually associated with external factors, such as poor health, widowhood, or retirement. In most cases, therefore, decreased life satisfaction is the normal response to adverse experiences and the social environment, not a symptom of a mood disorder (Thomae, 1980).

Loss of interest is a common symptom of depressive disorders in late life. This symptom is perhaps the single most useful symptom by which clinicians can distinguish melancholic from nonmelancholic depressed elders. Even if the depressed mood is only moderately severe, if the elder says, "I have everything to live for but I have no interest in doing the things I used to enjoy," the clinician should consider a melancholic depression and therefore biologic intervention. Impulses to cry are symptoms frequently exhibited by depressed older adults. Hustrup et al (1986) found no evidence of a decreased tendency to cry in a nonclinical sample of persons evaluated for depressive mood in late life compared with mid-life. Crying episodes apparently function for some individuals as an adaptive coping response to stress and, therefore, should not be interpreted as a sign or symptom of depression per se. In our current nomenclature (DSM-III-R, 1987), crying is a symptom of the dysthymic disorder but not of a major depressive episode.

Negative feelings toward the self were reported by 26% of severely depressed persons in Beck's sample (1967) but are not nearly as common in the elderly (Winokur et al, 1980). In contrast a sense of emptiness is frequently seen in severely depressed elders and is a concern to clinicians (Goldfarb, 1974). This feeling of emptiness is often associated with suicidal impulses.

Feelings of helplessness, hopelessness, and uselessness are experienced by persons suffering from depressive disorders at all stages of the life cycle. Demoralized and discouraged older adults, however, complain of a sense of hopelessness and helplessness about the future and may reflect a certain degree of reality considering the difficulties that they face. Physical illness and economic hardship can render the elder dependent on others and realistically discouraged about the future. Goldfarb (1974) describes an exaggeration of personal helplessness that is characteristic of depression in late life. The depressed elder may withdraw from social activities, which in turn leads to boredom and loneliness (Fassler and Gavirin, 1978).

Anxiety frequently accompanies depression in older persons being treated for depression (Blazer and Hughes, 1990). Balter (1982) found that, among persons between ages 65 and 79, psychic distress was experienced by 5.7% as a result of anxiety, 3.8% as a result of depression, and 9.5% as a result of mixed depression and anxiety. Therefore in both community and clinical settings the comorbodity of anxiety and depression is frequent. Yet this high comorbidity is not exclusive to the elderly. Alexopoulas (1990) found anxiety in older persons suffering depression less often than in younger depressed patients.

Cognitive Symptoms

Beck emphasized the importance of cognitive symptoms and depressive disorders (1967, 1979). He suggested that there has been a consistent lack of emphasis on the thought processes in depression that reflects the view that depression is an emotional disorder and that any impairment of thinking is a result of the emotional disturbance. Thoughts of a depressed older adult may be distortions or unrealistic conceptualizations that deviate from logical thinking about the self and the social environment, which in turn lead to a depressed affect.

Low self-esteem is the most characteristic cognitive symptom and was found in 81% of the severely depressed patients evaluated by Beck (1967). Low self-esteem is less common in the depressed elderly and tends to be replaced by other cognitive symptoms, such as unwarranted pessimism about the future. Statements such as "I have nothing to look forward to," "There is no sense in my doing anything," or "I will be dead within a matter of months" are often made by the depressed elderly.

Rumination about present and past problems is characteristic of depressed older adults. Such patients repeat their evaluations of feeling about particular events during successive therapeutic sessions. Rumination may be accompanied by delusions of uselessness. Delusions of unforgivable behavior or self-blame and criticisms are related to the egocentric notions of causality frequently seen in the elderly (Beck, 1967). Other investigators, however, have found that guilt is a less common symptom in the depressed elderly (Winokur et al, 1980; Blazer et al, 1987). Goldfarb (1974) found that paranoid reactions, such as "delusion of doubles," are occasionally seen in the depressed elderly. Rosenthal (1974) commented on the frequency of paranoid symptoms during the involutional period. Symptoms ranged from suspiciousness and irritability to frank delusions. The constellation of agitation, depression, and paranoia has been the cornerstone of diagnosis of involutional depression. However, this diagnostic category is no longer accepted among persons studying mood disorders across the life cycle. Most involutional depressive episodes are not the first onset episode or are followed by a recurrent episode later in life.

Winokur, Behan, and Schessler (1980) found that depressed patients older than 60 had suicidal thoughts less frequently than younger patients. These findings were confirmed by Blazer et al (1987). A more thorough discussion of suicide is found in Chapter 1. The frequency of cognitive impairment symptoms in depressed elderly is discussed in Chapter 15.

Physical Symptoms

Physical or endogenous symptoms are frequently associated with depression in late life. Wilson et al (1983) found that in primary care settings the somatic symptoms were common among persons suffering depression, regardless of age. The most common somatic symptoms were sleep problems (36%), fatigue (34%), dizziness (29%), appetite changes (21%), and gastrointestinal symptoms (20%). Casper et al (1985) suggest that the frequency and severity of somatic symptoms increase with the severity of depression among the elderly. They also found the classical somatic symptoms of depression to not be exclusive to endogenous nor melancholia depression. A number of investigators have confirmed Casper's findings (Berry et al, 1984; Zemore and Eames, 1967; Epstein, 1976).

Not everyone agrees with the theory that endogenous symptoms predominate in depression among the elderly. Gurland (1976) suggests that neurotic depression is relatively more common in the elderly than at other stages of the life cycle. Rapp and Vrana (1989) studied 150 elderly male inpatients. To establish whether the somatic symptoms of depression, such as appetite, weight loss, and disturbed sleep, influence more psychologic symptoms (e.g., worry and depressive affect) in the assignment of standardized Research Diagnostic Criteria diagnoses, they established two different diagnostic criteria. They found the correlation between somatic and nonsomatic symptoms to be low, yet the somatic symptoms correlate equally with all Research Diagnostic Criteria symptoms of depression. The new criteria, compared with the old criteria, gave fairly similar results in the diagnosis.

The debate about whether endogenous depression is more frequent in the elderly may center in part on the lack of adequate criteria, especially in epidemiologic studies for mild, endogenous depressions (i.e., depressive disorders that do not reach diagnostic criteria for major depression). Since depressive symptoms are basically unchanged in frequency across the life cycle (although the frequency of major depression is lower in late life), many elders with subsyndromal depressive episodes may experience endogenous symptoms. Snaith (1987) proposed a mild biogenic form of depression, likely to respond to antidepressant drug therapy and seen predominately by primary care physicians. He suggests that anhedonia is the central and most reliable symptom of mild depression. There has been little, if any, objective validation of a mild biogenic depressive syndrome. Snaith did not concentrate on the elderly. (See Chapter 11.)

A number of investigators have commented on the frequency of hypochondriac symptoms in the elderly (DeAlarcon, 1964; Brink, 1977; Goldfarb, 1974; Goldstein, 1979; Steuer et al, 1980). DeAlarcon found hypochondriac symptoms in 65.7% of the men and 62% of the women attending a geriatric clinic for depression. Of the patients with hypochondriac symptoms, only 19% showed a life-long concern for health; therefore the increased interest in health problems appeared to be related to the onset of the depressive symptoms. The digestive system was by far the most frequent locus of complaints. Headaches, complaint of urinary stricture, and falling out of the hair (especially in women) were among the other frequent complaints. Despite the high prevalence of cardiovascular disease in the elderly, complaints about the heart were less common than those related to the gastrointestinal system. Although Steuer et àl (1980) found numerous somatic symptoms in the depressed elderly, they found that somatic symptoms contribute less to depression than lack of hope, decreased activity, difficulty in doing things, feelings of uselessness, and problems in decision making. Musetti et al (1989) did not confirm the common clinical stereotypes that ascribe greater somatization, hypochondria, and agitation to the elderly depressed compared with younger depressed. Clinical presentation was relatively uniform across older and younger depressives in the study of 400 patients seen in outpatient clinics. All had a primary diagnosis of major depression according to DSM-III-R.

Williamson (1978) found severe localized pain to be an occasional symptom of depression in the elderly. Magni et al (1985) found chronic pain to be a more frequent complaint in the depressed elderly than in controls. Yet pain was more likely to be a symptom of a dysthymic disorder than major depression and was found less frequently in patients who admitted depression and anxiety. In the Williamson study the past personalities of patients who complained of pain as a primary symptom of depression were passive and demanding. For some patients, pain may be a means of inflicting self-punishment for guilt and frustration about one's past life.

Sleep difficulties are among the most common physical complaints of depressed elderly (Salzman and Shader, 1978b). Changes in sleep habits normally accompany aging, and these complaints may reflect a lack of understanding and tolerance of the normal physiologic changes, rather than symptoms induced by a depressive illness. Elderly depressed patients complain of sexual difficulties less often than do persons at other stages of the life cycle (Chessea, 1965; Winokur, Behan, and Schessler, 1980).

Volitional Symptoms

Volition is the constantly experienced striving impulse within an individual. Rather remarkable changes can occur in volition with the onset of depression. Beck (1967) noted that a striking feature of the depressed is regression. Many depressed patients withdraw from more demanding activities and are attracted to less demanding activities in terms of degree of responsibility or initiative required. This "paralysis of will" was found in 65% to 86% of the patients studied. Severe depression is often accompanied by complete paralysis of will, leading to almost total immobility associated with passive resistance to intervention by others. In a study of elder adults in the community, Gaitz and Scott (1972) reported that 37% of the elderly said that they "couldn't get going." This high percentage is secondary in part to residual physical disabilities, but motivational difficulty is a frequent cause of inability to initiate activity as well. Levins (1963) found apathy to be more common in the depressed elderly than in persons at other stages of the life cycle. According to Fassler and Gavirin (1978), older persons with depression tend to be more introspective and therefore withdraw from social activities. Yet Chessea (1965) found that the depressed elderly are more sociable than younger depressed patients.

■ SIGNS

On exam of the severely depressed older adult, the observable signs of depressive illness provide clues to the diagnosis not obtained through symptom review. Lehmann (1959) suggests that most cases of depression can be diagnosed by inspection. Sad expression, retardation or agitation, frequent crying, clinging, and other expressions of dependency and helplessness are characteristic of depression. Post (1968) found that the depressed elderly are often more agitated than persons at other stages of the life cycle. Weight loss has been found more common in the elderly depressed than in depressed persons younger than 60 years (Winokur, Behan, and Schessler, 1980; Blazer et al, 1987). Constipation can lead to an abdominal mass (impacted feces in the lower bowel) that can be found on physical examination. Older depressed patients often require enemas or manual reduction for bowel impaction.

In recent years, signs to depression have been less emphasized in the diagnostic workup than symptoms. Signs, however, may be important factors in diagnosing some types of depression, especially endogenous depression. For example, Nelson and Charrey (1981) found support for psychomotor signs (agitation and retardation) along with severity of mood, lack of reactivity, and delusions (compared with the distinct quality of the depressive mood, early morning awakening, and vegetative features) in distinguishing in-dividuals with melancholia or endogenous depression. Parker et al (1989) suggested psy-chomotor retardation, nonreactivity, distinct quality of mood, nonvariability of mood, and delusion/paranoid features as the most distinguishing signs of melancholia depres-sion. Parker et al emphasized the importance of observable signs, which can be as reli-able as self-reported symptoms. Observable signs may be especially relevant to older per-sons who may not volunteer their symptoms as easily or who may be so depressed that they are incapable of responding accurately to an interview.

Frequency of depressive symptoms

Numerous surveys of community, clinical, and institutional populations of the fre-quency of depressive symptoms have appeared in literature. Because of poor interrater reliability of clinician-based diagnoses of depression coupled with the expense of data gathering by clinicians in community studies, most of these surveys have used self-rating scales and symptom checklists for the identification of mood disorders. Five of the com-mon rating scales and the symptoms assessed by these scales are presented in Table 2-2. The Beck Depression Inventory (BDI), the Center for Epidemiologic Studies Depres-sion Scale (CES-D), and the Geriatric Depression Scale (GDS) are self-rating scales (Beck et al, 1961; Radloff, 1977; Yesavage et al, 1983). The Hamilton Depression Rat-ing Scale (HDRS) and the Montgomery Asberg Depression Rating Scale (MADRS) are rated by clinicians in semistructured interviews (Hamilton, 1960; Montgomery and As-berg, 1979). Other rating scales are available, but these five demonstrate the variety of symptoms assessed using such scales. The GDS was devised specifically to avoid somatic symptoms thought to complicate the identification of depression in the elderly with phys-ical illness. The intercorrelation in most studies between the scores using these various scales is quite high and therefore the frequency of depressive symptoms vary little from study to study, despite the use of different instruments.

How frequent are the symptoms of depression in community populations of the el-derly? The results of study of the Durham Epidemiologic Catchment Area (ECA) sam-ple of young and older adults is presented in Table 2-3. In general the symptoms of depression are less common in the elderly than in younger adults for the emotional and cognitive symptoms. The vegetative symptoms, on the other hand, are in general more common in the elderly than in younger persons. For the persons diagnosed as suffering from major depressive episode, some symptoms are more common in younger persons (e.g., crying spells), whereas others tend to be more common in the elderly (e.g., dif-ficulty concentrating). Vegetative symptoms appeared to be much more common in the elderly compared with younger persons in the community sample diagnosed with major depression. A comparison of symptom frequency for older and younger adults receiving treatment for major depression on a psychiatric inpatient service without complicating problems is presented in Table 2-4. Contrary to usual clinical lore, feelings of guilt were just as common in the elderly as in individuals of other stages of the life cycle. Suicidal ideation was less common and loss of appetite more common among older persons. In general, however, the similarities in symptom presentation between persons in mid-life and late life are more evident than the differences.

A comparison of factor analytic studies of persons 18 to 65 years old and those 65 years old and older, using the Center for Epidemiologic Studies Depression Scale (CSD),

TABLE 2-2. Comparison of Symptoms Assessed by Various Depression-Rating Scales

Symptoms	Beck (1967)	Hamilton (1960)	GDS Yesavage (1983)	CES-D Radloff (1977)	MA (1979)
Emotional					
Dejected mood	X	X	X	X	X
Negative feelings toward self	X	X			
Decreased life satisfaction	X	X	X		
Loss of interest	X	X	X		
Crying spells	X	X	X	X	X
Irritability	X	X	X	X	
Emptiness	X				
Fearfulness	X	X	X		
Boredom	X				
Cognitive					
Slowed thinking					
Low self-evaluation					
Negative expectations, hopelessness	X	X	X	X	X
Self-blame, self-criticism	X				
Worry	X	X			
Indecisiveness	X	X			
Guilt feelings	X	X			
Distorted self-image	X				
Loneliness		X			
Confusion	X	X	X	X	X
Preoccupation with health	X	X			
Helplessness	X				
Uselessness, sense of failure	X	X			
Worthlessness	X	X	X		
Sense of punishment	X	X			
Nihilistic					
Physical					
Fatigability	X	X	X	X	X
Sleep disturbance	X	X	X	X	X
Loss of appetite	X	X	X	X	X
Constipation	X				
Loss of libido	X				
Diurnal variation	X				
Weight loss	X	X			
Agitation	X	X	X		X
Retardation	X	X			
Volitional					
Paralysis of will	X				
Desire to withdraw socially	X	X	X		
Suicidal impulses (thoughts)	X	X	X		X

TABLE 2-3. Frequency (%) of Current Depressive Symptoms in Controls and Subjects with Symptoms Severe Enough to Meet DSM-III Criteria for Major Depressive Episode (MDE) and Dysthymia in Community Populations of the Elderly (60+) Compared with Younger Adults (<60)*

Symptoms	Elderly (n = 1286)	Young (n = 1674)	Elderly with MDE (n = 19)	Young with MDE (n = 36)	Elderly with Dysthymia (n = 28)	Younger with Dysthymia (n = 37)
Emotional						
Sadness	3.1	4.7	56	58	21	13
Crying spells	4.0	5.0	11	47	14	5
Cognitive						
Hopelessness	4.0	5.0	38	50		
Difficulty concentrating	3.8	2.7	67	40	67	40
Self-blame/guilt	1.6	2.1	33.3	38.9	33	39
Irritability	1.7	4.1	33	56	33	56
Suicidal thoughts	0.5	1.3	11	28	11	27
Vegetative						
Psychomotor retardation	2.5	2.4	67	39	26	3
Loss of appetite	3.9	1.7	78	28	11	2
Fatigue	7.1	7.9	75	56	75	56
Sleep difficulty	10.0	7.3	78	67	41	15
Restlessness/agitation	1.9	2.0	33	23	19	10
Constipation	14.4	4.7	56	17	25	10
Loss of libido	2.1	2.0	25	21.3	25	21

*Unpublished data from Duke Epidemiologic Catchment Area subjects from North Carolina.

is presented in Table 2-5. Results are presented for women only for persons 18 to 65 years old. The results for men are similar to those for women. Once again, the similarities in the factor analyses by age group are more evident than the differences. The CES-D factors into four subscales: depressed mood (factor 1); endogenous or vegetative factor (factor 2); positive affect or life satisfaction (factor 3); and an interpersonal factor (factor 4). Emotional and cognitive symptoms do not disaggregate in factor analytic studies, whereas vegetative symptoms do disaggregate. The CES-D does not contain items that assess volitional symptoms of depression. These factor analytic studies suggest that depressive symptoms cluster in community populations of older adults in a manner similar to their cluster in younger populations.

Yet another approach to determining the aggregation of depressive symptoms is grade of membership analysis (GOM). This multivariate classification technique can be used to examine whether the depressive symptoms and symptoms frequently associated with depressive disorders cluster into the recognizable syndromes that parallel traditional DSM-III-R psychiatric diagnoses. We used GOM to analyze symptom reports from all respondents in the Epidemiologic Catchment Area (ECA) project of the Piedmont Health region of North Carolina who reported suffering some depressive symptoms (n=446) at the second wave of the ECA study (Blazer et al, 1988). The analysis iden-

TABLE 2-4. Comparison of Symptoms (%) of Elderly and Middle-Aged Adult
Patients with Diagnosis of Major Depression with Melancholia
in Treatment.

Symptoms	Inpatients 60 + Years (n = 19)	Inpatients <60 Years (n = 18)
Emotional		
Sadness	100	100
Cognitive		
Feelings of guilt	74	89
Suicidal ideation	47	89*
Poor concentration	100	94
Vegetative		
Psychomotor retardation	84	83
Weight loss	74	39*
Sleep disturbance	95	94
Lethargy	79	94
Psychomotor agitation	37	39
Constipation	68	28
Diurnal variations of mood	42	67
Volitional		
Suicide attempts	10	7

From Blazer DG, Bachar JR, Hughes DC: *Journal of the American Geriatric Society* 35:927-932, 1987.

tified five profiles of symptoms that adequately described the interrelationship of symptoms reported by the sample. One profile included a set of symptoms nearly identical to the symptoms associated with DSM-III-R classification of major depression. Another, which was predominant among older persons, associated some vegetative symptoms of depression with cognitive impairment (Table 2-6). The existence of depressive syndromes identified by statistical techniques other than major depression and dysthymia may explain the discrepancy in epidemiologic literature between the high present prevalence of depressive symptoms and low prevalence of these two depressive disorders in community samples of older adults. One such syndrome may be a minor depression, as described previously in this chapter (see also Chapter 11).

Demoralization

Dohrenwend et al (1980), in yet another approach to determining the natural aggregation of depressive symptoms across the life cycle, reviewed screening instruments used in epidemiologic studies and noted that all of these instruments are similar in content and tend to correlate highly with each other (i.e., these instruments measure the same syndromes in community samples). A statistical analysis of these scales indicated that they have properties that meet the requirements for measuring a particular dimension, a dimension not specific from a clinical psychiatric viewpoint (i.e., the scales do not distinguish a known psychiatric disorder). Most of the items in these general screening scales are associated with affective distress but not depressive disorder. There is no good correlation between the scales and usual concepts of psychopathology (e.g., mania, major depression, hallucinations, or antisocial behavior) (Dohrenwend et al, 1979).

TABLE 2-5. Comparison of Factor Analytic Studies in Community Samples of Elderly Versus Younger Persons

Item	18-65* (n = 680, all female)				65+† (n = 2339, 58% female)			
	F1	F2	F3	F4	F1	F2	F3	F4
Blue	0.48	0.46	0.32	0.09	0.68	0.29	0.11	0.02
Bothered by things	0.40	0.36	0.13	0.05	0.38	0.47	0.03	−0.01
Depressed	0.54	0.45	0.33	0.18	0.65	0.35	0.25	0.01
Fearful	0.44	0.21	0.10	0.15	0.33	0.27	0.17	0.26
Lonely	0.36	0.31	0.33	0.27	0.65	0.21	0.17	0.11
Sad	0.63	0.21	0.28	0.25	0.74	0.21	0.20	0.11
Life a failure	0.45	0.12	0.35	0.12	0.26	0.17	0.45[a]	0.15
Crying spells	0.58	0.26	0.16	0.07	0.65	0.05	0.10	0.11
No appetite	0.36	0.44	0.14	−0.03	0.06	0.65	0.06	0.05
Trouble concentrating	0.30	0.41	0.14	0.05	0.28	0.38	0.07	0.13
Everything an effort	0.22	0.51	0.19	0.09	0.25	0.65	0.10	0.03
Trouble sleeping	0.27	0.40	0.13	0.08	0.22	0.49	0.18	0.05
Talk less	0.15	0.34	0.30	0.04	0.08	0.48	0.13	0.19
Cannot get going	0.10	0.59	0.12	0.17	0.17	0.60	0.23	0.03
Good as others	−0.09	−016	−039	−0.11	−0.07	−0.001	−0.59	−0.14
Hopeful	−0.09	−0.12	−0.43	−0.10	−0.02	−0.19	−0.67	−0.01
Happy	−0.20	−0.16	−0.75	−0.06	−0.32	−0.26	−0.62	−0.02
Enjoy life	−0.25	−0.14	−0.68	−0.03	−0.31	−0.14	−0.68	−0.06
People unfriendly	0.09	0.11	0.04	0.51	0.09	0.07	0.13	0.79
People dislike you	0.16	0.05	0.20	0.78	0.12	0.14	0.04	0.79

*From Berkman LF, Berkman CS, Kasl S, et al: *American Journal Epidemiology* 124:372-388, 1986.
†From Ross CE, Mirowsky J: *American Journal Epidemiology* 119:997-1004, 1984.

In a community survey of 200 adults in New York City, Dohrenwend et al (1980) administered an interview survey containing 25 symptom scales. In analysis, eight of these scales reflected a single dimension of nonspecific distress characterized by poor self-esteem, helplessness, hopelessness, dread, sadness, anxiety, confused thinking, psychophysiologic symptoms, and perceived poor physical health. The clustering of these symptoms is not unlike the symptoms encountered by the clinician treating the elderly depressed patient. Can this complex be equated with late life depressive disorder?

Many clinicians have described this psychologic state of distress within the constructs of diagnosable pathology (Dohrenwend et al, 1979). Foulds (1976) suggests the concept of *dysthymic states* as distinguished from neuroses and psychoses. Although dysthymic states can be found in conjunction with neuroses and psychoses, they exist as separate entities. Schmale (1972) has identified a given up-giving up syndrome frequently associated with physical illnesses. In addition to poor physical health, helplessness and hopelessness are part of the symptom.

Frank's discussion (1973) of demoralization (according to Dohrenwend, 1979) may best describe the symptom complex. Frank notes that a state of demoralization is characteristic of all persons seeking psychotherapy or other help, regardless of a particular diagnostic category. Demoralization occurs when a person "finds that he cannot meet the demands placed on him by the environment, and cannot extricate himself from this predicament." Particular environmental stressors that may precipitate demoralization include wartime experiences, genetic or inborn physical and psychologic defects, existen-

TABLE 2-6. Pure Types of Depressive Syndrome Based on Grade of Membership Analysis of Depressive Symptoms and Demographic Factors (Partial Presentation of Symptoms)

Symptoms	Pure Types (k = 5)				
	I	II	III	IV	V
Depressed 2 weeks	.226	.104	1.000	.229	.757
Decreased appetite	.036	.321	.531	.000	.472
Psychomotor retardation	.000	.000	1.000	.000	.438
Anxious	.146	.053	.485	.369	1.000
Cyclic irritability	.000	.000	.000	1.000	.000
Cyclic mood signs	.000	.000	.000	1.000	.000
Disoriented to time	.000	1.000	.000	.000	.193
Impaired short-term memory	.000	1.000	.472	.000	.210
Demographic Factors					
Age					
18-29	.177	.000	.000	.584	.313
30-59	.545	.000	.404	.416	.538
60-69	.162	.414	.524	.000	.149
Gender					
Male	.334	.337	.117	.000	.226
Female	.666	.663	.883	1.000	.774

From Blazer DG, Swartz M, Woodbury M, Manton KG, Hughes D, et al: *Archives for General Psychiatry* 45:1078-1084, 1988.

tial despair, physical illness (especially chronic physical illness), and crippling psychiatric symptoms. Dohrenwend et al (1979) suggest that the concept of demoralization fits the data from psychiatric surveys, although considerable inference is necessary when one jumps from community observations to clinical impressions.

How is the concept of demoralization to be used by researchers and clinicians? First, effort should be made to distinguish the psychiatric symptoms of known diagnostic entities, as outlined by the DSM-III-R and the upcoming DSM-IV, from symptoms of demoralization. The Diagnostic Interview Schedule (DIS), for example, surveys community populations for specific psychiatric disorders rather than the burden of psychic distress (Robins et al, 1981). Therefore the DIS would not be expected to identify a syndrome such as demoralization. Demoralization may also be distinct from traditional measures of function that have been used to predict health service use.

For the clinician, the concept of demoralization cuts across traditional boundaries of known psychologic, pharmacologic, and social therapies directed toward specific psychiatric syndromes. Is a construct, such as demoralization, amenable to psychiatric therapy? If community populations of older adults were surveyed for the symptom clusters proposed by Frank and studied by Dohrendwend et al, the prevalence of such clusters would be high among older adults (they are not necessarily high for other stages of the life cycle). Yet a high frequency of demoralization would not automatically lead to the assumption that depressive disorders are of greater frequency in older populations. The impact of broad-based service planning to address the symptoms and concurrent disability in the community should be carefully evaluated. Could it be that social, religious, and existential intervention are of more diagnostic and therapeutic benefit than traditional psychiatric intervention? Is intervention of any type necessary? These questions are discussed in more detail in Chapters 16 and 18.

REFERENCES

Alexopoulas GS: Anxiety-depression syndromes in old age, *International Journal of Geriatric Psychiatry* 5:351-353, 1990.

Balter MB (personal communication) cited in Crook T: Diagnosis and treatment of mixed anxiety-depression in the elderly, *Journal of Clinical Psychiatry* 43:35-43, 1982.

Beck AT: *Depression: Causes and Treatment.* Philadelphia, University of Pennsylvania Press, 1967.

Beck AT, Rush AJ, Shaw BF, Emery G: *Cognitive Therapy of Depression.* New York, John Wiley, 1979.

Beck AT, Ward CH, Mendelson M, Mock J, Erbaugh J: An inventory for measuring depression, *Archives of General Psychiatry* 4:561-571, 1961.

Berkman LF, Berkman CS, Kasl S, et al: Depressive symptoms in relation to physical health and functioning in the elderly, *American Journal of Epidemiology* 124:372-388, 1986.

Berry JM, Steorand TM, Coyne A: Age and sex differences in somatic complaints associated with depression, *Journal of Gerontology* 39:465-467, 1984.

Blazer DG, Bachar JR, Hughes DC: Major depression with melancholia: a comparison a middle-aged and elderly adults, *Journal of the American Geriatric Society* 35:927-932, 1987.

Blazer DG, George L, Landerman R: The phenomenology of late life depression. In Bebbington PE, Jacoby R (eds): *Psychiatric Disorder of the Elderly.* London, The Mental Health Foundation, 1984, pp. 143-152.

Blazer DG, Hughes DC, Fowler N: Anxiety as an outcome symptom of depression in elderly and middle-age adults, *International Journal of Geriatric Psychiatry* 4:273-278, 1989.

Blazer DG, Swartz M, Woodbury M, Manton KG, Hughes D, et al: Depressive symptoms and depressive diagnoses in a community population: a new procedure for analysis of psychiatric classification, *Archives of General Psychiatry* 45:1078-1084, 1988.

Bradley JJ: Severe localized pain associated with the depressive syndrome, *British Journal of Psychiatry* 109:741, 1963.

Brink PL: Depression in the aged: dynamics and treatment, *Journal of the National Medical Association* 69:891-893, 1977.

Casper RC, Redmond E, Katz MM, Schaffer CV, Davis JM, et al: Somatic symptoms in prior affective disorder: presence and relationship to the classification of depression, *Archives of General Psychiatry* 42:1098-1104, 1985.

Chessea ES: *A Study of Some Etiological Factors in the Affective Disorder of Old Age.* Unpublished Ph.D. dissertation. Institute of Psychiatry, University of London, 1965.

DeAlarcon RD: Hypochondriasis and depression in the aged, *Gerontology Clinic* 6:266-277, 1964.

Diagnostic and Statistical Manual of Mental Disorders (ed 3— revised). Washington, DC, American Psychiatric Association, 1987.

Dohrenwend BP, Oskenberg L, Shrout PE, Dohrenwend BS, Cook D: What brief psychiatries screen scales measure? In Sudman S (ed): *Proceedings of Third Biennial Conference on Health Survey Method.* Washington, DC, National Center for Health Statistics, 1979.

Dohrenwend BP, Shrout PE, Egri G, Mendelsohn FS: Non-specific psychological distress and other dimensions of psychopathologic measures for use in the general population, *Archives of General Psychiatry* 37:1229-1236, 1980.

Epstein LJ: Depression in the elderly, *Journal of Gerontology* 31:278-282, 1986.

Fassler LB, Gavirin M: Depression in old age, *Journal of the American Geriatrics Society* 26:471-475, 1978.

Foulds GA: *The Nature of Personal Illness.* New York, Academic Press, 1976.

Frank JD: *Persuasion and Healing.* Baltimore, John's Hopkins Press, 1973, pp. 312-318.

Gaitz C, Scott J: Age and measurement of mental health, *Journal of Health and Social Behavior* 13:55, 1972.

Goldfarb AI: Masked depression in the elderly. In Lesse (ed): *Masked Depression.* New York, Jason Aronson, 1974, pp. 236-249.

Goldstein S: Depression in the elderly, *Journal of the American Pediatric Society* 27:38-42, 1979.

Gurland, DJ: The comparative frequency of depression in various adult age groups, *Journal of Gerontology* 31:283-292, 1976.

Gross ML: *The Psychological Society.* New York, Random House, 1978.

Hamilton M: A rating scale for depression, *Journal of Neurology, Neurosurgery in Psychiatry* 23:56-62, 1960.

Hustrup JL, Baker JG, Kramer DL, Borstein RF: Crying and depression among older adults, *The Gerontologist* 26:91-96, 1986.

Lehmann AT: Psychiatric concepts of depression nomenclature and classification, *Canadian Psychiatric Association Journal* 4:51 (supp), 1959.

Leighton AH, Lambo T, Hughes C, Leighton B, Murphy J, et al: *Psychiatric Disorders among the Yuruba.* Ithaca, New York, Cornell University Press, 1963.

Levin S: Depression in the aged: a study of the salient external factors, *Geriatrics* 18:302, 1963.

Linn L: Clinical manifestations of psychiatric disorders. In Freedman AM, Kaplan HI, Sadock BJ (eds): *Comprehensive Textbook of Psychiatry* (vol 2). Baltimore, Williams and Wilkins, 1974, pp. 783-825.

Magni G, Schifano FD, Leo D: Pain as a symptom in elderly depressed patients: relationship to diagnostic subgroups, *Archives of Psychiatry in Neurological Sciences* 335:143-145, 1985.

Montgomery SA, Asberg M: A new depression scale designed to be sensitive to change, *British Journal of Psychiatry* 134:382-389, 1979.

Musetti L, Perugi G, Soriani A, Rassi VA, Cssano GB, et al: Depression before and after age 65: a reexamination, *British Journal of Psychiatry* 155:330-336, 1989.

Nelson JC, Charney DS: The symptoms of major depressive illness, *American Journal of Psychiatry* 138:1-13, 1981.

Parker G, Hadzi-Pavlovic D, Boyce P: Endogenous depression as a construct: a quantitative analysis of the literature and the study of clinical judgments, *Australian and New Zealand Journal of Psychiatry* 23:357-368, 1989.

Post F: The factor of aging and affective illness. In Oppen A, Wath A (eds): Recent developments of affective disorders, *British Journal of Psychiatry*, special publication No. 2, 1968, pp. 105-116.

Radloff LS: The CES-scale: a self-report depression scale for research in the general population, *Applied Psychological Measurement* 1:385-401, 1977.

Rapp SR, Vrana S: Substituting nonsomatic for somatic symptoms and the diagnosis of depression in elderly male medical patients, *American Journal of Psychiatry* 146:1197-1200, 1989.

Robins LN, Helzer JE, Croughan J, Ratcliff KS: The National Institute of Mental Health Diagnostic Interview Schedule: its history, characteristics and validity, *Archives of General Psychiatry* 38:381-389, 1981.

Rosenthal SH: Volitional depression. In Arieti S (ed): *American Handbook of Psychiatry* (vol 3). New York, Basic Books, 1974, pp. 694-709.

Ross CE, Malrowsky J: Components of depressed mood in married men and women: The Center for Epidemiologic Studies Depression Scale, *American Journal of Epidemiology* 119:997-1004, 1984.

Salzman C, Shader RI: Depression in the elderly. I. Relationship between depression, psychological defense mechanisms, and physical illness, *Journal of the American Geriatric Society* 26:253-260, 1978b.

Salzman C, Shader RI: Depression in the elderly. II. Possible drug etiologies and differential diagnostic criteria, *Journal of the American Geriatric Society* 26:303-308, 1978b.

Schmale AH: Giving up as a final common pathway to changes in health, *Advances in Psychosomatic Medicine* 8:20, 1972.

Snaith RP: The concepts of mild depression, *British Journal of Psychiatry* 150:387-393, 1987.

Steuer J, Bank L, Olsen EJ, Jervik LF: Depression, physical health and somatic complaints in the elderly: study of the Beck self-rating depression scale, *Journal of Gerontology* 35:683-688, 1980.

Thomae H: Personality and adjustment of aging. In Birren J, Sloane RB (eds): *The Handbook of Aging and Mental Health*. Englewood Cliffs, New Jersey, Prentice-Hall, 1980, pp. 285-309.

Watts CA: The mild endogenous depression, *British Medical Journal* 1:4, 1957.

Williamson J: Depression in the elderly, *Age and Aging* 7:35-40 (supp), 1978.

Wilson DR, Widmar RB, Cadrat RJ, Judiesch K: Somatic symptoms: a major feature of depression in a family practice, *Journal of Affective Disorders* 5:199-207, 1983.

Winokur G, Behan D, Schlesser M: Clinician and biological aspects of depression of the elderly. In Cole JO, Barrett JE (eds): *Psychopathology in the Aged*. New York, Raven Press, 1980, pp. 145-153.

Yesavage JA, Brink TL, Rose PL, Lum O, Huang V, et al: Development and validation of a geriatric depression screening scale: a preliminary report, *Journal of Psychiatry Research* 17:37-49, 1983.

Zemore R, Eames N: Psychic and somatic symptoms of depression among adults, institutionalized aged and noninstitutionalized aged, *Journal of Gerontology* 34:716-722, 1979.

3

Natural History

Depressive disorders in late life tend to recur or persist and change the course of a patient's life over time. Therefore clinicians working with depressed patients develop a relationship with those patients similar to the relationship of clinicians working with patients who have chronic physical illness. A major goal during the assessment of a depressed older adult is predicting the outcome or prognosis of the depressive disorder. Only with a knowledge of the natural history of the depressive disorder can clinicians, patients, and families accurately assess the value of any therapeutic intervention. An accurate prognosis also permits the patient and family to plan for and adapt to problems arising over time.

Clinicians must beware, since prognosis may become self-fulfilling prophecy. For example, a clinician who predicts that a patient's condition will not improve or even deteriorate may, through the expression of this opinion, alter the clinical course of the condition. However, even this risk does not negate the potential benefit of accurate prognosis.

Predicting the natural history of depressive illness in older adults is of additional benefit to the clinician and clinical investigator. Natural history is an important contribution to determining whether an assigned diagnosis is accurate. In other words, characterization of symptom complexes as diagnoses should predict the outcome of the symptom complexes. This validation element of the diagnostic process dates from the early stages of modern psychiatry. Kraeplin (1921) distinguished the mood disorders (which he labeled *manic depressive insanity*) from the schizophrenic disorders (which he labeled *dementia praecox*) primarily on the basis of their eventual outcome. Dementia praecox, by definition, was characterized by gradual deterioration over time. However, later studies demonstrated that schizophrenia does not always deteriorate, which led nosologists to reconsider the subgroups within the general category of schizophrenic disorder. Depressive illness, especially manic depressive or bipolar disorder, does not follow a uniform course, which suggests distinct subtypes, each with a potentially different outcome.

A number of measures are available to clinicians and clinical investigators to assess outcome or natural history of the depressive disorders. The onset and cessation of depressive episodes is the most basic measure of outcome. Natural history of episodes is usually described in terms of remission from and relapse into a depressive episode. Symptom severity at follow-up is another measure of outcome. Additional aspects of natural history include the patient's age at onset of the disorder and the effect of comorbidity (depression associated with other psychiatric and physical disorders). Did the depressive illness precede other physical and psychiatric problems, or did the illness follow another condition, such as an acute, severe physical illness? Many investigators are now exploring the relation of depression to disability, especially social and occupational disability. The impact of depressive symptoms over time on cognitive dysfunction in late life has been of interest. Finally, mortality studies of depression, especially studies of suicide in the elderly are important markers of natural history. Older persons, specifically older white males, are more likely to commit suicide and the majority of suicides result from depressive illness. Each of these topics is explored in this chapter via a review of the available data.

Age of Onset Studies

Many investigators have explored the relationship between the age of onset of depression among the elderly and natural history of the depressive illness. In these studies, older persons who experience their first onset depression in late life have usually been compared with older persons who experienced a recurrence of a depressive episode or continuation of depressive symptoms that first appeared earlier in life.

In a review of index cases of depression in clinical and community settings, approximately one half of subjects in late life report their first episode during late life and about one half report onset earlier in life. (Greenwald and Kramer-Ginsberg, 1988; Demalie, et al, in press). In these studies, age of onset of the first episode of depression does not appear to be a major factor in either the symptomatology of the depression or the natural history of the depression. Greenwald and Kramer-Ginsberg (1988) found that early onset (less than 60 years of age) and late onset (more than 60 years of age) of the first episode of depression did not significantly differentiate symptomatology, cognitive impairment, physical illness, family history, or treatment responsiveness in a group of 71 depressed in patients 60 years of age and older. Herrmann et al (1989) reviewed the records of 55 psychiatric inpatients with an average age of 77 years. There was no association between age and psychosis, severe cognitive impairment, positive family history, length of hospitalization, prescribed treatment, or treatment response. When the cases were regrouped on the basis of age of first admission, only the rates of family history were significantly different (i.e., older depressed patients were less likely to report a positive family history of depression). In a community sample of over 2000 persons, Lewinsohn et al (1986) did not find the duration of an episode of depression to increase with age.

A common clinical impression is that late onset of depression is associated with a greater likelihood of delusional depression or psychotic depression. In a sample of patients over the age of 60 suffering a primary diagnosis of unipolar manic depression, Nelson et al (1989) found the mean age of onset was not significantly different in 39 delusional and 79 nondelusional unipolar depressed patients. This finding does not contradict the finding that delusional depressions are more common in late life but does suggest that age of the first episode is not a factor in the increased prevalence of delusional depression in late life.

The most consistent finding in the literature regarding age of onset is an inverse relationship between age of onset of depression in probands and the risk of depression in their relatives (Mendlewicz, 1976; Hopkinson, 1964). Yet these family history differences do not appear to contribute significantly to either the symptom presentation of depression in late life or the biologic correlates of late life depression (Meyers and Alexopoulos, 1988).

Another area of interest regards the nature of symptomology of bipolar affective disorder by age of onset. A study by Carlson et al (1977) provides some insight. These investigators studied a group of early onset bipolar patients (most of them were in adolescence) and compared them with patients whose illness onset was after the age of 45 (a late onset for individual experiencing manic-depressive illness). Results indicated that a late age of onset was not a factor in the course and prognosis of the manic-depressive illness.

A review of the literature, therefore, suggests that age of depression onset in late life is not a significant predictor of symptoms nor the natural history of late life depression.

Clinical Course Depressive Symptoms

A number of studies have emerged in the literature over the past 15 years that document the clinical course of depressive symptoms across the life cycle. To place the studies devoted to late life depression in context, a review of studies devoted to clinical course earlier in life, especially of unipolar and bipolar disorders, is necessary. The studies available can be divided into long-term and short-term outcome studies.

Perhaps the most in-depth long-term study was a prospective longitudinal study lasting 15 years of unipolar, bipolar, and schizoid affective patients by Angst (1980). Unipolar depressions followed a much more favorable course than bipolar and schizoid affective depressions. Unipolar depressions began on the average when the patient was 45 years old, whereas the average ages of onset of bipolar disorder was 35 and 32 for the schizoid affective psychoses. Duration of unipolar depressions was an average of 6 months, whereas bipolar diseases last for 4.4 months and schizoid affective psychosis for 4.7 months. Chronicity, a duration of an episode exceeding 1 to 2 years, was often observed. The probability at the last episode reported by this prospective cohort being chronic was 24.5% for the unipolars, 17.9% for the bipolars, and 18% for the schizoid affectives.

Perhaps the most troubling aspect of the data reported by Angst for older depressives is the time spacing of successive phases or cycles of affective illness. He found a systematic reduction in the time between cycles with increasing age. Initially, time between episodes was more than 5 years in unipolar subjects and about 4 years in bipolar subjects, but this shortened quickly (exponentially) until "a certain limit value, which is intra-individually different, had been attained." All patients, however, did not continue to suffer relapses. Approximately 44% of the unipolar patients, 17% of the bipolar patients, and 37% schizoid affective patients had 5-year disease-free intervals at the time of follow-up. The majority of the cases of disease, regardless of diagnosis, were still active at an average age of 60 (the average age at which this follow-up was completed).

Overall, complete remissions were seen in 41% of unipolar cases, 36% of bipolar cases, and in 27% schizoid affective cases. Approximately 10% of the depressed subjects committed suicide over the 15-year period.

Lehmann et al (1988) reported an 11-year follow-up of 110 depressed patients in Montreal, Canada. The mean duration of the index and subsequent episodes in this cohort was approximately 12 months. At least one recurrence after the index episode was reported by 78% and at least four recurrences were reported by 19%. Sixty percent were depressed for at least 1 year and 31% for at least 2 years of the 11 years of follow-up. Approximately 10% of the cohort committed suicide after the 11-year follow-up.

Kiloh et al (1988) reported a 15-year follow-up of 145 patients with a primary depressive illness who were hospitalized between 1966 and 1970 in Australia. During the follow-up period, 7% had committed suicide, 12% had remained incapacitated by illness, and 12% had remained continuously well. Patients for whom the index admission was not their first were especially likely to be readmitted during the follow-up. The majority of the subjects, 63%, reported episodes.

In summary, the long-term follow-up of individuals with bipolar or unipolar mood disorder across the life cycle from large university–based cohorts suggests a chronic course for mood disorders. Few subjects recover from an episode and remain recovered through the follow-up period. Most subjects recover and then suffer a subsequent relapse. Approximately 20%, however, remain continuously ill, therefore the depression becomes a chronic disorder lasting for many years. In addition, the risk for suicide is high, 10%, in subjects suffering recurrent mood disorders.

In recent years a number of studies have emerged in the literature that have documented, in much greater detail, the outcome of mood disorders prospectively for shorter duration. The results from the Psychobiology of Depression group (Keller et al, 1982a and Keller et al, 1982b; Keller et al, 1981) are the most frequently quoted studies in the literature. Data from the psychobiology of depression studies reveal that in 1 year of follow-up, 50% of a cohort of persons diagnosed with major depression 59 years of age and younger recovered but that the annual rate of recovery after 1 year decreased to 28% during the second year and 22% in the third year. Therefore recovery from an index episode of major depression is most likely to occur within the year after diagnosis of the episode. Among those individuals who recover, 24% will suffer a relapse within 3 months. Of the 101 subjects in this study, 16% remained ill throughout the year, 63% recovered with 12% having almost complete recovery. Eight percent had a partial remission and 36% of those with complete or almost complete recovery suffered a relapse. Five percent had more than one relapse. Twenty-four percent had some recurrence of symptoms but no relapse.

Rounsaville et al (1980) followed 72 ambulatory patients for 12 months. These investigators found at follow-up 30% asymptomatic, 36% gradually improving, 13% still depressed or becoming more depressed, and 21% who experienced recovery but who also suffered one or more relapses during the 12-month follow-up. Three percent of this sample made a suicide attempt during follow-up. In a 1-year follow-up of patients with an average age of 55, Goodnich (1987) found that despite remission, there were significant symptoms of mania and depression at each follow-up visit. In a community sample of over 2000 subjects, Lewinsohn et al (1989) found that the probability of relapse among those subjects identified as suffering from a unipolar depressive disorder was positively related to the number of previous episodes of unipolar depression, female gender, and severity of episode but not age of onset. Keller et al (1981) found that coexistent dysthymic disorder was a poor prognostic sign for recovery and remaining well from major depression.

In summary the short-term, intense studies of the clinical course of unipolar depressive disorders confirm the findings of the long-term studies. Depressive disorders are chronic illnesses and, to some extent, the "rule of thirds" applies. Approximately one third of subjects recover and remain recovered during a follow-up. Another one third exhibit a pattern of recovery and relapse during follow-up. The final one third do not recover or experience only a partial recovery during follow-up. Suicides are infrequent in short-term follow-up studies (as would be expected) but in the short-term study by Rounsaville et al (1980), 3% of the cohort made suicide attempts during the 12-month follow-up.

Outcome studies of bipolar disorders are less frequent. In a recent study by Broadhead and Jacoby (1990), manic patients over the age of 60 were compared with manic patients below 40 years of age. The elderly bipolars were clinically distinguished from younger bipolars in that elderly patients with bipolar disorder appeared to experience more "fragile recovery," since significantly more elders relapsed into a depressive episode between resolution of their manic illness and discharge from the hospital. In general, among patients suffering bipolar disorder, about 15% of the episodes of mood disorders they experience are manic episodes (Carlson et al, 1974). Chronicity in bipolar disorders appears even greater than in unipolar patients. After a 2-year follow-up, according to Winokur et al (1969), about one third of the subjects remained chronically ill after the index episode. Bipolar patients who recover from an episode of major depression are also more likely to relapse than unipolar patients (Coryell et al, 1987). Across the life span, the probability of unipolar recurrent depressives becoming bipolar is approximately 5% (Dunner et al, 1976).

In summary, bipolar disorder is a disorder that usually has its onset early in life, although a first manic episode can occur in the elderly. Unipolar disorders that have been chronic through the life span are unlikely to revert to a bipolar disorder in late life. Early onset bipolar disorders, on the other hand, persist into late life. Ziss and Godwin (1979), following a cohort of depressed subjects across the life cycle, found that a later age of onset of both bipolar and unipolar disorder correlates with shorter first and subsequent intervals between episodes. They also found that the probability of relapse within 24 months increases with age for both unipolar and bipolar patients (i.e., from about 30% in the twenties to about 70% in the sixties for bipolar and from about 20% in the twenties to about 80% in the fifties for unipolar). Yet these findings have not been replicated. In general the extant data do not suggest that bipolar disorder worsens with aging. On the contrary, Angst (1981) found that burning out (three or less episodes over 5 years) was seen in 29% of bipolars and 42% of unipolars as they entered old age.

A review of studies documenting the clinical course of depression among older adults is presented in Table 3-1. The results from these studies, when compared with the studies reported in previous sections, suggest that, except for the increased mortality rate observed in elderly depressive (e.g., the Murphy [1983] and Robinson studies), the natural history is similar to that reported for the young and middle-aged. In other words, the rule of thirds also applies to depression in late life. The studies by Post (1962) and

TABLE 3-1. Outcome Studies of Depression in Late Life

Author	Sample	Follow-up Period	Results
Post, 1962	100	6 years	31% well throughout follow-up period, 28% suffered at least one relapse but recovered, 23% had a poor recovery with invalidism, and 17% were ill throughout the follow-up period.
Murphy, 1983	124	1 year	14% died, 35% had good outcome, 48% had poor outcome, and 3% developed dementia.
Baldwin and Jolly, 1986	100	42-104	22% well throughout the follow-up period, 28% recovered and relapsed, and 33.7% did not recover.
Cole, 1985	60	2-6 years (outpatients)	18% fully recovered, 52% partially recovered, and 30% not recovered.
Kivela et al, 1991	199 elderly with dysthymia and 42 with major depression	Mean duration of 15 months	43% of dysthymic men, 38% of dysthymic women, 39% of major depressive men, and 48% of major depressive women had a good outcome.
Borville et al, 1991	103 elderly depressives	12 months	Outcome good in 32% to 47% of cases. Increased mortality in men. No obvious clinical correlates of poor outcome.
Demalie et al, in press	47 elders and 678 middle-aged with major depression	12 months	55% recovered at 6 months and an additional 9% recovered at 12 months for both age groups. Social factors associated with recovery in midlife but not late life.

Murphy (1983) illustrate the similarity. Post (1962), in a 6-year follow-up of 100 consecutive cases of late life depression, found only 19% achieved recovery both of satisfactory quality and of extended duration. Approximately 35% of the subjects had improved social and psychologic adaptation after the depressive episode, 28% demonstrated little change, and 18% showed definite deterioration of the symptoms at sixth-year follow-up. Factors associated with better long-term recovery were age of less than 70 years, absence of physical illness, good social adjustment, and a symptom complex approximating the manic-depressive symptom pattern (in contrast to the study by Angst that suggests a manic-depressive symptom complex is associated with worse prognosis). Patients did less well if they developed their first symptoms after the age of 50 years, suggesting that late-onset depression, in contrast to manic-depressive disorder, may be less likely spontaneously remit or respond to therapy. This finding was previously reported by Lunguist (1945).

Roth (1955), however, describes a more favorable prognosis. He suggests that individuals with late-onset depression have better outcomes than those with illnesses occurring at an earlier age. In a 2-year follow-up study he found that, of 253 institutionalized patients with affective disorders, 64% had been discharged, 19% were dead, and 17% remained as inpatients.

Murphy (1983), using Research Diagnostic Criteria for major depression, replicated the study of Post (1972). In a 1-year prospective study of 124 elderly depressed patients, only one third of the group had a favorable outcome. Poor outcome was associated with severity of initial illness, those with depressive delusions having a particularly poor outcome. The outcome was also influenced by physical health problems and severe life events during the follow-up year. There was no evidence that an intimate relationship protected against relapse. The mortality rate was especially high, yet only 14.5% of the patients had no physical health problems, and 38% had major physical health problems.

A particularly troublesome problem during the course of depression, regardless of age, is the development of a rapid cycling disorder. Rapid cycling has been defined as four or more mood episodes (manic-depressive episodes) occurring in a year (Dunner and Fieve, 1974). Rapid cycling has been associated with poor thyroid functioning (Cowdry et al, 1983) and long-term use of medications (Wehr, 1979). Rapid-cycling major depression is one of the most difficult clinical challenges today and occurs in late life as it does at other stages of the life cycle. Angst et al (1990) have described a variant of rapid-cycling depression (i.e., recurrent brief depression). In a cohort of young adults a substantial proportion met all criteria for major depression except duration. The mood changes would occur for as short as 2 to 3 days but occurred at least one to two times per month during the year of follow-up. Although these subjects reported a euthymic mood most of the time, the depressive symptoms were severe enough to lead to considerable impairment in social and occupational functioning. This entity may also be present among the elderly.

■ COMORBID STUDIES

The natural history of depressive disorders across the life cycle is affected in large part by other disorders that accompany the depressive episode (see box on p. 50). In a 2-year follow-up study, Keller et al (1983) found that approximately 25% of inpatients with an index diagnosis of major depression suffered a preexisting chronic depression of at least a 2-years duration. Chronic depression reduced the apparent effect of the known predictors of recovery and relapse from major depressive disorders and predicted a more negative outcome. If the subject reported suffering from a chronic depression after recovering from the index episode, the probability of a relapse into another major depres-

---

Factors Associated with a Less Favorable Outcome from Major Depression in Late Life

Comorbid dysthymic disorder
Comorbid generational anxiety and passive
Psychotic depression
Comorbid medical problem
Comorbid personality disorder
Impaired social support
Stressful life events during the period of follow-up
Comorbid cognitive impairment
Multiple previous episodes of depression
Bipolar disorder

---

sive episode was increased. This coexistence of major and chronic depression (dysthymia) is often called *double depression* and is as frequent in late life as during other stages of the life cycle.

The coexistence of the symptoms of generalized anxiety and major depression is also recognized to predispose to a poor outcome of the depressive disorder (Paykel, 1972). VanValkenburg et al (1984) found that patients with both depression and panic attacks reported a poorer outcome than patients suffering from depression alone. Anxiety is a frequent symptom accompanying depressive disorders, occurring in as many as 75% of subjects. Blazer et al (1989), reported early-morning anxiety at follow-up in 32% of 131 elderly and middle-aged patients hospitalized for major depression 1 to 2 years after hospitalization. Most of the patients who complained of early-morning anxiety at follow-up also complained of anxiety at other times of the day. Early-morning anxiety in this sample appears to be a variant of a more severe anxiety disorder that persisted in approximately 30% of the subjects. Seventy-three percent of the sample suffered the symptoms of generalized anxiety (symptoms of anxiety lasting for at least 1 month) at baseline and the comorbid frequency of anxiety did not vary by age. Only 15% reported that the anxiety preceded the depressive episode. Therefore it is difficult to determine whether coexistence anxiety is a comorbid state (major depression and generalized anxiety) or a symptom of the depressive episode per se.

Psychotic features also affect the prognosis of affective disorders across the life cycle. Coryell et al (1990), in a 5-year follow-up of patients from the Psychobiology of Depression Study, found that patients with schizoid affective disorder, manic type, experienced a poorer follow-up than patients with a pure manic episode. In the same study (Coryell et al, 1990b), factors that predicted a poor outcome included being single rather than married, social impairment as adolescent, and a history of schizophrenic-like psychotic features temporally disassociated from affective symptoms. In another study, Coryell and Tsuang (1982) found no differences between delusional and nondelusional groups with primary unipolar depressions in terms of marital, residential, and occupational outcome status or death by suicide in a 40-year follow-up study.

Aronson et al (1988), in a naturalistic study, followed a cohort of 52 patients with delusional depression and found that over 80% relapsed an average of two times during the 32-month follow-up. The majority of relapses occurred while patients were either medication-free or on prophylactic doses of psychotherapeutic medications during combination treatment with antidepressants and lithium carbonate. Baldwin (1988) tested the hypothesis that delusional and nondelusional depressive illnesses are distinct entities during late life in a prospective follow-up study. During the index admission, deluded older patients were significantly more depressed and/or in the hospital for a longer period of time, responded less well to antidepressants alone, and required more physical treatments (especially electric convulsive therapy and major tranquilizers). Only the deluded group experienced delusional relapses. The outcome status was similar for both groups, such as the relapse rates and the persistence of depressive symptoms over 42 to 104 months. These findings do not concur with other reports of a poor outcome for delusional depression in late life (Murphy, 1983).

The outcome of major depression has also been shown to be less positive when patients suffer from significant medical illnesses. Shulberg et al (1987), in an investigation of 274 patients suffering depressive symptoms, found that the coexistence of depression and physical problems at baseline were strong predictors of persistent depression at follow-up. They also found that the number of assigned medical diagnoses, rather than the physician's recognition and treatment of the depression during the index episode, were the strongest predictors of a continued depressive illness. Keitner et al (1991) compared patients admitted to a psychiatric service with pure major depression to patients with major depression compounded by coexisting medical or other psychiatric conditions. The recovery rate of the patients with compounded depression was significantly worse than for pure depression.

In another study, however, Lustman et al (1988) reported a 5-year follow-up study of depression among adult diabetics. Among patients diagnosed with major depression and reinterviewed 5 years later, 64% had experienced an episode of major depression within the previous 12 months, most of these episodes satisfying criteria for a major depressive episode. Patients reporting recurrent depression had an average of four depressive episodes over the 5-year period, a recurrence rate not unlike subjects without medical illness.

Stoudenine et al (in press) followed two groups of medically ill elders diagnosed with major depression, one with cognitive impairment and one without. In patients with normal pretreatment cognitive functioning, cognition remained stable (even among these subjects receiving ECT) and improved in many subjects. Relapse was frequent, however, and 26% were rehospitalized during the year after the index episode.

Personality factors have also been associated with the prognosis of major depression. Pfohl et al (1987) found that the presence of personality disorders in a series of 78 nonpsychotic inpatients with major depression predicated an especially poor prognosis. Depressed inpatients who met more than the average number of personality disorder criteria among the entire group of subjects were approximately one half as likely to show improvement at discharge and at 6-month follow-up as patients with less than the average number of criteria. Shea et al (1990), in a study deriving from the NIMH Treatment of Depression Collaborative Research Program, found that, among 239 outpatients with major depression randomly assigned to one of four 16-week treatment conditions, the majority (74%) were found to have notable personality disturbance on one or more of the DSM-III disorders on assessment at pretreatment. Personality disordered patients had a significantly worse outcome than patients who did not suffer personality disorders and also were more likely to report residual symptoms of depression at follow-up regardless of the treatment assigned.

Although most of the studies of comorbidity and the outcome of depression have not been directed specifically to the elderly, there is no evidence from the literature that the patterns of comorbidity and poor prognosis found at earlier stages of the life cycle do not apply to the elderly. Therefore comorbid generalized anxiety, dysthymic disorder (chronic minor depression), major medical problems, or major personality dysfunction all contribute to a poor prognosis of major depression in late life. More studies should be directed, in the future, to determine the specific role of comorbidity in late life, especially for those comorbid factors known to be of increased prevalence among the depressed elderly, such as medical illness and organic mental disorders. There is little evidence that dysthymic disorder, generalized anxiety, or personality disorders (the most frequently described comorbid psychiatric disorders that lead to poor prognosis) are more common in late life (they may be less common). Psychotic depressions are more prevalent in late life than during other stages of the life cycle. Psychotic depressions are more likely to predict psychotic depressions in the future but do not necessarily suggest a poor prognosis overall for functioning of the older depressed adult.

Cognitive impairment has also been associated with a poor prognosis for the outcome of depressive disorders. In a 2-year follow-up of 16 patients with mixed symptoms of depression and dementia, Reynolds et al (1986) found one half exhibiting clinical improvement and the other half deterioration. Improvement at 2-year follow-up was associated with the following baseline measures: a Mini-Mental State Score of 21 or greater, a Hamilton depression score 21 or greater, and sleep efficiency of less than 75%. This finding suggests that among the elderly with mixed symptoms of depression and dementia, a more favorable outcome is associated with initially greater depressive symptoms and moderate sleep continuity disturbance, specifically early morning awakening. Carl and Emory (1989) followed 44 elderly patients (a mean age of 77) experiencing depression and dementia who were initially treated for depression. Most of these patients exhibited an improvement in cognitive function initially. Patients were retested at 6-month intervals for an average of 8 years. At the end of the observation period, 89% had developed a dementia syndrome of the Alzheimer's type.

■ DEPRESSION, DISABILITY, AND SOCIAL FUNCTIONING

No study of the natural history and clinical course of depressive disorders in the elderly would be complete without investigating social functioning of depressive elders subsequent to experiencing a depressive episode. Wells et al (1989), in a well-publicized study of over 11,000 outpatients in general medical facilities, found that patients with either current depressive disorder or depressive symptoms in the absence of disorder experienced worse physical, social, and role functioning, as well as worse perceived current health and greater bodily pain, than patients with no chronic conditions. The poor functioning uniquely associated with depressive symptoms, with or without depressive disorder, was comparable with or worse than that associated with eight other chronic medical conditions, such as hypertension, diabetes, arthritis, and lung problems. Data were not stratified by age, but the average age of the subjects was 48 years old and there was no upper age limit of the sample.

Barrett et al (1989) reported data on the outcome of depressions seen in a rural primary care setting. Depressed patients were more likely, compared with those without depression and those with anxiety disorders, to report new complaints at follow-up to their primary care physicians. Minor depressives as a group had more new complaints per visit and more visits to their primary care providers. The complaints of minor depression may be appropriately treated with antidepressive medications. The investigators did not disaggregate this sample by age, but many of the subjects were 65 years of age and older.

Broadhead et al (1990) performed a study in North Carolina similar to the study by Wells reported previously. In a sample of nearly 3000 North Carolina community residents, compared with asymptomatic individuals, persons with major depression had nearly five times greater risk of disability days and days lost from work during the year after diagnosis. Persons with minor depression with mood disturbance but not major depression had 1.5 times greater risk. Because of its relatively greater prevalence, minor depression was associated with two times as much disability among community-dwelling residents as major depressives during follow-up. Minor depressions were also at increased risk of having a concomitant anxiety disorder, of developing major depression within the year after which they were identified, and of suffering from minor depression at follow-ups. Major depression was much less common in the elderly in this sample compared with young persons and those in middle-age, whereas minor depression was more common in the elderly than during other stages of the life cycle.

Kennedy et al (1991) studied the relationship of disability and poor health to persistence or remission of depressive symptoms in a community sample of older adults (n = 1577). They compared the characteristics of community residents whose depressive symptoms persisted over 24 months with a group whose symptoms remitted. Decline in health status, older age, sleep disturbance, poor social support, and serious illness accounted for more than 30% of the variance between the persistently depressed and the remission groups.

Tsuang et al (1979a and b) have reported on the long-term outcome of major psychoses. In this 30- to 40-year follow-up of 200 schizophrenic, 100 manic, 225 depressive, 160 psychiatrically symptom-free surgical patients, the investigators found that, overall, patients with schizophrenia and affective disorders had notedly poorer outcomes than patients psychiatrically healthy. Schizophrenic patients fared more poorly than patients with affective disorders. Twenty-two percent of manic patients had poor ratings for marital status, 14 for residential status, 24 for occupational, and 29 for psychiatric status. Among depressed patients, 9% were rated at outcome for poor marital status, 12% for poor residential status, 70% for poor occupational status, and 22% for poor psychiatric status. As these subjects were in late mid-life or late life at follow-up (mean age of surviving patient over 62 years), these data provide significant insight into the effects of psychiatric illness on functioning among older adults.

■ MORTALITY STUDIES

Late life depression has been associated with increased mortality. In this section, studies are reviewed regarding the association of bereavement and mortality, major depression and mortality, and suicide among the elderly.

Bereavement and Mortality

Outcome studies of the elderly have consistently revealed associations between bereavement and mortality. Jacobs and Ostfeld (1977) reviewed the epidemiologic evidence for such an association. Data suggest that mortality is increased among the bereaved during the first year after a loss for all age groups (Cocco, 1940; Cox and Ford, 1964; Young, et al, 1963), yet the association is higher for younger than older persons. This may reflect the observation that death of a spouse or other loved one in late life is an expected event (Neugarten, 1970) and therefore may not be as stressful. Cumming and Henry (1961) stated that social isolation is a typical and expected result of the aging process. The process of disengagement takes place at approximately age 65 years and this results in "mutual severing of ties between a person and others." Therefore reactions to grief may not be as severe for the elderly. Maddox (1963), however, is one of many researchers who refute this notion.

Since the review of Jacobs and Ostfeld (1977) a significant study has appeared in the literature (Levav et al, 1988). These investigators studied the health consequences of parental bereavement in which mortality in two groups of bereaved Israeli parents were compared with the general population. One cohort comprised the parents of over 2500 soldiers killed in the Yon Kippur War of 1973 (soldiers between the ages 18 and 40) and the second consisted of parents of over 1000 men between 18 and 30 years of age who died in accidents between 1901 and 1975. The 10-year age-adjusted data exhibit a mortality risk higher among fathers whose sons died in accidents rather than in war, but mortality did not differ significantly between the two groups of mothers. Overall, the investigators found no excess mortality among the bereaved parents as compared with the general population. The findings do not provide support for the hypothesis that the loss of an adult son is associated with increased short-term mortality in married parents.

Other Mortality Studies

A number of population studies have emerged in the literature documenting the impact of depression on mortality. Kaplan and Reynolds (1983) studied the association between depressive symptoms, cancer incidence, and mortality from noncancer causes in nearly 7000 persons free of cancer at initial contact. They demonstrated an association between depressive symptoms at baseline and death from noncancer causes but no association with either cancer incidence or cancer mortality. Murphy et al (1987), in a 16-year prospective study of a general population sample, found that sample members who reported depression and/or anxiety disorder at baseline experienced 1.5 times the number of deaths expected. Increased risk of death was found to be significantly associated with affective but not physical disorders and with depression but not generalized anxiety.

In another community sample of older adults, Bruce and Leaf (1989) found the odds of dying from an affective disorder over 15 months in persons 55 years of age and older to be four times greater than for others in the sample, controlling for age, gender, and physical health. Fredman et al (1989), however, did not confirm this result. In a study of over 1600 persons 60 years of age and older in the epidemiologic area study in North Carolina, neither depressive diagnosis (major depression and/or dysthymic) nor depressive symptoms were associated with higher mortality when individuals were followed for 24 months.

Increased mortality for individuals suffering from depression have also been documented in clinical base studies. Tsuang et al (1980) found a significant increase in mortality rates for individuals suffering affective disorders (both mania and depression) compared with controls and the overall general population. Excess causes of death were suicides, accidents, infections, and circulatory system diseases. As with the study by Kaplan and Reynolds, Tsuang et al did not find mortality because of neoplasm significantly higher among depressives than the general population.

Murphy et al (1988) studied 4-year mortality of 124 elderly depressed patients. Even when physical illness was controlled, depressed patients had a significantly higher 4-year mortality, especially from cardiovascular disease. Rabins et al (1985) found, among 62 elderly depressed patients followed for 1 year after discharge from the hospital, that 13% had died, a nearly 75% greater than expected mortality rate. Patients dying in this study were more likely to carry a diagnosis of cardiovascular disease.

Rouner et al (1991) examined the relationship between depression and mortality in nursing homes. Major depressive disorder, but not depressive symptoms, was a risk factor for mortality over 1 year, independent of the health status of the respondents. Major depression increased the likelihood of death by 59%.

Suicide

By far the most tragic outcome of depressive disorders in late life is suicide. According to Stengel (1983), "a suicidal act is any deliberate act of self-damage that the person committing the act could not be sure to survive." Successful suicides are usually considered acute, such as when an individual commits a violent act that results in his or her own death. Menninger (1938) pointed out that suicides may also be chronic. Many behaviors are forms of indirect self-destruction, such as asceticism, martyrdom, neurotic invalidism, alcohol addiction, antisocial behavior, psychosis, self-mutilation, malingering, polysurgery, purposive accidents, impotence, rigidity, and even certain physical illnesses. Stengel warned, however, that self-destruction is not always inherent in the suicidal acts. Attempted suicide may serve as a warning and therefore has the effect of an appeal for help. Other persons may make suicidal gestures (acts in which the elder clearly does not expect to die) to gain attention.

The overall suicide rate for older adults has decreased steadily during the latter twentieth century until recently (Centers for Disease Control, 1985; Meechan et al, 1991). Suicide rates from 1980 through 1986 increased among white males by 23% and among black males by 42% (Meechan et al, 1991). Two peaks in rates (during the years before World Wars I and II) have occurred during this century. Since World War II, the rates have declined steadily until the recent upturn. If investigators disaggregate suicide rates by age, the rates for the young during the past 20 years have increased compared with the decrease in rates for the elderly (Murphy and Wetzel, 1980; Manton et al, 1987). Nevertheless, suicide rates remain higher for persons in later life than for those at other stages of the life cycle. The recent upturn in rates is therefore disturbing. Yet older persons made fewer suicide attempts than any other age group (Grollman, 1971).

Parkin and Stengel (1965), in a 2-year survey of hospitals and general practitioners, found that the ratio of suicide attempts to successful suicides in persons 60 years of age and older was 4 to 1, whereas the ratio of attempts to suicides for persons younger than 40 was 20 to 1. Bock (1972) found that older persons communicate the intentions to commit suicide less frequently, and Maris (1969) found that older persons are more likely to use weapons to commit suicide. A number of investigators have found that older persons in general are more successful at suicide attempts than younger persons (Resnick and Cantor, 1970; Sendbuehler and Goldstein, 1977). Between the ages of 65 and 69, male suicides outnumber female suicides 4 to 1. By age 85 years, this ratio increases to approximately 12 to 1 (National Center for Health Statistics, 1977).

When compared with all adults, the frequency of expressed thoughts about death and desire to die among the elderly was similar to the frequency in younger adults studied in an epidemiologic survey within North Carolina (Blazer et al, 1986). More than 7% of the overall sample versus 3.5% of the elderly, however, reported having thoughts about suicide sometime during their life. More than 1% of the entire sample, versus 0.3% of the elderly, had attempted suicide.

Suicide by older persons is difficult to predict (Miller, 1979). An inability to cope with loss is not enough to explain the increased rate of suicide among the elderly. Barraclough (1971) confirms the experience of many clinicians that depressive symptoms among the elderly who attempt suicide may not appear severe. However, depression, insomnia, tension, and agitation are nearly always present in older persons who do make suicide attempts. Suicide in late life is frequently an impulsive act. Family members of persons who commit suicide often report that the elders appeared no different on the day of the suicide than on any other day and that they spoke of plans for the future earlier in the day of the suicide. Although many of these persons express considerable psychic and psychophysiologic discomfort, Batchelor (1957) noted that physical illness is not a cause of the majority of late life suicides.

In general, psychiatrists and other physicians are poor at predicting suicide in individual patients that they are treating. Nevertheless, studies of attempted and successfully completed suicide suggest a number of risk factors to clinicians in estimating suicidal potential. The overall increased risk of suicide with age has never been adequately explained, however. Miller (1979) suggests that the loss of family and social ties leads to increased potential for suicide. This theory dovetails with the early work of Durkheim (1951) who stated that "suicides occurring at the crisis of widowhood . . . are really due to domestic anomie resulting from the death of husband or wife. . . . The survivor . . . has not adapted to the new situation in which he finds himself and accordingly offers less resistance to suicide."

A brief discussion of other risk factors that interact with age can be of benefit to clinicians in assessing the risk for suicide (Blazer, 1991). Gender is a risk factor of suicide that interacts with age. For all age groups, males have reported higher suicide rates than females. Older white males commit suicide at higher rates than any other group by age and race. Race is a risk factor of suicide that tends to be overlooked when only overall trends in suicide rates are examined. Monk (1987) reported that black males have experienced a tripling of suicide rates in the past 25 years in the over 85 age group. During the same period, suicide rates for white men 85 years of age and older did not change although the rates for white men continue to be three times higher than for black men in the over 85 age group. This increased rate in suicide among the oldest black males parallels an increased rate among younger men for both races in the 15-to-24 age group.

Marital status varies as a risk factor for suicide by age (Smith et al, 1988). At all ages, married persons have the lowest suicidal rates and the widowed and divorced have the highest rates. Yet the increased risk among the single, divorced, and widowed is less for the elderly than at earlier stages of the life cycle. Young widowed males have an exceptionally high rate of suicide. Marshall (1978) compared suicide rates in the middle of this century for the impact of economic status. Income status exerted a significant buffer on aged white male suicides in the post-World War II era. Other social variables, such as employment status and divorce rate in wartime, did not appear to be associated with suicide.

Psychiatric disorders, especially depression, are associated with an increased risk of suicide, regardless of age. Miles (1977), in a review of over 100 longitudinal studies of psychiatric patients, concluded that nearly all suicides in the United States are committed by persons with a mental disorder. He found a marked increase of suicide among persons suffering mood disorders, and especially among individuals with a mood disorder that was comorbid with alcohol problems and/or organic mental disorder. The risk of suicide secondary to psychiatric disorder appears to be greater in men than in women.

Suicide attempts are yet another risk factor for suicide across the life cycle. Regardless of age, most suicide attempts do not result in a successful suicide; yet the attempt does place the individual at much greater risk for suicide during the months and years that followed the attempt. Dorpat and Ripley (1960) reviewed 15 studies that compared successful suicides among persons who had made suicide attempts. Between 0.03% and 22% had committed suicide at follow-up depending primarily on the length of time to follow-up. These rates are over 100 times greater than rates of suicide in the general population.

In his survey of vital statistics in London, Sainsbury (1962) found that bereavement had been experienced by 16% of individuals who committed suicide. Paykel et al (1975) found that 21% of persons who committed suicide had reported bereavement within 6 months before suicide, as compared with 4% of a group of matched controls. The majority of grief episodes at all stages of the life cycle, however, are not accompanied by suicide attempts. Isolation and aloneness are other risk factors that should be considered. In the same study, Sainsbury reported that 39% of elderly persons who committed suicide had been living alone. Batchelor and Napier (1953) found aloneness in a majority of individuals who made suicide attempts. In contrast, O'Neal et al (1956) did not find loneliness to be a significant contributing factor.

In summary, age, male gender, white race, comorbid physical and psychiatric illness, divorce or widowhood, bereavement, alcohol and drug problems, low income, and a history of suicide attempts all render the older adult greater risk for suicide (see box on p. 58). When the clinician, during the process of evaluation of the depressed older adult, sees these factors begin to cluster, he/she should seriously consider intervention strategies to decrease the risk, such as hospitalization or constant supervision by family and friends during the initial period.

Risk Factors for Suicide in the Elderly Depressed

Older age (e.g., 75+ years)
Male gender
White race (difference in rates between white and black men is decreasing)
Low income (greater risk for males than females with low income)
Social isolation
Divorce or widowhood
Bereavement
Comorbid physical illness
Comorbid psychiatric illness (e.g., depression plus panic disorder)
Alcohol abuse/dependence
Drug abuse/dependence
History of suicide attempt(s)
Impulsive behavior

REFERENCES

Angst J: Clinical indications for a propel active treatment of depression. In Mendlewicz J, Coppen A, Van-Prag H (eds): *Depressive Illness-biological and Psycho Pharmacological Issues*. Symposium Amsterdam 1980 Advances in Biological Psychiatry, (vol 7), Basel, Kerger, 1981 pp. 218-229.

Angst J: Course of unipolar depressive, bipolar manic-depressive, and schizoid affective disorders. Results of a prospective longitudinal study, *Fortschritte Der Neurologie-Psychiatrie* 48:3-30, 1980.

Angst J, Merikangas K, Scheidegger P, Wicki W: Recurrent brief depression: a new subtype of affective disorder, *Journal Affective Disorders* 19:87-98, 1990

Aronson PA, Shukla S, Gujavarty K, Hoff A, DiBuono M, et al: Relapse and delusional depression: retrospective study of the course of treatment, *Comprehensive Psychiatry* 29:12-21, 1988.

Baldwin RC, Jolley DJ: The prognosis of depression in old age, *British Journal of Psychiatry* 149:574-583, 1986.

Barett J, Oxman T, Barett J, Gerver P: *Outcome of Depressions in a Primary Care Practice*. Paper presented at the Annual Meeting of the American Psychiatric Association, May 11, 1989, San Francisco, California.

Barraclough BM: Suicide in the elderly. In Key DWK, Walk A (eds): *Recent Development in Psycho Geriatrics*. London, Headley Brothers, 1971.

Batchelor IRC: Suicide in old age. In Sehnidman E, Farburow N (eds). *Clues to Suicide*. New York, McGraw-Hill, 1957 pp. 143-152.

Batchelor IRC, Napier M: Attempted suicide and old age, *British Medical Journal* 2:1186, 1953.

Blazer D: Suicide risk factors int he elderly: an epidemiologic study, *Journal of Geriatric Psychiatry* 24:175-190, 1991.

Blazer DG, Bachar JR, Manton KG: Suicide in late-life: reviewing commentary, *Journal of the American Geriatrics Society* 34:519-525, 1986.

Blazer D, Hughes DA, Fuller N: Anxiety as an outcome symptom of depression in elderly in middle-age adults, *International Journal of Geriatric Psychiatry* 4:273-278, 1989.

Bock E: Aging and suicide, *The Family Coordinator* 21:71, 1972.

Broadhead J, Jacoby R: Mania in old age: at first prospective study, *International Journal and Geriatric Psychiatry* 5:215-222, 1990.

Broadhead WE, Blazer DG, George LK, Tse CK: Depression, disability days, and days lost from work in a prospective epidemiologic survey, *Journal of American Medical Association*, 264:2525-2528, 1990.

Bruce ML, Leaf PJ: Psychiatric disorders in 15-month mortality in a community sample of older adults, *American Journal of Public Health* 79:727-730, 1989.

Burvill PW, Hall WD, Stampfer HG, Emerson JP: The prognosis of depression in old age, *British Journal of Psychiatry* 158:64-71, 1991.

Carlson GA, Davenport YB, Jemison K: A comparison of outcome in adolescence-and late-onset bipolar manic-depressive illness, *American Journal of Psychiatry* 134:919-922, 1977.

Carlson GA, Kotin J, Davenport YD, Adland M: Follow-up of 53 bipolar and manic-depressive patients, *British Journal of Psychiatry* 124:134-139, 1974.

Centers for Disease Control. *Suicide Surveillance, 1970-1980.* Atlanta, 1985.

Cocco A: The mortality of husbands and wives, *Human Biology* 12:508, 1940.

Cole MG: Age, age of onset in course of primary depressive illness in the elderly, *Canadian Journal of Psychiatry* 28:102-104, 1983.

Cole MG: The course of elderly depressed outpatients, *Canadian Journal of Psychiatry* 30:217-220, 1985.

Coryell W, Andreasen NC, Endicott J, Keller M: The significance of past mania or hyper mania in the course and outcome of major depression, *American Journal of Psychiatry* 144:309-315, 1987.

Coryell W, Keller M, Lavori P, Endicott J: Affective syndromes,psychotic features, in prognosis: I. Depression, *Archives of General Psychiatry* 47:651-657, 1990a.

Coryell W, Keller M, Lavori P, Endicott J: Affective syndromes, psychotic features, in prognosis: II. Mania, *Archives of General Psychiatry* 47:658-662, 1990b.

Coryell W, Tsuang MT: Primary unipolar depression and the prognostic importance of delusions, *Archives of Journal Psychiatry* 39:1181-1184, 1982.

Cowdry RW, Wehr TA, Ziss AP, Godwin FK: Thyroid abnormalities associated with rapid cycling bipolar illness, *Archives of General Psychiatry* 40:414-420, 1983.

Cox PR, Ford JR: The mortality of widowers shortly after widowhood, *Lancet* 1:163, 1964.

Cumming E., Henry W: *Growing Old.* New York, Basic Books, 1961.

Demalie DA, Blazer DG, Hughes DC: Symptoms and correlates of major depression in natural history study: an age comparison, (in press).

Dorpat TL, Ripley HS: A study of suicide in the Seattle area, *Comprehensive Psychiatry* 1:349-359, 1960.

Dunner DL, Fieve RR: Clinical factors in lithium carbonate profolax failure, *Archives of Journal Psychiatry* 30:229-233, 1974.

Dunner DL, Fleiss J, Fieve RR: The course of development of mania in patients with recurrent depression, *American Journal of Psychiatry* 133:905-908, 1976.

Durkheim E: *Suicide* (translated by JA Spalding and G Simpson). New York, Free Press, 1951.

Fredman L, Schoenbach VJ, Kaplan BH, Blazer DG, James SA, et al: The association between depressive symptoms and mortality among older participants in the epidemiologic captured area-Piedmont Health Survey, *Journal of Gerontology* 44:S149-S156, 1989.

Gallagher-Thompson D, Hanley-Peterson P, Thompson LW: Maintenance of gains versus relapse following brief psychotherapy for depression, *Journal of Consulting in Clinical Psychology* 58:371-374, 1990.

Goodnich PJ, Fieve RR, Schlegel A, Kaufman K: Enter-episode major and subclinical symptoms and affective disorder, *Actas Psychiatric and Scandanivica* 75:597-600, 1987.

Greenwald BS, Kramer-Ginsberg E: Age onset in geriatric depression: relationship to clinical variables, *Journal of Affective Disorders* 15:61-68, 1988.

Grollman E: *Suicide: Prevention, Intervention and Postvention.* Boston, Beacon Press, 1971, pp. 57, 58, 132-134.

Herrmann N, Lieff S, Silberfeld M: The effect of age onset on depression in the elderly, *Journal of Geriatric Psychiatry Neurology* 2:182-187, 1989.

Hopkinson GA: Genetic study of affective illness in patients over 50, *British Journal of Psychiatry* 110:244-254, 1964.

Jacobs S, Ostfeld A: An epidemiologic review of the mortality of bereavement, *Psychosomatics Medicine* 39:344, 1977.

Kaplan GA, Reynolds P: Depression and cancer mortality and morbidity: prospective evidence from the Alameda county study, *Journal of Behavioral Medicine* 11:1-13, 1988.

Keitner GI, Ryan CE, Miller IW, Kohn R, Epstein NB: Twelve-month outcome of patients with major depressive and comorbid psychiatric or medical illness (compound depression), *American Journal of Psychiatry* 148:345-350, 1991.

Keller MB, Lavori PW, Endicott J, Coryell W, Klearman GL: "Double depression": two-year follow-up, *American Journal of Psychiatry* 140:689-694, 1983.

Keller MB, Shapiro RW, Lavori PW, Wolfe N: Recovery in major depressive disorder: analyses with the life table and regression models, *Archives of General Psychiatry* 39:905-910, 1982a.

Keller MB, Shapiro RW, Lavori PW, Wolfe N: Relapse in major depressive disorder: analyses with the life table, *Archives of General Psychiatry* 39:911-915, 1982.

Keller MB, Shapiro RW: Major depressive disorder: initial results from a one year, prospective, naturalistic follow-up study, *Journal of Nervous and Mental Diseases* 169:761-768, 1981.

Kennedy GJ, Kelman HR, Thomas C: Persistence in remission of depressive symptoms in late life, *American Journal of Psychiatry* 148:174-178, 1991.

Kiloh LG, Andrews G, Neilson M: The long-term outcome of depressive disorders, *British Journal of Psychiatry* 153:752-757, 1988.

Kivela S, Pahkala K, Laippala P: A one-year prognosis of disthymic disorder and major depression in old age, *International Journal of Geriatric Psychiatry* 6:81-87, 1991.

Kraeplin E: *Manic-depressive Insanity and Paranoia* (edited and translated by R Barkley). Edinburgh, ES Livingston, 1921.

Kral VA, Emery OB: Long-term follow-up of depressive dementia of the aged, *Canadian Journal of Psychiatry* 34:45, 46, 1989.

Lehmann HE, Fenton FR, Deutsch M, Feldman S, Engelsman F: An eleven-year follow-up study of 110 depressed patients, *Actas Pyschiatric and Scandanivica* 78:57-65, 1988.

Levav I, Friedlander Y, Kerk JD, Peritz E: An epidemiologic study of mortality among bereaved parents, *The New England Journal of Medicine* 319:457-461, 1988.

Lewinsohn PM, Fenn DS, Steinton HA, Franklin J: Relation of age of onset to duration of episodes in unipolar depression, *Journal of Psychology in Aging* 1:63-68, 1986.

Lewinsohn PM, Zeiss AM, Duncan EM: Probability of relapse after recovery from an episode of depression, *Journal of Eminolo Psychology* 98:107-116, 1989.

Lunguist G: Prognosis and course of manic depressive psychosis: a follow-up study of 319 of first admissions, *Actas Psychiatrica Neurologica* (supp) 35:1945.

Lustman PJ, Griffith LS, Clouse RE: Depression in adults with diabetes: results five-year follow-up study, *Diabetes Care* 11:605-612, 1988.

Maddox G: Activity and morale: a longitudinal study of selected elderly subjects, *Social Forces* 42:195, 1963.

Manton KG, Blazer DB, Woodbury MA: Suicide in middle age and later life: sex- and race-specific life table and cohort analyses, *Journal of Gerontology* 42:219-227, 1987.

Maris R: *Age and the Suicide Rates.* Homewood, Illinois, Dorsey Press, 1969, pp. 93-96, 98-100.

Marshall JR: Changes in aged white male suicide: 1948-1972, *Journal of Gerontology* 33:763-768, 1978.

Mendlewicz J: The age factor in depressive illness: some genetic contributions, *Journal of Gerontology* 31:300-303, 1976.

Menninger K: *Man against Himself.* New York, Harcourt, Brace and World, 1938.

Meechan PJ, Salzman LE, Satin RW: Suicides among older United States residents: epidemiologic characteristics and trends, *American Journal of Public Health* 81:1198-1200, 1991.

Meyers BS, Alexopoulos G: Age of onset and studies of late-life depression, *National Journal of Geriatric Psychiatry* 3:219-228, 1988.

Miles CP: Conditions predisposing to suicide: a review, *Journal of Nervous and Mental Diseases* 164:231-246, 1977.

Miller M: *Suicide after Sixty: The Final Alternative.* New York, Springer, 1979.

Monk M: Epidemiology of suicide, *Epidemiologic Reviews* 9:51-69, 1987.

Murphy E: The prognosis of depression in old age, *British Journal of Psychiatry* 142:111-119, 1983.

Murphy E, Smith R, Lindesy J, Slattery J: Increased morality rates in late-life depression, *British Journal of Psychiatry* 152:347-353, 1988.

Murphy GE, Wetzl RD: Suicide risk by birth cohort in the United States, 1949-1974, *Archives of General Psychiatry* 37:519-523, 1980.

Murphy JM, Monson RR, Olivier DC, Sobol AM, Mighton AH: Affective disorders and mortality: a general population study, *Archives of the General Psychiatry* 44:473-480, 1987.

National Center for Health Statistics. *Final Mortality Statistics,* 1975, vol. 25, 1977.

Nelson JC, Conwell Y, Kim K, Mazure C: Age of onset in late-life delusional depression, *American Journal of Psychiatry* 146:785-786, 1989.

Neugarten DL: Adaption and the life cycle period, *Journal of Geriatric Psychology* 4:71, 1970.

O'Neal P, Robins E, Schmidt EH: A psychiatric study of attempted suicidal persons over 60 years of age, *Archives of Neurology and Psychiatry* 75:275, 1966.

Parkin D, Stengel E: Incidence of suicide attempts in an urban community, *British Medical Journal* 2:133, 1965.

Paykel ES: Depressive topologies in response to emtripline, *British Journal of Psychiatry* 120:147-156, 1972.

Pfohl D, Coryell W, Zimmermann M, Stangl D: Prognostic validity of self-report and interview measures of personality disorders and depressed inpatients, *Journal of Clinical Psychiatry* 48:468-472, 1987.

Post F: The management and nature of depressive illness in late life, a follow through study, *Journal of Psychiatry* 121:393, 1972.

Post F: *The Significance of Affective Symptoms at Old Age.* Maudsley Monograph 10. London, Oxford University Press, 1962.

Rabins PV, Hervis K, Koven S: Half mortality rates of late-life depression associated with cardiovascular disease, *Journal Affective Disorders* 9:165-167, 1985.

Resnick HLP, Cantor J: Suicide and aging, *Journal of the American Geriatric Society* 18:152, 1970.

Reynolds CF, Kupfer DJ, Hoch CC, Stack JA, Houck PR, Sewitzh DE: Two-year follow-up of elderly patient with mixed depression and dementia: clinical and electrographic sleep finding, *Journal of the American Geriatrics Society* 34:793-799, 1986.

Robinson JR: The natural history of mental disorder and old age: a long-term study, *British Journal of Psychiatry* 154:793-789, 1989.

Roth M: Natural history of mental disorders and old age, *Journal of Mental Sciences* 101:281, 1955.

Rouner BW, German PS, Branth J, Clark R, Burton L, et al: Depression and morality in nursing homes, *Journal of American Medical Association* 265:993-996, 1991.

Rounsaville BJ, Prusoff BA, Padian N: The course of nonbipolar, primary major depression: Prospective 16-month study of ambulatory patients, *Journal of Nervous and Mental Diseases* 168:406-411, 1980.

Sainsbury P: Suicide in later life, *Gerontologia Clinica* 4:161, 1962.

Schulberg HC, McClelland M, Goding W: Six-month outcomes for medical patients with major depressive disorders, *Journal of Internal Medicine* 2:312-317, 1987.

Sendbuehler JM, Goldstein S: Attempted suicide among the aged, *Journal of the American Geriatrics Society* 25:245, 1977.

Shea MT, Pilqonis PA, Beckham E, Collins JF, Elkin I, et al: Personality disorders and treatment outcomes int he NIMH Treatment Depression Collaborative Research Program, *American Journal of Psychiatry* 147:711-718, 1990.

Smith JC, March JA, Conn JM: Marital status in the risk of suicide, *American Journal of Public Health* 78:78-80, 1988.

Stengel E: *Suicide and Attempted Suicide.* New York, Bengoin Book, 1973.

Stoudemire A, Hill C, Morris R, Martino-Saltzman D, Markwaiter H, et al: Cognitive outcome following tricyclic and electroconvulsive treatment of major depression in the elderly, *American Journal of Psychiatry* 148:1336-1340, 1991.

Tsuang MT, Wilson RF, Fleming JA: Premature death and schizophrenia and affective disorders: In an analyses of survival curves and variables affecting to shorten survival, *Archives of the General Psychiatry* 37:979-983, 1980.

Tsuang MT, Wollson RF, Fleming JA: Long-term outcome of major psychosis I. Schizophrenia and affective disorders compared with psychiatrically symptom-free surgical conditions, *Archives of General Psychiatry* 36:1295-1301, 1979.

VanValkenburg C, Akiskal HS, Puzantian V, Rosenthal T: Anxious depressions: clinical, family history, and naturalistic outcome-comparisons with panic and major depressive disorders, *Journal of Affective disorders* 6:67-82, 1984.

Wehr TA, Godwin FK: Rapid cycling in manic-depressive induced by tricyclic antidepressant, *Archives of Journal Psychiatry* 36:555-559, 1979.

Wells KB, Stewart A, Hays RD, Burnam A, Rogers W, et al: The functioning and well-being of depressed patients: results from the medical outcomes study, *Journal of the American Medical Association* 262:914-919, 1989.

Winokur GW, Clayton PJ, Reich T: *Manic Depressive Illness.* St. Louis, Mosby–Year Book, 1969.

Young M. Benjamin B, Willis C: The mortality of widowers, *Lancet* 2:454, 1963.

Ziss AP, Grof P, Godwin FK: The natural course of affective disorders: Implications for proflaxis. In Croll BJ (CD): *Lithium: Controversies in Unresolved Issues: Proceedings of the International Lithium Conference.* Amsterdam, Excerpta Medica, 1979, pp. 381-398.

The Origins of Late Life Depression

4

BIOLOGIC ORIGINS OF DEPRESSION IN LATE LIFE

The concept that fluctuations in mood can be caused by biologic changes is almost as old as the history of medicine. A Hippocratic physician stated the following:

> . . . and men should know that from nothing else but from the brain come joys, delights, laughters and jest, and sorrows, griefs, despondency and limitations. And by this . . . we require wisdom and knowledge . . . and by the same organ we become mad and delirious and fears and terrors assail, some by night and some by day, and dreams and untimely wanderings and cares that are not suitable and ignorance of present circumstances, desuetude and unskillfullness. All these things we endure from the brain, when it is not healthy, but more hot, more cold, more moist or more dry than natural, or when it suffers any other preternatural and unusual affliction (Adams, 1939).

Hippocrates also suggested that disorders of the mind were accounted for by the four humors of ancient biochemistry, melancholia being caused by black bile (Adams, 1939).

In more recent years, we have learned that late life depressions are often associated with biologic changes (Lipton and Nemeroff, 1978; Veith and Raskind, 1988; Ferrier and McKeith, 1991). Even Freud recognized that "melancholia takes on various clinical forms (some with somatic rather than psychogenic affections) but does not seem to definitely warrant production to unity" (Freud, 1950). The current understanding of brain function suggests that organized behavior results from impulse transmission through intricate networks of neurons in the brain. Interconnections are extensive and consist primarily of chemical synapses, each of which offers a potential site for establishing or modifying a neuronal circuit (Brodie and Sack, 1975; Roberts and Hammerschlag, 1972). Synapses have been the major focus of interest in biologic psychiatry investigation. They appear to be the anatomic loci for information transfer. Therefore both emotion and cognition potentially have a biologic substrate—the transmission of information from one nerve cell to another.

Two tasks are undertaken in this chapter. First, the basic neurophysiology of the nervous system is reviewed, with attention directed toward changes with aging. Second, the relationship between normal changes with aging within the central nervous system and pathologic changes in depression are explored. The accumulated data have begun to converge toward an overall psychobiologic model of depression across the life cycle.

■ BASIC NEUROPHYSIOLOGY AND AGING

Physiologic, morophologic, and behavioral characteristics are determined to varying degrees by biologic processes that are "gene directed" (Kessler, 1975). At conception each individual possesses a constellation of genes that influences behavior by affecting the development and functioning of the organism. Yet genetic determination does not proceed blindly, since the intracellular and intercellular milieu of the body, as well as the external environment, modulate gene function. The state of the organism at any point in the life cycle depends on its ability to assess feedback from the internal and external environment and to regulate physiologic processes accordingly.

The nervous and endocrine systems and circadian rhythms have been well established as the regulators of physiologic processes throughout the body. Extracellular factors, such as neurotransmitters and hormones, are known to play an important role as regulators. Although the individual steps in many of the important metabolic pathways have been identified, complex mechanisms by which these systems react and interact remain unknown. Before the current hypotheses about neurophysiology of aging and mood disorders are explored, the gross neuroanatomic, the intracellular, and intercellular mechanisms by which information transfer and regulation occur within the central nervous system, the endocrine system, and circadian rhythms are briefly described.

Although heredity determines the formation and growth of the central nervous system, there is little evidence for genetically controlled changes in the morphology of the central nervous system that lead to depression in late life. Nevertheless the complex and varied ways in which the genome controls the organism throughout life has not been applied specifically to the psychiatric disorders in late life. The few studies that examine the genetic basis of depression in late life are reviewed next.

Structural Brain Changes with Aging

There is considerable evidence for changes in brain structure with aging. The advent of magnetic resonance imaging (MRI) techniques has made it possible to examine the brain in much greater detail than previously in vivo (Krishnan, [in press]). In general, brain volume decreases with aging and cerebral spinal fluid volume increases. This leads to cortical atrophy and enlarged lateral ventricles, which can be seen when scanning. In addition, periventricular white matter hyperintersities increase in prevalence with aging; subcortical gray matter hyperintensities in the basal ganglia, thalamus, and pons also increase. In one study, these hyperintsensitives were correlated with the previous history of risk factors for ischemic cerebral vascular disease and hypertension. Sullivan et al (1990) found these changes to be associated with both age and a history of stroke.

In cross-sectional studies, comparisons of specific brain structures indicate evidence of change with age as well. Krishnan et al (1990) found that the caudate nucleus declines steadily in size with age. Other investigators have found similar changes in the putamen, with the decline in volume of the cerebral hemisphere being much smaller than the change in volume of the basal ganglia and had a moderate decline in the midsagittal corpus callosum area with aging (McDonald et al, [in press]; Doraiswamy et al [in press]).

Microscopic Brain Changes and Aging

The neuron is the basic anatomic and functional microscopic unit for the central nervous system. Transfer of information from one neuron to another is the major function of neurons, and this information transfer has been the subject of most microscopic investigations in neurobiology. Multiple connections between neurons through their dendritic processes allow an almost infinite number of potential patterns of transmission. Information transfer between neurons is mediated by chemical substances called *neurotransmitters*. This contrasts with the transfer of information within a neuron, which is mediated by the polarization of the nerve cell membrane by an action potential leading to change in the flux of sodium, potassium, and calcium. When the depolarized impulse reaches the periphery of the axon (the nerve cell terminal), a change in calcium concentration appears to be critical in releasing the chemical neurotransmitters. The transmission takes place at a structure called the *synapses*. The synapses consist of the nerve terminal, the postsynaptic membrane, and a discontinuity called a *synaptic cleft*.

Polarization of the nerve terminal membrane initiates diffusion of storage vessicles containing the neurotransmitter substance to the membrane of the nerve terminal. These substances then extrude into the synaptic clefts, diffuse across the cleft, and interact with postsynaptic receptors (as well as presynaptic receptors). The action of these transmitters may enhance either depolarization of the postsynaptic membrane (resulting in excitation of the second neuron) or hyperpolarization (resulting in an inhibition of impulse transfer) (Ciaranello and Patrick, 1977). The events leading to depolarization of the postsynpatic membrane after the binding of the neurotransmitter are not fully understood. In recent years, investigators have focused on the role of cyclic adeneline monophosphate (AMP) as a "second messenger" in the effects mediated by the biogenic amines (Brodie and Sack, 1975). Adenyl cyclase, which catalyzes the formation of cyclic AMP, may be activated by the biogenic amines. Cyclic AMP in turn provokes depolarization of the postsynaptic neuron.

After neurotransmitter substances have entered the synaptic cleft, they are subject to inactiviation through a number of processes. First, neurotransmitters can be metabolized by enzymes within the synaptic cleft, such as acetylcholine. Second, the nerve terminal or presynaptic membrane may reabsorb the neurotransmitter substances, such as norepinephrine and serotonin. Third, the substances may be blocked by the competitive action of either internal or external agents, such as other neurotransmitters or antidepressant agents (Figure 4-1).

Virtually all studies of the processes of neurotransmission by age have considered age-related declines in either presynaptic or postsynaptic concentrations of neurotransmitters and receptors (Morgan and May, 1990). There is no evidence that the process of

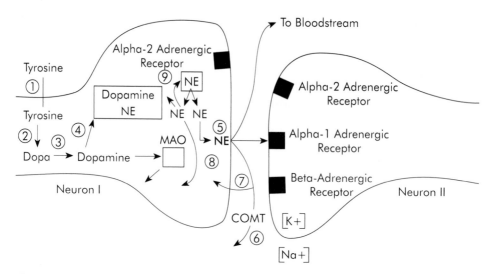

Figure 4-1. Biochemistry of synaptic transmission. (1) Uptake of tyrosine into cell; (2) conversion of tyrosine into dopa; (3) conversion of dopa to dopamine; (4) uptake of dopamine into vesicle; (5) release of norepinephrine at synapse; (6) deactivation of norepinephrine by COMT; (7) reuptake of norepinephrine into cell; (8) deactivation of norepinephrine by MAO; (9) uptake of norepinephrine into storage granule.

neurotransmission is interrupted with aging, and Cotman (1990) concludes that the brain retains its plastic capabilities throughout life. The number of synaptic connections between neurons decreases with aging, although the aged brain exhibits a continued capacity to mobilize axon sprouting and to make new synapses even in the course of age-related neurodegenerative diseases.

Neurotransmitter receptors are likened at times to a lock for which the transmitter is the key (Willner, 1985). The receptor is a membrane-bound protein, and when combined with the neurotransmitter the shape of the protein is thought to change, resulting in a series of intracellular events. These events include changes in ionic permeability of the cell membrane that will either increase or decrease the likelihood that an action potential will be generated during neurotransmission. There are at least three types of receptors for the norepinephrine system, alpha-1 adrenergic receptors, alpha-2 adrenergic receptors, and beta-adrenergic receptors (see Figure 4-1). Alpha-1 and beta-adrenergic blocking agents inhibit the effects of sympathetic nerve stimulation and the action of exogenously administered norepinephrine. In contrast, presynaptic alpha-2 receptors appear to facilitate adrenergic activity.

Significant data have accumulated that illuminate the major neurotransmitters found in the central nervous system and their changes with aging. To better understand how these neurotransmitters may contribute to the development of affective disorders, one should briefly review some of the general aspects of their synthesis and metabolism. Figure 4-2 shows the major neurotransmitters in the central nervous system, their metabolic pathways, and the enzymes associated with their synthesis and breakdown.

Acetylcholine is synthesized from choline in the nerve terminals of cholinergic neurons. As with other neurotransmitters, acetylcholine is stored in microgranules in the nerve terminal, where it is released by a nerve impulse to activate the postsynaptic

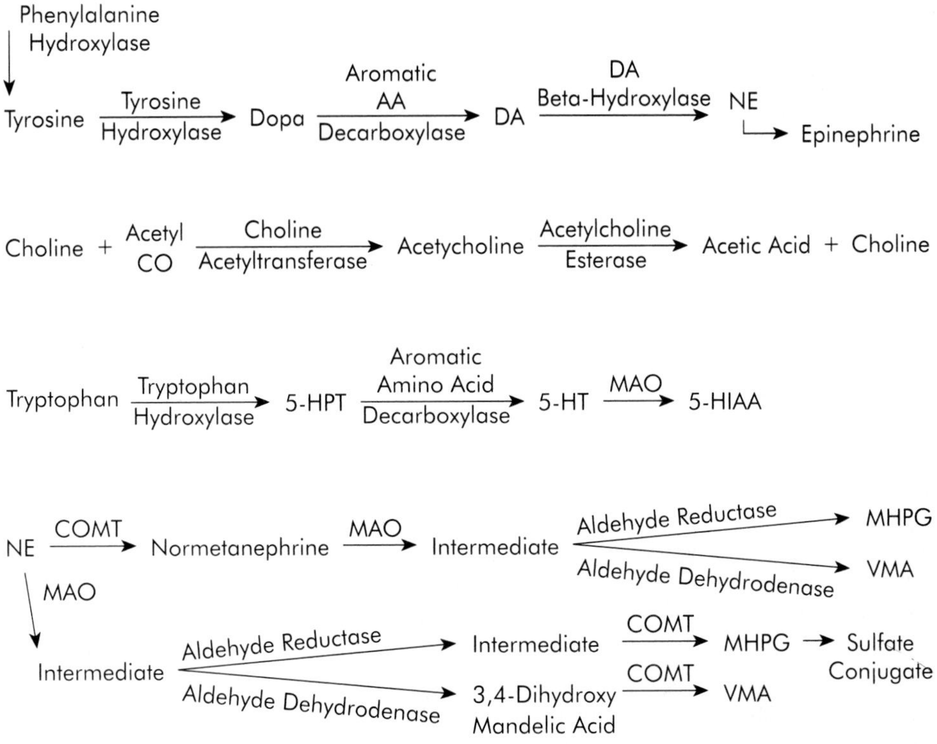

Phenylalanine
| Hydroxylase

Tyrosine $\xrightarrow[\text{Hydroxylase}]{\text{Tyrosine}}$ Dopa $\xrightarrow[\text{Decarboxylase}]{\text{Aromatic AA}}$ DA $\xrightarrow{\text{DA Beta-Hydroxylase}}$ NE $\longrightarrow$ Epinephrine

Choline + Acetyl CO $\xrightarrow[\text{Acetyltransferase}]{\text{Choline}}$ Acetycholine $\xrightarrow[\text{Esterase}]{\text{Acetylcholine}}$ Acetic Acid + Choline

Tryptophan $\xrightarrow[\text{Hydroxylase}]{\text{Tryptophan}}$ 5-HPT $\xrightarrow[\text{Decarboxylase}]{\text{Aromatic Amino Acid}}$ 5-HT $\xrightarrow{\text{MAO}}$ 5-HIAA

NE $\xrightarrow{\text{COMT}}$ Normetanephrine $\xrightarrow{\text{MAO}}$ Intermediate $\xrightarrow{\text{Aldehyde Reductase}}$ MHPG / $\xrightarrow{\text{Aldehyde Dehydrodenase}}$ VMA

| MAO

Intermediate $\xrightarrow{\text{Aldehyde Reductase}}$ Intermediate $\xrightarrow{\text{COMT}}$ MHPG $\rightarrow$ Sulfate / $\xrightarrow{\text{Aldehyde Dehydrodenase}}$ 3,4-Dihydroxy $\xrightarrow{\text{COMT}}$ VMA Conjugate Mandelic Acid

Figure 4-2. Metabolic pathways of major neurotransmitters.

nerve terminal, where it is released by a nerve impulse to activiate the postsynaptic receptors. Metabolism of acetylcholine occurs through the action of acetylcholinesterase, which hydrolyzes the neurotransmitter; subsequently choline is taken back up into the presynaptic nerve terminal.

Normal aging in humans does not appear to be associated with increased central nervous system cholinergic activity (Veith and Raskind, 1988). Data available suggest either no change or perhaps a decrease in the integrity of the presynaptic cholinergic neurons and postsynaptic cholinergic receptors with aging.

Serotonin, or 5-hydroxytryptamine (5-HT), like other brain transmitters, is present in many parts of the body. Serotonin is synthesized from tryptophan, which enters the nervous system via active uptake from the plasma. When taken back from the synaptic cleft into the presynaptic neuron, serotonin is metabolized by the enzyme monoamine oxidase (MAO), which converts the substance into 5-hydroxyindoleacetic-acid (5-HIAA) through a process of deamination. Norepinephrine, epinephrine, and dopamine are collectively called the *catecholamines* and are derived from a common amino acid phenylalanine. Dopamine, norepinephrine, and epinephrine may be synthesized after conversion of phenylalanine to tyrosine. Two enzymes are of importance in the metabolic breakdown of the cathecholamines, MAO and catechol-O-methyltransferase (COMT).

In the study of neurotransmitters and depression in late life in recent years the role serotonin of 5-HT receptors has received the most attention. There are many different subtypes of 5-HT receptors, the main ones being 5-HT1, 5-HT2, and 5-HT3 (Trickle-bank, 1987; Ferrier and McKeith, 1991).

The changes in central nervous system serotonin with aging have not been inten-sively investigated (Veith and Raskind, 1988). Some studies indicate that aging is asso-ciated with a substantial reduction in the concentration of serotonin and its synthetic enzyme, tryptophan hydroxylase. In the nuclei of the brain stem, Wong et al (1984) (using positron emission tomography [PET]) reported a linear reduction in human serotonin-2 receptor binding in multiple brain segments from 19 to 73 years of age. Re-garding changes in central nervous system norepinephrine activity of the aging, the an-swer is also unclear. Aging is associated with a loss of neurons in the locus ceruleus and there is a significant age-related reduction in norepinephrine in human brain tissue (Mc-Geer, 1978). The catabolic enzyme, MAO, is increased in tissues of older persons (Mc-Geer, 1978), which may further reduce central nervous system norepinephrine activity (Veith and Raskind, 1988). Yet Raskind et al (1989) have shown that cerebral spinal fluid norepinephrine is increased in normal old men compared with normal young men, thus suggesting an increased, rather than decreased brain norepinephrine activity and turnover.

The synthesis and metabolism of the neurotransmitters (described previously and out-lined in Figure 4-2) suggest that neurotransmitter function may be altered in a number of ways. Changes in the amount of certain enzymes could either increase or decrease the concentrations of these transmitters at the postsynaptic receptor. Increased dietary intake of the precursors of these enzymes may increase the availability of the precursors in the nerve terminal. These neurotransmitters may also be competitively replaced at the postsynaptic junction by substances that have a strong affinity for the postsynaptic receptor but that are ineffective in potentiating information transfer. Enhanced metab-olism of neurotransmitters in the synpatic cleft may be yet another means of decreasing the concentration of the neurotransmitter at the nerve terminal. Increased activity of metabolic enzymes inhibit neurotransmitter function by increasing the rate of their me-tabolisms. Changes in receptor numbers and actions also contribute to changes in neu-rotransmission.

Studies of depression with aging have centered on changes in function within the limbic system and the hypothalamus as putative sites for the development of mood dis-orders. Norepinephrine is essentially a peripheral compound but is within the central nervous system and is found most abundantly in the hypothalamus and brain stem. Do-pamine, on the other hand, is found in highest concentrations in the corpus striatum and substantia nigra. The tuberoinfundibular system is also mediated by dopamine as it projects down to the hypophyseal portal vessels. Serotonin can be found in the pineal gland and the hypothalamus and in quite high concentrations in a group of mesence-phalic pontine and raphe nuclei. Epinephrine is a major neurotransmitter outside the central nervous system, especially in the adrenal medulla, and can be found in the cen-tral nervous system, especially in limbic sites.

Brain Physiology and Aging

The physiologic activity of the brain, overall, has been investigated by determining the electrical activity through the electroencephalogram (EEG) and metabolism through PET, or cerebral blood flow. The normal human EEG undergoes a progressive change with age beginning at birth (Busse, 1989). Alpha rhythms, an 8 to 12 per second rhythmic sine wave, decrease gradually as age increases for both genders. Scattered slow waves (beta and delta waves) begin to appear in the EEG tracing with increased age. Almost 7% of the EEGs in older persons manifest a dominant frequency of 6 to 8 cycles per second. These slower waves have been correlated with cerebral blood flow (Obrist et al, 1963). In addition, frequent focal abnormalities appear with increased age. Busse et al (1954) found 30% to 40% of apparently healthy older persons to have temporal focal abnormalities predominately on the left side of the brain. Goodin and Aminoff (1986) studied long-latency, auditory-evoked potentials in normal individuals and in demented patients. The response to a rare tone was complex, and certain components the N1, N2, and P3 became progressively longer with increased age. They suggested these findings reflected a slowing of neuronal transmission with increased age.

One of the more persistent changes with aging reported in the gerontology literature is the decrease in cerebral blood flow with increasing age (Busse, 1989). Significant differences have also been found between the cerebral blood flow in normal individuals and aged-matched persons suffering from psychiatric disorders throughout the life cycle. Mathew et al (1985) found that the age-related reduction in cerebral blood flow was most marked in the frontal region. Women, regardless of age, had higher cerebral blood flow than men. Differences were most significant in the frontal region.

PET is an important new technique for clinical investigation and clinical assessment. The metabolism of different compounds can be compared across different anatomic regions within the brain, using the quantitative PET technique. Persons with psychiatric disorders exhibit changes from normal individuals overall in cerebral metabolism when viewed using PET scanning. Rapaport (1986) reported that age differences were not present for the regional metabolic rates for glucose metabolism, as measured by PET. Asymmetry in cerebral metabolism, on the other hand, appears early in Alzheimer's disease (i.e., patchy areas of the brain exhibit decreased metabolism).

Endocrine System Changes with Aging

The endocrine system is the regulating system in the human body that complements the nervous system. In contrast with the nervous system the endocrine system responds more slowly to internal and external environmental changes. At least three pituitary hormones (ACTH, growth hormone, and TSH) and two target organ hormones (cortisol and the thyroid hormones) are influenced by stress. The portion of the endocrine system most relevant to depression is the hypothalamic-pituitary-adrenal (HPA) axis. Both physical and psychologic stressors stimulate the HPA axis in humans and animals (Mason, 1974). The response of the HPA axis to stressors appears to be relayed through the HPA axis (Everitt, 1973) (Figure 4-3).

Biogenic amine neurotransmitters, especially dopamine, norepinephrine, and serotonin, play a major role in regulation of pituitary function. Regulation occurs via an influence on hypothalamic releasing and inhibiting factors, which are excreted from nerve terminals in the hypothalamus into the pituitary portal circulation. For example, norepinephrine may stimulate ACTH release via its stimulation of corticotrophin-releasing factor (CRF). Older theories suggest that norepinephrine is the main inhibitor rather than a stimulus for CRF release. A dual system of releasing factors, consisting of one inhibitory factor and one excitory factor, regulates the release of growth hormone. The

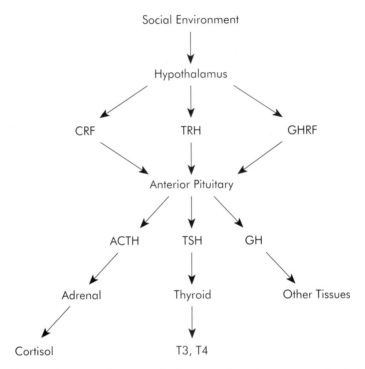

Figure 4-3. Neuroendocrine pathways in which changes have been associated with late life depression.

release of these hormones is facilitated by both dopaminergic and noradrenergic alpha-receptor stimulation.

Regarding the HPA axis, age is positively associated with basal plasma cortisol concentration (Veith and Raskind, 1988; Davis et al, 1984). The HPA axis can be tested by the administration of a synthetic steroid, dexamethasone (the Dexamethasone Suppression Test or DST). There appears to be no consistent change in the influence by dexamethasone on plasma cortisol in normal adults with increasing age, although post-dexamethasone cortisol is found in higher concentration on average in older adults (Tourigny-Rivard, 1981). An age-related decrease in the activity and density of noradrenergic neurons in the central nervous system may play a role in the increased basal level of cortisol of older persons and may, in turn, account for the association between age and plasma cortisol responses to yohimbine and alpha-2 antagonist (Price et al, 1986).

The thyroid-stimulating hormone (TSH) response to thyroid-releasing hormone (TRH) has been shown to decrease in older men with increasing age but not in older women (Snyder and Utiger, 1972a and b). Meites et al (1976) reported a significant decrease in the magnitude of TRH-induced TSH response in old rats as compared with young rats. Therefore some impairment in the thyroid axis analogous to that described for the HPA axis may be present, such as an alteration in receptor sensitivity.

Growth-hormone secretion is regulated by the hypothalamic growth-hormone releasing factor (GHRH) and somatostatin (Veith and Raskind, 1988). Growth hormone exerts many effects, especially in regulating the growth of the skeleton, muscle tissue, and connective tissue. There has been consistent evidence that growth hormone is dysregulated in depression, with the usual finding that secretion has decreased in response to provocative stimuli. There is inconsistent evidence of increased growth-hormone basal secretion in depression. Age is a most important determinant of growth hormone activity (Veith and Raskind, 1988). Growth-hormone secretion appears to decrease with increasing age (Zadik et al, 1985). In addition, growth-hormone responses to provocative stimuli decrease with increased age.

Circadian Rhythm Changes with Aging

Another normal regulating process that changes both in depression and aging is that of circadian rhythms. During any 24-hour period, individuals exhibit marked variation in biologic and physiologic activities (e.g., body temperature, cortisol secretion, urine volume, and the sleep-wake cycle). These biologic rhythms often become dysregulated with increasing age, such as the lowest level of cortisol secretion occurring earlier in the morning. Periodicities in the clinical manifestations of psychiatric illness have been recognized for many years and related to these circadian rhythms (Kraepelin, 1913). Much investigation of mood disorders is based on the hypothesis that disturbances in the normal periodic biologic processes may contribute to episodic depression.

Perhaps the most significant circadian changes with aging are changes in sleep. Sleep changes characteristic of normal aging are similar to those that occur in depression (Prinz et al, 1979; Reynolds, 1987). With increasing age, persons experience more episodes of wakefulness during the night, have more difficulty falling asleep, and exhibit reduced slow wave (or stage 4) sleep. Total REM (rapid eye movement) sleep is reduced and the REM latency is decreased. Sleep changes with age are related to neurotransmitter changes as well. Prinz (1979) found a relationship between increased 24-hour plasma norepinephrine in older persons and problems with REM sleep.

Evidence is emerging that, overall, the circadian clock shortens with age in some animals (including humans), yet significant differences exist between species (Richardson, 1990). One consequence of this shortened circadian cycle in humans is that the system advances to earlier hours. Therefore older persons tend to be more active and energetic in the morning, awaken earlier, experience a phase advance of their temperature cycle and a phase advance of the circadian cortisol cycle. This phase advance may be just an entrainment artifact, not an endogenous neuroendocrine rhythm phase advance. The reason for this phase advance is not well known, but some investigators suggest that the vasopressinergic neurons within the suprachiasmic nucleus (SCN), which are important in the generation of circadian rhythmicity, are selectively lost in older animals and humans.

■ BIOLOGIC THEORIES OF DEPRESSION AND AGING

Genetic Theories

The strongest evidence for a genetic contribution to the etiology of depression in the elderly comes from twin and family studies (Slater and Cowie, 1971). The average risk for affective disorders among relatives of individuals with bipolar disorder is 14.3% for parents, 14.8% for children, and 12.9% for siblings, about four times higher than for the general population. According to one twin study, if one monozygotic twin develops the disorder, the risk is 68% for the other and 23% for dizygotic twins (Price, 1972). The monozygotic concordance rates are much higher than for the dizygotic twins. Another finding that supports a genetic contribution is the relatively higher prevalence of affective disorders in women, suggesting possible transmission on the X chromosome (Slater and Cowie, 1971). The genetic risk of unipolar depressive disorder is much lower (Perris, 1966), suggesting that genetic factors play less of a role in unipolar disorder than in bipolar disorder.

Extant studies suggest that the genetic contribution to depressive disorders in late life is weaker than at younger ages (Hopkinson, 1964; Mendlewicz, 1976; Schulz, 1951). Hopkinson (1964) found the risk for immediate relatives of patients whose onset of depression occurred after age 50 years to be 8.3% as compared with 20.1% for the relatives of patients whose onset occurred earlier. Schulz (1951) found the risk for parents of depressed individuals with late onset depression to be 9.3% and 15.7% for patients of those with early onset. Stenstedt (1959) found the risk of depression in late life to be lower than the risk among younger relatives of manic-depressive probands. Mendelwicz and Baron (1981) compared the risk for depressive illness in relatives of patients whose episodes started before the age of 40 with patients whose episodes started after the age of 40. They found the morbidity risk was lower in late-onset depressives.

Stone (1989), in a study of 92 patients 65 years of age and older who were admitted to a hospital with mania, found that patients with a family history of affective disorder had a significantly earlier age of onset and approximately 25% of these patients overall reported a positive family history.

One would expect the frequency of affective disorders in relatives to be lower with late-onset depressive and manic episodes than with early-onset episodes. Genetic determinism should initiate its influence before late life, and environmental contributors to depression should become relatively more important with advancing age.

An exception is the expression of the genetic predisposition to Alzheimer's disease in late life. However, these findings must be considered with caution. Family data collected from older persons are less reliable because of declining memory of subjects and the death or geographic separation of relatives, rendering accurate family history data much more difficult to obtain (Mendlewicz, 1976). Genetic factors may also contribute to depressive disorders indirectly in late life, specifically through cell loss. Hayflick (1965) reported that normal human fibroblasts, when cultured in an optimum medium, undergo a finite number of cell divisions and then die. This suggests that intrinsic (i.e., genetic) mechanisms within each cell program the cell to cease functioning at some point in the future. Whether this finding of genetically determined cell death can be applied to non-dividing cells in the central nervous system remains undetermined. Cell loss and the accumulation of cell toxins with aging may in turn lead to abnormal performance of cells in critical areas within the central nervous system, thus contributing to the development of depression and manic-depressive illness. Nielsen (1978) and Jarvik (1975) demonstrated that older women with primary degenerative dementia have a higher frequency of hypodipolody, a loss of chromosones, than normal persons. In addition, the clear genetic relationship between dementia and family history suggests that genetics may influence disease onset during the later decades of life.

■ NEUROANATOMIC CHANGES AND DEPRESSION IN THE ELDERLY

As described previously, 30% of patients over the age of 60 exhibit patchy deep white matter lesions (PDWML) of abnormal signal intensity with T2 weighted images on MRI (Bradley et al, 1984). These foci are rare in individuals below the age of 45. In 35 middle-aged and elderly patients, Krishnan et al (1988) found that one fourth of the patients below the age of 45 with major depression had PDWML and that nearly 60% of patients above the age of 45 exhibited these lesions. When patients 60 years of age and older with depression were examined, 85% had PDWML. The frequency of PDWML in elderly patients with depression was greater than found in elderly patients with Alzheimer's disease. Coffey et al (1988) replicated these findings. Of 36 patients who had MRI scanning, only three were normal. Subcortical grey matter abnormalities were also observed in many of the patients with PDWML. Twenty-three of the 31 patients exhibited lacunae in either the basal ganglia, thalamus, or pons. Fifteen patients had basal ganglia lesions. Thalamic lesions were seen in 8 of these patients and pontine lesions in 13. Most of these patients also exhibited cortical atrophy and ventricular enlargement.

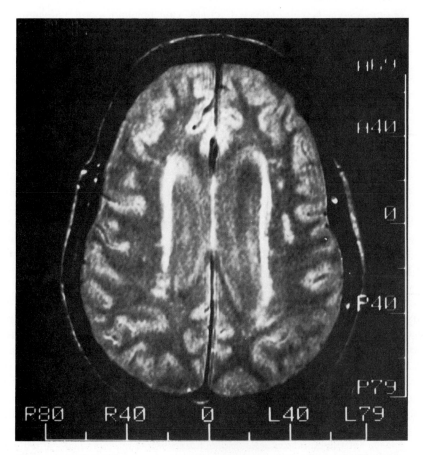

Figure 4-4. Cortical magnetic resonance imaging scan of a depressed older adult.

Krishnan (in press) summarized the MRI changes in late life depression as enlargement of the lateral ventricles; cortical atrophy; increased incidence of periventricular hypertensity deep white matter lesions, basal ganglia lesions; a smaller caudate nucleus, and a smaller putamen. He suggests that, even though the clinical significance of leukoencephalopathy is unclear, some interesting postulates may be derived from these studies. His postulates include the following:

- Patients at risk for cerebral vascular disease (hypertension or diabetes) are also at greater risk for developing mood disorders.
- The biologic depression of the elderly is related to the sum of the risk of cerebral vascular disease, life stresses, and genetic factors.
- Patients with leukoencephalopathy are more sensitive to side effects of medications and electroconvulsive therapy.
- Patients with leukoencephalopathy have a poorer response to treatment. The fact that the prevalence of leukoencephalopathy is greater in patients referred for electroconvulsive therapy than for depressive patients in general would support this hypothesis.
- Patients with leukoencephalopathy have a poor long-term prognosis.
- Pontine lesions may be reflected in low catecholamines and indolamine turnover (a recent study has demonstrated that a decreased latency of REM during sleep of elderly depressed patients is associated with pontine lesions) (Erwin et al, 1989).
- Leukoencephalopathy in depressed older adults is related to cognitive impairment (Steingart et al, 1986).

Cerebral Blood Flow and Metabolism

Although the results have been mixed, it appears that depressive episodes are associated with decreased cerebral blood flow and metabolic activity, and manic episodes are associated with an increase in activity (Joyce, 1991). Studies of cerebral metabolism generally fall into two categories—those that study cerebral blood flow using xenon as a photon-emitting radio tracer (Obrist, 1967) and studies of regional glucose metabolism (PET) (Reivich et al, 1979). According to Joyce (1991), many studies document a decreased function of the frontal cortex in depression. Baxter et al (1985) studied regional glucose-metabolism during both depressive and manic episodes in rapid-cycling subjects and found a significant increase in hemispheric glucose metabolism during the manic phase.

Joyce (1991) suggests that if decreased metabolism of the frontal-striatal axis is associated with depression, then antidepressant efficacy may enhance neurotransmission in noradrenergic and serotonergic systems, which in turn increases metabolism in these areas. An alternative possibility is that boosting the outflow of normal neurotransmission might, temporarily, reverse dysfunction in these areas. Since normal aging is associated with a decrease in metabolism in these same areas of the brain, it is possible that older persons are more susceptible to an increase of depressive syndromes. Imaging of both dopamine and serotonin receptors has revealed an age-related reduction in receptor binding in the caudate nucleus and frontal cortex (Veith and Raskind, 1988; Wong et al, 1984). Yet these findings are not conclusive. Although a gradual age reduction in average cerebral metabolic rate for glucose has been demonstrated, the rates were pronounced in the superior and posterior inferior frontal cortex, and one study did not document a corresponding reduction in oxgen use (Kuhl et al, 1984; Veith and Raskind, 1988).

Noradrenergic and Serontonergic Depletion/Dysfunction and Depression

The locus ceruleus is a major structural component of the norepinephrine system, since the dorsal norepinephrine system derives from its cell bodies. Changes in the concentration and function of the catecholamine neurotransmitters may be related to structural changes in the locus ceruleus. Schildkraut (1965) introduced the catecholamine hypothesis of depression, which essentially states that depression is associated with an absolute or relative depletion of catecholamines, particularly norepinephrine, at functionally important adrenergic receptor sites in the brain. In contrast, mania is presumed to be associated with an absolute or relative increase in these neurotransmitters. Evidence for the catecholamine hypothesis includes the following:

- Drugs that deplete brain catecholamines, such as reserpine, cause depression in humans (Goodwin and Bunney, 1973).
- Drugs used to treat depression increase the level of available catecholamines in the brain (Mendels et al, 1976).
- Drugs known to increase the level of catecholamines in the brain lead to increased activity and alertness in experimental animals (Schildkraut, 1973).

In a number of studies of manic-depressive patients the urinary excretion of norepinephrine has been found to be lower during periods of depression than during periods of manic or after recovery from the depression (Bunney et al, 1970; Bunney and Davis, 1965). Only a small fraction of the urinary norepinephrine orignates in the brain, however, because there is an effective blood-brain barrier to norepinephrine (Maas and Landis, 1966). Therefore researchers have given more attention to the metabolites of norepinephrine, such as urinary 3-methoxy-4-hydroxy-phenylglycol (MHPG). About 30% of MHPG in the urine is thought to come from the metabolic degradation of norepinephrine in the central nervous system. Like norepinephrine, this metabolite has been found in lower concentrations in depressed patients and to return to normal after treatment with tricylic antidepressants (Fawcett et al, 1972). In some studies, however, subgroups of depressed persons appear to have elevated plasma and urinary MHPG concentrations (Jimerson et al, 1983). Veith and Raskind (1988) suggest that elevations of plasma urinary MHPG observed in subgroups of depressed patients may represent increased peripheral sympathetic nervous system activity rather than changes in the central nervous system.

Cerebral spinal fluid studies of central nervous system norepinephrine have not provided consistent evidence indicating a change in norepinephrine concentrations in depressed patients (Post et al, 1984). Mann et al (1986) found a significant increase in beta-adrenergic receptors in the frontal cortex of suicide victims who were drug free. They suggested that decreased concentrations of norepinephrine near these receptors might account for the increase in receptor numbers in these subjects.

Enzymes involved in the synthesis and metabolism of brain neurotransmitters in humans have been studied more thoroughly than the neurotransmitters themselves. These enzymes are more stable, less likely to be diffused through the brain, and more easily measured (Samorajski and Hartford, 1980). Levels of MAO, an enzyme that breaks downs norepinephrine, increase markedly with age in the human brain, platelets, and plasma (Robinson et al, 1972). Women have a significantly higher average platelet and plasma MAO activity than do men of the same age, however. Estrogen is an MAO inhibitor, which may account for the increased levels of MAO in postmenopausal women. The second major metabolic enzyme of norepinephrine and dopamine, catechol-O-methyl-transferase (COMT), does not appear to change with aging (Robinson et al, 1977). Since MAO increases with age in both animal and human brains and COMT activity remains constant, it may be assumed that oxidative amination rather than methylation is the increasingly predominant pathway for the metabolism of the biogenic amines in the central nervous system of aging animals and humans (Samorajski and Harford, 1980).

Zubenko et al (1990) studied the brains of 37 demented patients with or without major depression and 10 controls with no history of dementia or depression. In these subjects, demented patients with major depression exhibited a tenfold to twentyfold reduction in the level of norepinephrine in the cortex, along with a relative preservation of choline and choline acetyl transferase (CAT) activity in subcortical regions, compared with demented patients who were not depressed. They also found serotonin levels to be reduced in all areas of the brain (but this reduction did not reach statistical significance) and an increase of dopamine levels in the entorhinal cortex of the depressed-demented patients. They concluded that the development of major depression in comorbid dementia and depression was associated with a series of neurochemical changes consistent with the existing neurochemical hypotheses of idiopathic affective disorders and distinct from that associated with primary dementia. Alexopoulos et al (1984; 1987) found that platelet MAO in depressed older women was significantly lower among those whose illness began at 55 years of age or older than in those who had an early onset of depression and controls. They also found that platelet MAO activity was higher in demented patients with and without depression and depressed patients with dementia than in nondemented depressed patients. These data suggest that abnormally high platelet MAO activity may predispose individuals to development of the depression-dementia syndrome. Platelet MAO activity has often been used as a marker of monoaminergic neurotransmission and has been suggested to be increased in patients with unipolar depression (Marbach et al, 1981).

Recent attention has been directed to the role of serotonin in the development of depressive disorders. The urinary excretion of 5-hydroxy-indoleacetic acid (5-HIAA), and metabolite of serotonin, may differentiate subtypes of depressive illness (Asberg et al, 1976). A number of investigators have found reduced cerebral spinal fluid levels of 5-HIAA in depression, suggesting decreased central nervous system serotonin activity (Post et al, 1984). Serotonin levels and levels of 5-HIAA have been found to be decreased in the brain stems of suicide victims in other studies (Pare et al, 1969).

The relationship of serotonin depletion to depression can be studied indirectly by the study of radioisotope labeled or tritated imipramine binding (TIB) sites. Binding sites for the antidepressant imipramine are found both in brain tissue and platelets and are closely associated with serotonin uptake sites on presynaptic serotonergic neurons. The number of TIB sites has been shown to be reduced in the frontal cortex of suicide victims (Stanley and Mann, 1983). There is also a significant decrease in the number of platelet-TIB sites in elderly depressed patients, compared with elderly controls and individuals suffering from Alzheimer's disease (Nemeroff et al, 1988). In the Nemeroff et al study, there was no correlation between a reduced number of platelet-TIB sites and post-DST plasma cortisol concentrations. Similar to the DST, however, platelet-TIB site reduction appears to be a state phenomenon in depressive episodes. Langer et al (1986) found that, after electroconvulsive therapy, the number of TIB sites increased. Severson et al (1985) found aging associated with an increased density of specific binding sites for tritiated-imipramine in mouse brains. Yet, as noted previously, there have been reports of age-related reduction in serotonin-2 receptor binding in the frontal context (Mann et al, 1985).

Sympathetic Nervous System Hyperactivity

Veith and Raskind (1988)suggest that a major correlate of depression across the life cycle is increased peripheral sympathetic nervous system activity. In their review of the literature, they note that venous plasma norepinephrine is increased in depressed patients, is higher in melancholic than non-melancholic patients, and is related to DST nonsuppression. In addition, investigators have reported a decreased beta-adrenergic stimulation of adenylate cyclase in lymphocytes and subsequent shift to a subsensitivity of these beta-receptors in response to higher circulating plasma norepinephrine levels. These higher norepinephrine levels may also produce a subsensitivity of the peripheral alpha-1 and postsynaptic alpha-2 adrenergic receptors that mediate constriction of peripheral blood vessels. They suggest, in view of the inhibitory effect of norepinephrine on brain-stem mechanisms regulating sympathetic nervous system outflow, that decreased central nervous system or brain-stem norepinephrine activity could result in increased sympathetic nervous system outflow.

Normal aging in humans is associated with an elevation in blood pressure and plasma norepinephrine. (Veith et al, 1986) Therefore older persons may be more likely to exhibit yet another biologic marker of depression, increased peripheral sympathetic nervous system outflow.

■ DYSREGULATION OF THE NEUROENDOCRINE SYSTEM

The Hypothalamic-Pituitary-Adrenal Axis

Clinical investigators have recoginized for years that persons with an increased secretion of cortisol are more prone to depression. The high percentage of patients with Cushing's syndrome coupled with the increased incidence of mood disorders after the use of steroid compounds has established the relationship between hypothalamic-pituitary-adrenal (HPA) activity and depression. Dysregulation of the HPA axis is a particularly attractive construct of depression, since it necessarily includes interaction of depressive symptoms, biologic functioning, and the environment. Sachar et al (1967) demonstrated that the diurnal curve of cortisol secretion is different in depressed persons from normal persons, showing more peaks during the 24-hour cycle, lower amplitude, and an overall basal increase in cortisol secretion, especially during the night.

Hyperactivity of the HPA axis is also reflected by the DST (i.e., resistance to suppression of cortisol by dexamethasone), a snythetic glucocorticoid (Carroll et al, 1981). Cortisol secretion is higher in older persons after the administration of dexamethasone compared with younger persons (Weiner et al, 1987). Among individuals with a clinical diagnosis of major depression, the percentage with abnormal DST results increases with aging (Davis et al, 1984).

Major depression also appears to be associated with increased secretion of corticotrophin-releasing hormone (CRH) into the cerebral spinal fluid and a decreased response of adreno-corticotrophin hormone (ACTH) on administration of exogenous CRH (Veith and Raskind, 1988; Nemeroff et al, 1984; Gold et al, 1986). This finding has not been consistent across all studies, however. Various neurotransmitter abnormalities have been suggested to account for the dysregulation of the HPA axis in depression (Veith and Raskind, 1988). These include a decreased norepinephrine input into the hypothalamus or pituitary and increased cholinergic activity. The aged-related reduction in the activity and density of noradrenergic neurons in the central nervous system, as noted previously, could lead to the increased basal cortisol levels in older individuals and therefore predispose them to develop depressive disorders, if the older theory that norepinephrine inhibits CRF release is correct.

Dysregulation of the HPA axis, however, may not be specific to the depressive disorders. Considerable literature has emerged suggesting that elevated postdexamethasone cortisol is likely to be found in demented patients and in patients suffering from depression. Jenike and Albert (1984) found that, in a group of demented subjects without depressive symptoms, DST results were abnormal in few of the mildly impaired but in a majority of the moderate to severely impaired dementia patients. Krishnan et al (1988) found that, in a group of early-onset Alzheimer's patients, DST findings were not related to the presence of depression, however. In contrast to Jenike and Albert, they did not find a relationship between the severity of dementia and postdexamethasone cortisol concentration. The age difference between the patients in these studies may explain the differences in results, however. Most investigators recommend that the nonspecificity of the DST in distinguishing depression from moderate-to-severe dementia precludes its use as a specific diagnostic test to distinguish the two syndromes (Gierl et al, 1987; Katona, 1988).

Dysregulation of the Thyroid Axis

The association between the thyroid function and depression has received considerable attention in the literature (Whybrow and Prange, 1981). Patients suffering from hypothyroidism exhibit many of the symptoms and signs of major depression, such as an apathetic mood, slow movement, and difficulty concentrating. In addition, nearly one fourth of depressed patients exhibit a blunted thyrotrophin (TSH) response to thyrotrophin-releasing hormone (TRH) when the latter is administered exogenously (Loosen and Prange, 1982). Thyroid hormone (especially triiodothyronine or T3), given as a supplement, may reduce the period between the onset of therapy with tricylic antidepressants and the response to those drugs (Prange et al, 1969). Thyroid dysfunction is a frequent finding among psychiatric inpatients admitted for severe depression (Gold et al, 1982). Sternbach (1983) found that, among 44 consecutive outpatients referred to a psychiatric hospital for evaluation of depression and anergia, 43% exhibited a blunted TSH response to protirelin. One patient had a low T4 level and three patients had elevated basal TSH levels. Nevertheless, nearly 15% of these patients had an augmented TSH response, indicating some degree of hypothyroidism. Most of these patients were found to have elevated antithyroid antibodies.

Nemeroff et al (1985) assessed the presence of antithyroid (both antimicrocosomal and antithyroglobulin) antibodies in 45 psychiatric inpatients with significant depressive symptoms, most of whom were diagnosed with major depression. Twenty percent had detectable titers of antithyroid antibodies, considerably higher than the 5% to 10% observed in the normal population.

Veith and Raskind (1988) conclude that TRH release is increased in depressed patients and blunted TSH responses to TRH may result from increased cortisol levels. This attenuated TSH response may also be secondary to increased secretion of growth hormone. Decreased norepinephrine or serotonin input to the hypothalamus may also attenuate the TSH response, since increased levels of norepinephrine provide negative feedback to the release of TRH.

Growth Hormone

In recent years, investigators have focused on the secretion of growth hormone in depressed patients. Growth-hormone secretion is regulated by both stimulatory and inhibitory factors in the hypothalamus, similar to corticotrophin-releasing hormone and thyroid-releasing hormone. The inhibitory factor of growth hormone is somatostatin (Krishnan et al, 1988). Both norepinephrine and serotonin may stimulate growth-hormone secretion.

In one study a blunted growth-hormone response to clonidine, a pharmacologic stimulus to growth-hormone secretion, has been reported in patients with depression (Krishnan, 1988). This blunted response to clonidine has led investigators to suggest that there is a decreased central alpha-2 adrenergic receptor sensitivity in depression.

Yet another factor, however, has been suggested to explain change growth-hormone secretion in the depressed, (i.e., cholinergic input). Changes in centrally active cholinergic agonists or cholinesterase inhibitors that stimulate growth-hormone release may explain the changes in growth-hormone response in depression (Veith and Raskind, 1988; Casanueva et al, 1984).

Normal aging does not appear to be associated with either an increase or a decrease in CNS cholinergic activity. As noted previously, growth-hormone activity definitely diminishes with increased age. Therefore the increase in growth hormone associated with depression is in contrast to the decreased 24-hour hormone secretion normally seen in aging.

■ NEUROPEPTIDES

A large number of neuropeptides are known to be present in the mammalian central nervous system. Their anatomic location and chemical structure, as well as pharmacologic properties, render them likely candidates for modulating normal and abnormal behavior. For example, neuropeptides and monoamines are often located in the same area of the brain, such as the joint localization of substance P and serotonin. Consistent changes in the concentration of two peptides have been found in Alzheimer's disease (somatostatin and corticotrophin-releasing factor). There is little evidence, however, that somatostatin decreases with aging, except perhaps in striatum (Morgan and May, 1990). There is some evidence that beta endorphin decreases in concentration in the hypothalamus with aging.

The role of neuropeptides in mood disorders is questionable as well. Alexopoulous et al (1983) found, in a group of middle-to-late life older adults suffering from major depression, plasma beta-endorphin levels were similar to age- and gender-matched controls. After electroconvulsive therapy, there was a transient increase in plasma beta-endorphin levels, suggesting, possibly, a transient elevation in adrenal corticotrophic hormone levels (ACTH). Yet plasma levels of beta endorphin may have no relationship to brain neuropeptides.

■ EEG CHANGES AND EVOKED POTENTIAL CHANGES IN DEPRESSION

Depressed patients, compared with control subjects, exhibit differences in quantitative EEG activity. Actively depressed patients have been demonstrated to exhibit larger EEG amplitude, greater alpha amplitude, and more asymmetric beta activity (Shagass et al, 1982; VonKnorring et al, 1983; Perris et al, 1981). Pollock et al (1988) found the topographic EEG differences that distinguish normal elderly subjects from elderly depressives to be similar to those changes that distinguish younger adult depressed patients from normal subjects. Older subjects with past histories of depression show higher amplitude of alpha activity (especially in the frontal and temporal areas).

EEG tracings have also been suggested to differentiate depressive illness from other psychiatric disorders, usually based on evoked potentials. Heyman et al (1991) evaluated waking EEGs in 61 elderly depressed patients without cognitive impairments and not receiving psychotropic medications. Conventional visual EEG analysis revealed no significant differences in the mean alpha rhythm, incidents of abnormal rhythms, or types of EEG abnormalities. Computerized spectral EEG analysis also did not differentiate between the early- and late-onset depressives.

Much interest has emerged in the use of evoked potentials to differentiate depressive elderly patients from dementia patients. Kraiuhin et al (1990) found that, although the average P300 latency in Alzheimer's patients was greater than that of depressed patients, which in turn was greater than that of older aged normals, none of the group differences in latency were statistically significant. They concluded that the performance of a single tone discrimination task requiring button-press response did not sufficiently tax those cognitive functions impaired in the early stages of Alzheimer's dementia to result in abnormally slow cognitive processing of the kind reflected in P300 latency.

■ DISRUPTION OF BIOLOGIC RHYTHMS

Disruption of Circadian Rhythms

One of the more persistent changes observed biologically in persons suffering from severe depression, regardless of age, is some form of electroencephlographic-verified sleep disturbance (Veith and Raskind, 1988; Reynolds and Kupfer, 1987). According to Reynolds and Kupfer (1987), the most common sleep changes associated with depression are: (1) problems with sleep continuity—for example, a prolonged sleep latency (the period of time from turning out the lights to sleep onset); (2) multiple awakenings and early morning awakening; (3) a decrease in the relative percentage of stage 3 and stage 4 sleep; (4) a shortened REM latency; and (5) a shift of REM sleep to the first half of the night. Kupfer et al (1981) found the most consistent of these changes to be shortened REM latency. In addition, when the depressed are treated with tricyclic antidepressants, both a prolongation of REM latency and a suppression of REM sleep early in treatment were predictive of clinical response.

The sleep changes characteristic of depression are similar to those found with normal aging, as described previously. Nevertheless, Reynolds et al (1988) found that through quantitative assessment of the EEG, normal elderly subjects could be discriminated from the elderly depressed and elderly demented patients. In Alzheimer's disease, there is more sleep continuity disturbance, a greater reduction in both slow wave and REM sleep, and decrements in REM sleep that parallel the degree of cognitive dysfunction. Sleep in the depressed elderly is marked by an increased REM sleep pressure, whereas extreme old age and dementia are characterized by a decrease in REM sleep pressure (Reynolds et al, 1990).

Reynolds et al (1990) explored the effects of a two-night REM sleep-deprivation procedure on electroencephalographic sleep and mood in elders with dementia, depression, and normal controls. Compared with control subjects, both patient groups obtained a higher amount of REM sleep and REM activity during REM sleep deprivation. Depressed patients showed little rebound in REM sleep after the deprivation procedure. This contrasted with the rebound in REM sleep activity in control subjects. The authors concluded that these findings demonstrate a greater plasticity of REM regulation in the healthy elderly control subjects with high REM pressure in depressed patients. In contrast, patients with dementia appeared to have an impaired capacity to respond to the challenge of REM sleep deprivation.

In contrast the circadian changes and activity with depression are the opposite of those found with normal aging. As noted previously, evidence is emerging that suggests a phase advance of activity and mood with aging. In other words, older persons tend to feel more active and in a better mood in the morning compared with the middle-aged. In contrast the marked diurnal variation seen in the more severe depressive disorders renders the older person less active and more depressed during the morning hours. Healy and Williams (1988) suggested an interesting association between the circadian disruption in depression and learned helplessness. The disruption in circadian rhythms, the sleep disturbance, and changes in activity cycles during the day may render the depressed person more dysphoric and feeling less in control of his or her activities.

Seasonal Rhythm Disturbances

Seasonal affective disorder (SAD) has been recognized as a psychiatric disorder than can affect people across the life cycle. SAD is a disturbance of mood and behavior that can resemble seasonal changes seen in lower mammals (Jacobsen et al, 1987). Criteria for a SAD include the following: (1) a history of depression meeting the criteria for major depression; (2) a history of at least 2 consecutive years of fall or winter depressive episodes that remit in the spring or summer; and (3) the absence of other disorders that would explain the seasonal mood changes. The recognition of seasonal changes in mood has led to the introduction of exposure to light for maintaining mood during the winter months when light exposure may be decreased. Exposure to bright artificial lights of high intensity in the home or work place have therefore been suggested as means for treating SAD.

TABLE 4-1. Psychobiologic Correlates of Aging, Mood Disorders in Mid-Life, and Mood Disorders in Late Life.

	Aging	Mid-Life Depression	Late Life Depression
Genetic predisposition to depression	NA	++	+
Genetic predisposition to mania	NA	+++	++
Neuronanatomic changes			
Periventricular white matter lesions	++	0 to +	+++
Deep grey matter nuclei lesions	++	0 to +	+++
Gross neurophysiologic changes			
Cerebral blood flow decrease	++	+++	
Glucose metabolism decrease	++	++	++
CNS norepinephrine function			
Brain NE content decrease	0 to +	0 to +	0 to +
Beta-adrenergic receptor binding increase	?	+	?
CNS serotonin (5HT) function			
Brain 5HT context	0	0 to +	?
Platelet tritiated imipramine binding decreased	0	+	+
Hypothalamic-pituitary adrenal (HPA) activity	+	++	+++
Decreased responsiveness to TRH	+	++	++
Growth hormone secretion	0	+	+
Disruption of biologic rhythms			
Sleep regulation			
REM latency decline	+	+	++
Sleep discontinuity	+	+	++
stage 3-4 sleep decrease	+	+	++
Activity cycle			
Mood and activity increased in AM	++	0	0

Typical symptoms of depression in SAD include decreased activity, sadness, anxiety, carbohydrate craving, daytime drowsiness, increased sleep (in contrast to usual depressive disorders), and work or interpersonal difficulties (Jacobsen et al, 1987). The age of onset of SADs is usually in the twenties. Nevertheless, SAD is found among older adults.

In a telephone survey in Maryland, using the Seasonal Assessment Pattern Questionnaire, investigators found that 92% of the survey subjects noticed seasonal changes of mood and behavior to various degrees. For 27% of this sample, seasonal changes were a problem and 4% to 10% rated the problem severe enough to qualify for SAD diagnosis. The prevalence of SAD gradually declined with age for both males and females, explained predominantly by the very high frequency of SADs among young women (Kasper et al, 1989).

■ CONCLUSIONS

A summary of the psychobiologic correlates of aging, mood disorders in mid-life, and mood disorders in late life are presented in Table 4-1. That the more severe depressive disorders are strongly influenced by psychobiologic phenomona is undisputed today. As can be observed, many of the psychobiologic changes that occur with aging are parallel to those that occur in depression. Therefore older persons may be at greater risk for developing a depressive disorder psychobiologically than persons at earlier stages of the life cycle. No comprehensive theory has yet emerged to explain varied psychobiologic changes that are described in this chapter. Nevertheless, the interactions of these changes with psychologic and social factors undoubtedly contribute, in a complex way, to the outset of depression in late life.

REFERENCES

Adams F (ed and translator): *The Genuine Works of Hippocrates*. Baltimore, Williams and Wilkins, 1939.

Alexopoulos GS, Inturrisi CE, Lipman R, Frances R, Haycox J, et al: Plasma immunoreactive beta-endorphin levels in depression, *Archives of General Psychiatry* 40:181-183, 1983.

Alexopoulos GS, Lieberman KW, Yung RC, Shamoian CA: Platelet MAO activity in age and onset of depression in elderly depressed women, *American Journal of Psychiatry* 141:1276-1278, 1984.

Alexopoulos GS, Yung RC, Lieberman KW, Shamoian CA: Platelet MAO activity in geriatric patients with depression and dementia, *American Journal of Psychiatry* 144:1480-1483, 1987.

Asberg M, Thoren P, Traskman L, Bertillson L, Ringberger V, et al: Serotonin depression: a biochemical subgroup within the affective disorders? *Science* 191:478, 1976.

Baxter L, Phelps M, Mazziotta J, Schwartz M, Gerner RH, et al: Cerebral metabolic rates for glucose in mood disorders, *Archives of General Psychiatry* 42:441-447, 1985.

Bradley WG, Waluch V, Brandt D, Zawadski M, et al: Patchy, periventricular white matter lesions in the elderly: a common observation during NMR imaging, *Non-Invasive Medical Imaging* 1:35-41, 1984.

Brodie HKH, Sack RL: Promising directions in psychopharmacology. In Hamburg DA, Brodie HKH (eds): *American Handbook of Psychiatry* (vol VI). New York, Basic Books, 1975, pp. 533-551.

Bunney WE, Davis JM: Norepinephrine and depression reaction: a review, Archives of General Psychiatry 13:483-494, 1965.

Bunney WE, Murphy DL, Goodwin FK: The switch process from depression to mania: relationship to drugs which alter brain amines, *Lancet* 1:1022, 1970.

Busse EW: Cerebral metabolism and electrical activity. In Busse EW, Blazer DG (eds): *Geriatric Psychiatry*. Washington, DC, American Psychiatric Press, 1989, pp. 135-161.

Busse EW, Barnes RH, Silverman AJ: Studies of the processes of aging: factors that influence the psyche of elderly persons, *American Journal of Psychiatry* 110:897-903, 1954.

Carroll BJ, Feinberg M, Greden JF, Terika J, Albala RF, et al: A specific laboratory test for the diagnosis of melancholia: standardization, validation, and clinical utility, *Archives of General Psychiatry* 38:15-22, 1981.

Casanueva FF, Villanueva L, Cabaranes JA, Kabazas A, Cerrato J, et al: Cholinergic mediation of growth hormone secretion elicited by arginine, clonidine, and physical exercise in man, *Journal of Clinical Endocrinological and Metabolism* 59:526-530, 1984.

Ciaranello RD, Patrick RL: Catecholamine neuroregulation. In Barchas JD, et al (eds): *Psychopharmacology: From Theory to Practice.* London, Oxford University Press, 1977, pp. 16-32.

Coffey CE, Figiel GS, Djang WT, Cress M, Saunders WB, et al: Leukoencephalopathy in elderly depressed patients referred for ECT, *Biological Psychiatry* 24:143-161, 1988.

Cotman CW: Synaptic plasticity, neurotrophic factors, in transplantation in the aged brain. In Schneider EL, Rowe JW (eds): *Handbook of the Biology of Aging* (ed 3). New York, Academic Press, 1990, pp. 255-274.

Davis KL, Davis BM, Mathe AA, Mohs RC, Rothpearl AB, et al: Age and the dexamethasone suppression test in depression, *American Journal of Psychiatry* 141:872-874, 1984.

Doraiswamy PM, Figiel GS, Husain MM, McDonald WM, Shah SA, et al: Aging of the human corpus collosum: MR imaging in normal volunteers, *Journal of Neuropsychiatry and Clinical Neurological Sciences* 3(4):392-397, 1991.

Erwin CW, Coffey CE, March GR: Polysomnographic findings in elderly depressed patients with unsuspected MRI abnormalities of the pons, *Sleep Research* 18:174, 1989.

Everitt AV: The hypothalamic-pituitary control of aging and age-related pathology, *Experimental Gerontology* 8:265-274, 1973.

Fawcett J, Mass JW: Depression and MHPG excretion: response to dextroamphetamines and tricyclic antidepressants, *Archives of General Psychiatry* 26:246, 1972.

Ferrier IN, McKeith IG: Neuroanatomical and neurochemical changes in affective disorders in old age, *International Journal of Geriatric Psychiatry* 6:445-451, 1991.

Freud S: Mourning and melancholia (originally published in 1917). In *Collected Papers* (vol IV). London, Hogarth Press, 1950, pp. 152-172.

Gierl B, Groves L, Lazarus LW: Use of the dexamethasone suppression test with depressed and demented elderly, *Journal of the American Geriatrics Society* 35:115-120, 1987.

Gold MS, Pottash ALC, Extein I: "Symptomless" autoimmune thyroiditis in depression, *Psychiatric Research* 6:261-269, 1982.

Gold PW, Loriaux DL, Roy A, Kling MA, Calabrese JR, et al: Responses to corticotrophin-releasing hormone in the hypercortisolism of depression in Cushing's disease. Pathophysiologic and diagnostic implications, *New England Journal of Medicine* 314:1329-1335, 1986.

Goodin DS, Aminoff MJ: Electrophysiological differences between subtypes of dementia, *Brain* 109:1103-1113, 1986.

Goodwin FK, Bunney WE: A psychobiological approach to affective illness, *Psychiatric Annals* 3:19, 1973.

Hayflick L: The limited in vitro lifetime of human diploid cell strains, *Experimental Cell Research* 37:614, 1965.

Healy D, Williams JMG: Dysrhythmia, dysphoria, and depression: the interaction of learned helplessness and circadian dysrhythmia in the pathogenesis of depression, *Psychological Bulletin* 103:163-178, 1988.

Heyman RC, Brenner RP, Reynolds CF, Houck PR, Ulrich RF: Age and initial onset of depression in waking EEG variables in the elderly, *Biological Psychiatry* 29:994-1000, 1991.

Hopkinson G: A genetic study of affective illness in patients over 50, *British Journal of Psychiatry* 110:244-254, 1964.

Jacobsen FM, Wehr TA, Sack DA, James SP, Rosenthal NE: Seasonal affective disorder: a review of the syndrome and its public health implications, *American Journal of Public Health* 77:57-60, 1987.

Jarvik LF: The aging central nervous system: clinical aspects. In Brodie H, Harmon D, Ordy JM (eds): *Aging.* New York, Raven Press, 1975.

Jenike MA, Albert MS: The dexamethasone suppression test in patients with presenile and senile dementia of the Alzheimer's type, *Journal of the American Geriatrics Society* 32:441-444, 1984.

Jimerson DC, Insel TR, Reus VI, Kopin IW: Increased plasma MHPG in dexamethasone-resistant depressed patients, *Archives of General Psychiatry* 40:173-176, 1983.

Joyce EM: Cerebral blood flow and metabolism in affective disorders, *International Journal of Geriatric Psychiatry* 6:423-430, 1991.

Kasper S, Wehr TA, Bartko JJ, Geist PA, Rosenthal NE: Epidemiological findings of seasonal changes in mood and behavior: a telephone survey of Montgomery County Maryland, *Archives of General Psychiatry* 46:823-833, 1989.

Katona CLE: The dexamethasone suppression test in geriatric psychiatry (editorial), *International Journal of Geriatric Psychiatry* 3:1-3, 1988.

Kessler S: Psychiatric genetics. In Hamberg DA, Brodie HKH (eds): *American Handbook of Psychiatry* (vol VI). New York, Basic Books, 1975, pp. 352-384.

Kraepelin E: Manic-depressive insanity and paranoia. In Kreplin E: *Textbook of Psychiatry* (translated by RM Barclay). Edinburgh, Livingstone, 1913.

Kraiuhin C, Gordon E, Coyle S, Sara G, Rennie C, et al: Normal latency of the P300 event-related potential in mid-to-moderate Alzheimer's disease in depression, *Biological Psychiatry* 28:372-386, 1990.

Krishnan KRR: *Neuropathology of Late Life Depression, Journal of Geriatric Psychiatry and Neurology* (in press).

Krishnan KRR, Goli V, Ellinwood EH, France RD, Blazer DG, et al: Leukoencephalopathy in patients diagnosed as major depressive, *Biological Psychiatry* 23:519-522, 1988.

Krishnan KRR, Heyman A, Ritchie JC, Utley CM, Dawson DV, et al: Depression in early-onset Alzheimer's disease: clinical and neuroendocrine correlates, *Biological Psychiatry* 24:937-940, 1988.

Krishnan KRR, Husain MM, McDonald WM, Doraiswamy PM, Figiel GS, et al: In vivo stereological assessment of caudate volume in man: effect of normal aging, *Life Sciences* 47:1325-1330, 1990.

Krishnan KRR, Manepalli AN, Ritchie JC, Rayasam K, Melville ML, et al: Growth hormone response to growth hormone-releasing factor in depression, *Peptides* 9 (supp 1):113-116, 1988.

Kuhl DE, Metter EJ, Reige WH, Hawkins RA: The effect of normal aging on patterns of local cerebral glucose utilization, *Annals of Neurology* (supp) 15:S133-S137, 1984.

Kupfer DJ, Spiker DG, Coble PA, Neil JF, Ulrich NR, et al: Sleep and treatment prediction in endogenous depression, *American Journal of Psychiatry* 138:429-434, 1981.

Langer SZ, Sechter D, Loo H, Raisman R, Zarifian E: Electroconvulsive shock therapy and maximum binding of platelet tritiated imipramine binding in depression, *Archives of General Psychiatry* 43:949-952, 1986.

Lipton MA, Nemeroff CB: The biology of aging and its role in depression. In Usden G, Hofling CK (eds): *Aging: The Process and the People.* New York, Brunner/Mazel, 1978, pp. 47-95.

Maas JW, Landis DH: Techniques for assaying kinetics of norepinephrine metabolism in central nervous system in vivo, *Psychosomatic Medicine* 28:247, 1966.

Mann JJ, Petito C, Stanley M, McBride PA, Chin J, et al: Amine receptor binding and monoamine oxidase activity in post mortem human brain tissue: effect of age, gender, and post mortem delay. In Burrows GD, Norman TR, Dennerstein L (eds): *Clinical and Pharmacologic Studies in Psychiatric Disorders.* London, John Wiley, 1985, pp. 37-39.

Mann JJ, Stanley M, McBride A, McEwen BS: Increased serotonin 2 and beta adrenergic receptor binding in the frontal cortices of suicidal victims, *Archives of General Psychiatry* 43:954-959, 1986.

Mason J: Specificity in the organization of neuroendrocrine response profiles. In Seeman P, Brown G (eds): *Frontiers in Neurology and Neuroscience Research.* Toronto, The University of Toronto Press, 1974, pp. 68-80.

Mathew RJ, Margolin RA, Kessler RM: Cerebral function, blood flow and metabolism: a new vista in psychiatric research, *Intergrative Psychiatry* 3:214-225, 1985.

McDonald WM, Husain MM, Doraiswamy PM, Figiel GS, Boyko OB, et al: A magnetic resonance imaging study of age-related changes in human putamen nuclei, *Neuroreports* 2(1):57-60, 1991.

McGeer EG: Aging and neurotransmitter metabolism in the human brain. In Katzman R, Terry RD, Bick KL: *Alzheimer's Disease: Senile Dementia and Related Disorders* (Aging, vol VII). New York, Raven Press, 1978, pp. 427-440.

Meites J, Huang HH: Relation of the hypothalamo-pituitary-gonadal system to decline of reproductive functions in aging female rats, *Current Topics in Molecular Endocrinology* 3:3-20, 1976.

Mendels J, Stern S, Frazer A: Biochemistry of depression, *Diseases of the Nervous System* 37:3, 1976.

Mendelwicz J: The age factor in depressive illness: some genetic considerations, *Journal of Gerontology* 31:300, 1976.

Mendelwicz J, Baron M: Morbidity risk in subtypes of unipolar depressive illness: differences between early and late onset forms, *British Journal of Psychiatry* 139:463-466, 1981.

Morgan DG, May PC: Age-related changes in synaptic neurochemistry. In Schneider EL, Rowe JW (eds): *Handbook of the Biology of Aging* (ed 3). New York, Academic Press, 1990, pp. 219-254.

Nemeroff CB, Knight DL, Krishnan KRR, Slotkin TA, Bissette G, et al: Marked reduction in the number of platelet-tritiated imipramine binding sites in geriatric depression, *Archives of General Psychiatry* 45:919-923, 1988.

Nemeroff CB, Simon JS, Haggerty JJ, Evans DL: Antithyroid antibodies in depressed patients, *American Journal of Psychiatry* 142:840-843, 1985.

Nemeroff CB, Widerlov E, Bissette G, Walleus H, Karlsson I, et al: Elevated concentrations of CSF corticotrophin-releasing factor-like immunoreactivity in depressed patients, *Science* 226:342-343, 1984.

Nielsen J: Chromosomes in senile dementia, *British Journal of Psychiatry* 114:303, 1968.

Nurnberger JI, Jr, Jimerson DC, Bunney WE, Jr: A risk factor strategy for investigating affective illness, *Biological Psychiatry* 18:903-908, 1983.

Obrist WD, Sokoloff L, Lassen NA, et al: Relationship with EEG to cerebral blood flow and metabolism in old age, *Electroencephalographic Clinical Neurophysiology* 15:610-619, 1963.

Obrist WD, Thompson HK, King CH, Wang HS: Determination of regional cerebral blood flow by inhalation of 133 xenon, *Circulation Research* 20:124-135, 1967.

Pare CMB, Yung DPH, Price K, Stacey RS: Five-hydroxy tryptamine, noradrenaline, and dopamine in brain stem, hypothalamus, and caudate nucleus of controls and patients committing suicide by coal-gas poisoning, *Lancet* 2:113-135, 1969.

Perris C: A study of bipolar (manic-depressive) and unipolar recurrent depressive psychoses, *Acta Psychiatrica Scandinavica* 194:1 (supp), 1966.

Perris C, von Knorring L, Cumberbatch J, Marcino F: Further studies of depressed patients by means of computerized EEG, *Advances in Biological Psychiatry* 6:41-49, 1981.

Pollack VE, Schneider LS, Zemansky MF, Sloane RB: Tomographic EEG in recovered depressed elderly. In *Proceedings of the International Psychogeriatric Association Meeting,* Chicago, 1988, pp. 41-43.

Post RM, Ballinger JC, Goodwin FK: Cerebral spinal fluid studies of neurotransmitter function in manic and depressive illness. In Post RN, Ballinger JC: *Neurobiology of Mood Disorders.* Baltimore, Williams and Wilkins, 1984, pp. 685-717.

Prange AJ, Wilson IC, Rabon AM, Lipton MA: Enhancement of imipramine antidepressant activity by thyroid hormone, *American Journal of Psychiatry* 126:457-469, 1969.

Price JS: Genetic and phylogenetic aspects of mood variation, *International Journal of Mental Health* 1:124, 1972.

Price LH, Charney DS, Rubin L, Heninger GR: Alpha-2 adrenergic receptor function in depression, *Archives of General Psychiatry* 43:849-858, 1986.

Prinz PN, Halter J, Benedetti C, Raskind M: Circadian variation of plasma catecholamines in young and old men: relation to rapid eye movement and slow wave sleep, *Journal of Clinical Endocrinology and Metabolism* 49:300-304, 1979.

Rapaport SI: Positron emission tomography in normal aging and Alzheimer's disease, *Gerontology* 32 (suppl 1):6-13, 1986.

Raskind MA, Peskind ER, Vieth RC, Beard JC, Gumbrecht G, et al: Increased plasma and cerebrospinal fluid norepinephrine in older men: differential suppression by clonidine, *Journal of Clinical Endocrinology and Metabolism,* 66(2):438-443, 1988.

Reivich M, Kuhl D, Wolf A, Greenberg J, Phelps M, et al: The [18F] fluorodeoxyglucose method for measurement of local cerebral glucose utilization in man, *Circulation Research* 44:127-139, 1979.

Reynolds CF, Busse DJ, Kupfer DJ, Hoch CC, Houch PR, et al: Rapid eye movements, and sleep deprivation as a probe in elderly subjects, *Archives of General Psychiatry* 47:1128-1136, 1990.

Reynolds CF, Kupfer DJ: Sleep research in affective illness: state of the art circa 1987, *Sleep* 10:199-215, 1987.

Reynolds CF, Kupfer DJ, Houck PR, Hoch CC, Stack JA, et al: Reliable discrimination of elderly depressed and demented patients by electroencephalographic sleep data, *Archives of General Psychiatry* 45:258-264, 1988.

Richardson GS: Circadian rhythms in aging. In Schneider EL, Rowe JW (eds): *Handbook of the Biology of Aging* (ed 3). New York, Academic Press, 1990, pp. 275-305.

Roberts E, Hammerschlag R: An overview of transmission. In Ables RW (ed): *Basic Neurochemistry*. Boston, Little, Brown and Company, 1972, pp. 83-88.

Robinson DS, Nies A, Davies JN, Bunney WE, Davis JM, et al: Aging, monoamines and monoamine oxidase levels, *Lancet* 1:290, 1972.

Robinson DS, Sourkes TL, Nies A, Harns LS, Spector S, et al: Monoamine metabolism in human brain, *Archives of General Psychiatry* 34:89, 1977.

Sachar EJ: Corticosteriods in depressive illness. I. A re-evaluation of control issues and the literature. II. A longitudinal psychoendocrine study. *Archives of General Psychiatry* 17:544-567, 1967.

Sachar EJ, Finkelstein J, Hellman L: Growth hormone responses in depressive illness. I. Response to insulin tolerance test. *Archives of General Psychiatry* 25:263, 1981.

Samorajaski T, Hartford JM: Brain physiology of aging. In Busse EW, Blazer DG (eds): *Handbook of Gertiatric Psychiatry*. New York, Van Nostrand/Reinhold, 1980, pp. 46-82.

Schildkraut JJ: Norepinephrine metabolites as biochemical criteria for classifying depressive disorders and predicting responses to treatment: preliminary findings, *American Journal of Psychiatry* 130:695, 1973.

Schultz B: Auszahlunger in der vervandtschaft von nach erkrankrankungsaltr und geschlecht grupierpen manisch-depressien, *Archiv Fur Psychiatrie und Nervenkrankheiten* 186:560-576, 1951.

Severson JA, Marcusson JO, Osterburg HH, Finch CE, Winblad B: Elevated density of [3H] imipramine binding in aged human brain, *Journal of Neurochemistry* 45:1382-1389, 1985.

Shagass C, Roemer R, Straumanis J: Relationships between psychiatric diagnoses and some quantitative EEG variables, *Archives of General Psychiatry* 39:1423-1435, 1982.

Slater E, Cowie V: *The Genetics of Mental Disorders*. London, Oxford University Press, 1971.

Snyder PJ, Utiger RD: Response to thyrotropin releasing hormone (TRH) in normal man, *Journal of Clinical Endocrinology and Metabolism* 34:380-385, 1972.

Snyder PJ, Utiger RD: Thyrotropin response to thyrotropin releasing hormones in normal females over 40, *Journal of Clinical Endocrinology and Metabolism* 34:1096-1098, 1972.

Stanley M, Mann JJ: Serotonin-2 binding sites are increased in the frontal cortex of suicide victims, *Lancet* 1:214-216, 1983.

Steingart A, Lau K, Fox A, Diaz F, Fishman M, et al: Significance of white matter lucencies on CT scan in relation to cognitive impairment, *Canadian Journal of Neurological Science* 13:383-384, 1986.

Stenstedt A: Involutional melancholia: an etiologic, clinical and social study of endogenous depression in later life with special reference to genetic factors, *Acta Psychiatrica Neurologica Scandinavica*, 1959: (suppl) 127:5-71.

Sternbach HA, Gold MS, Pottash AC, Extein I: Thyroid failure and protirelin (thyrotrophin-releasing hormone) test abnormalities in depressed outpatients, *Journal of the American Medical Association* 249:1618-1620, 1983.

Stone K: Mania in the elderly, *British Journal of Psychiatry* 155:220-224, 1989.

Sullivan P, Pary R, Telang F, Rifai AH, Zubenko GS: Risk factors for white matter changes detected by magnetic resonance imaging in the elderly, *Stroke* 2:1424-1428, 1990.

Tourigny-Rivard MF, Raskind M, Rivard D: The dexamethasone suppression test in an elderly population, *Biological Psychiatry* 16:1177-1184, 1981.

Tricklenbank MD: Subtypes of 5HT receptors, *Journal of Psychopharmacology* 1:222-226, 1987.

Veith RC, Featherstone JA, Linares OA, Halter JB: Age differences in plasma norepinephrine kinetics in humans, *Journal of Gerontology* 41:319-324, 1986.

Veith RC, Raskind MA: The neurobiology of aging: does it predispose to depression? *Neurobiology of Aging* 9:101-117, 1988.

von Knorring L, Parris C, Goldstein L, Kemali B, Monakhof K, et al: Intercorrelations between different computer-based measures of the EEG alpha amplitude and its variability over time and their validity in differentiating healthy volunteers from depressed patients. In Mendlewicz J, Van Praag H (eds): *Advances in Biological Psychiatry* (vol 13). New York, Karger, 1983.

Weiner MF, Davis BM, Mohs RC, Davis KL: Influence of age and relative weight on cortisol suppression in normal subjects, *American Journal of Psychiatry* 144:646-649, 1987.

Whybrow TC, Prange AG: A hypothesis of thyroid-catecholamine-receptor interactions: its relevance to affective illness, *Archives of General Psychiatry* 38:106-113, 1981.

Willner P: *Depression: A Psychobiological Synthesis*. New York, John Wiley and Sons, 1985, p. 13.

Wong DFHN, Wagner Jr RF, Dannals JM, Links J, Frost J, et al: Effects of age on dopamine and serotonin receptors measured by positron tomography in the living human brain, *Science* 226:1393-1396, 1984.

Zadik ZS, Chalew SA, McCarter RJ, Meiscas M, Kowarski AA: The influence of age on the 24-hour integrated concentration of growth hormone in normal individuals, *Journal of Clinical Endocrinology and Metabolism* 60:513-516, 1985.

Zubenko GS, Moosy J, Kopp U: Neurochemical correlates of major depression and primary dementia, *Archives of Neurology* 47:209-214, 1990.

5

Psychologic Origins

The psychiatric literature is replete with discussions of the psychologic etiology and psychodynamics of depression, regardless of age (Beck, 1967; Freud, 1917-1950; Mendelsohn, 1960). Central to these discussions of psychologic etiology is the belief in continuity of mental processes from early childhood throughout the life cycle. The persistence of early patterns of human behavior, such as unresolved conflicts, will therefore be expressed in depressed symptoms during one's later years. Two major questions underlie most of the observations and studies reported in this chapter. Is there a difference between the origin of depression with onset in late life and depression with onset at earlier stages of life? What are the psychologic origins of late life depression?

Cameron (1956), in his discussion of the neuroses of late life, states that there is no significant psychologic difference between neuroses of the elderly and those of middle-aged persons. Biologic characteristics and changing social status or conditions contribute to the observed modifications in symptoms. When elderly persons are faced with decreasing physical vigor and endurance, disorders of multiple organ systems, impairment of perception, and loss of emotional support through isolation, increased anxiety and despair may emerge as the predominant affective tone. Personality characteristics, such as independence and autonomy, that once enabled individuals to master self and environment or to gain prestige in early and middle years may hinder adaptation in later life. Resultant symptoms include neurotic aggression, hypochondriacal complaints, withdrawal and resignation, or demands for constant care. Older persons are also subject to the prejudicial influences of society. As children's sexual interest and activity were repressed and ignored before Freud's discovery of psychosexual development, sexuality after the middle years has been underestimated and misunderstood. Therefore psychologic reactions may occur to real or perceived declining sexual potency and/or societal prohibition including aggression, guilt, fear, and anxiety.

Although Freud (1924) believed that "near or above the 50s the elasticity of the mental processes, on which treatment depends, is as a rule lacking—older people are no longer educable," his pessimism about the adaptability of older people is challenged by recent theorists and counted by much data from cognitive psychology. Erikson (1950), following the psychoanalytic tradition, suggests that persons must face a series of challenges throughout the life cycle. Depending on the age of the individual, the crises and adaptation to these crises vary. The challenge of late life is to integrate one's entire life. Successful resolution of the challenge leads to wisdom, and maladaptation leads to despair. Today most researchers and clinicians agree with the latter assumption, namely, that age-specific intrapsychic and psychosocial changes occur throughout life and that inability to adapt to these challenges definitely contributes to the symptoms, etiology, and outcome of late life depression.

What changes occur in psychologic processes with aging and what are the mechanisms of late life depression? Attention is directed in this chapter to the psychologic changes in late life often associated with depression: changes in motivation and cognition; intrapsychic changes; and changes in overall life satisfaction. Changes in memory and other cognitive processes are reviewed in Chapter 15. Changes with aging usually do not contribute to depression in the elderly, such as changes in motivation, yet the differentiation of a depressive affect from these usual changes with aging is not always easily accomplished. Next, the psychologic theories of depression most prevalent in the literature are discussed as they relate to late life depression. Most of these theories derive from a rich, long-standing literature on the psychodynamics of depression coupled with a more recent literature on cognitive changes in depression. Personality and behavioral changes associated with depression are also discussed. Finally, changes in morale and life satisfaction during the transition from middle to late life are reviewed.

■ MOTIVATION

Motivation may be defined as those energizers of behavior and the sources of energy in a particular set of responses that keep those responses dominant over others and that account for behavioral continuity and direction (Hebb, 1955). Wigdor (1980) has published a thorough review of this subject. She suggests that needs, drives, incentives, and goals may all be included under the general heading of motivation. Drive is the energy and impetus arising from basic physiologic and psychologic needs coupled with external stimulation that results in heightened arousal. Drives tend to lead to activity but interact with other factors, such as incentives and goals.

Researchers who have examined the evidence of slowing of the central nervous system and concomitant shrinkage and atrophy of cortical and subcortical structures with aging conclude that the amount of stimulation needed for arousal is probably higher for the elderly (Wigdor, 1980). The "drive centers" of the central nervous system (including the reticular activating system, hypothalamus, and lymphic system) are discussed in Chapter 4. Yet these physiologic changes do not explain changing behaviors of the aging. For example, Strelu (1970) suggests that a more aroused central nervous system is less reactive to external stimuli. The elderly may have an over-aroused autonomic nervous system, which may explain some of their difficulty in performing certain tasks (Eisdorfer et al, 1970).

Drives may be conceptually divided into primary drives (i.e., drives that originate within the person that must be satisfied, usually on a physiologic level) and secondary drives (i.e., needs that develop in the individual secondary to learning that take place at an interpersonal level, leading to particular motivational situations for the individual), as well as those general societal reinforcers that stem from cultural influences (Wigdor, 1980). It is frequently difficult to distinguish primary drives from secondary drives and even more from complex motivators of behavior. A consideration of drives frequently affected by depressive symptoms of aging is helpful. Hunger and thirst are primary drives that must be satisfied. Although there is evidence of reduced drive or activity related to food or drink consumption with aging, there is little evidence to suggest that psychologic needs for food and drink decrease significantly with aging. Older persons often tend to eat less. Weight loss with aging is expected and even desired, given the increased ratio of fat-to-muscle tissue with aging. Modifications in behavior related to food consumption can be based on the person's interaction with the environment or decreased enjoyment of food because of changes in taste perception (Schiffman, 1977). However, weight loss may also signal the onset of a depressive disorder.

Women experience a sudden and significant alteration in endocrine function at menopause. Aging men do not experience this dramatic change in hormone levels, but there appears to be a decline in the ability of the Leydig cells of the testes to produce testosterone in response to gonadotrophin. Sexual drive has never been ascribed to a particular hormone, but much interest has been directed to testosterone in both men and women as a marker of sexual drive. In the Duke Longitudinal Studies of Aging, sexual interest in men and women did not decline over a 10-year period (Pfeiffer et al, 1969). This contrasted markedly with the decline in sexual activity for both groups during the same 10-year period. Sexual interest cannot be equated with sexual drive, because interest interacts with a number of cultural and physiologic variables. Sexual activity, on the other hand, is not always related to biologic capability; instead the availability of a partner, social expectations, marital conflict, and depression may determine activity.

Hebb (1955) has shown that activity and exploratory behavior are basic drives of healthy animals and that these drives appear to be reduced in older animals. A lowered energy level in the elderly organism may lead to a higher proportion of the available energy being used to fulfill the basic animal drives for food and drink, leaving less energy available for exploratory behavior (Wigdor, 1980). Healthy persons, however, continue to seek activity and stimulation, even when elderly (Maddox, 1968).

Not only do humans need to explore the environment, they also need to effect change within the environment (Buck, 1976). Some authorities believe that the need to achieve and to experience competence in the physical and social environment is a primary need that may be thwarted or distorted by negative feedback or lack of reinforcement. Others suggest that this need for competence, achievement, and control is a secondary need determined by learning in a society that values competitive striving and achievement (Wigdor, 1980). Anthropologic studies are replete with examples of societies in which achievement is valued highly and societies in which it is not (Benedict, 1934). Competence and control of the environment would appear to be primary drives that may be channeled into a drive for achievement, depending on societal expectations.

Rodin (1986) suggests that changes in options for control may affect emotional health, possibly by influencing stress resistance, physiologic responses, and behavior relevant to health. Experiences related to control, she noted, become more apparent in old age and/or have a different social meaning. For example, the loss of a friend may affect options for living in late life more profoundly than at earlier stages of the life cycle. Older persons, for example, are not as successful as younger persons in anticipating and managing events associated with moving that may result from the loss of a loved one. The reaction to these losses may be fueled by gradual loss of control in other areas, such as money, transportation, physical mobility, and social infuence. Data do not clearly document, however, that perceived control decreases with increased age.

Beck (1967) has emphasized the changes in motivation that occur in depressed patients according to his cognitive theory of depression (discussed later). He classifies these changes into four groups: paralysis of the will; escapist and avoidant wishes; suicidal wishes; and intensified dependency wishes. The loss of spontaneous motivation, or paralysis of the will, has been considered a core symptom of depression in traditional psychiatric literature. Loss of motivation may be viewed as the result of the patient's hopelessness and pessimism. As long as the patient expects a negative outcome from a behavior, there is little internal stimulation to do anything.

■ LEARNING AND BEHAVIORISM

A number of investigators hypothesize a relationship between environmental reinforcement and depression. Learning experiences may be a primary cause of depression symptoms or may interact with biologic and social factors. Lewinsohn et al (1969) argue that dysphoria results directly from reduction in the rate of response-contingent positive reinforcement. Dysphoria has been postulated to occur when there is little environmental reinforcement or when available reinforcers are not contingent on the person's behavior.

Perhaps the best-known behavioral model of depression is the model of *learned helplessness* (Seligman, 1974). The term *learned helplessness* was first used to describe the behavior of dogs produced by inescapable shock and the process believed to underlie the behavior (Seligman and Maier, 1967). Dogs given repeated inescapable shocks gradually performed less well at escaping shock in an escapable situation. The inescapable-shocked animals appeared to give up and passively accept the shock. Even when they occasionally did escape the shock, they failed to learn this behavior. In other words the dogs failed to learn from exposure to a shock-determination contingency. The main behavioral symptoms of learned helplessness are failure to initiate responses and difficulty in learning that a particular response is effective.

Seligman (1974) reviewed the similarities between behaviors characteristic of learned helplessness and symptoms of depression. Since learned helplessness is caused by learning that response is independent of reinforcement, the model suggests that the cause of depression is the expectation that initiating action in the social environment is futile. Experiences with uncontrollability are in many ways similar to those experiences that are classically considered precipitants of depression, such as loss of a loved one or loss of one's role because of, for example, forced retirement. These events cannot be controlled, and the elder comes to learn that his or her own behavior does not appreciably change the event, relieve suffering, bring gratification, or provide nurturance. In other words the individual is helpless.

Many researchers, including Schmale (1958), emphasize the roles of helplessness, hopelessness, illness, and death in rendering individuals more susceptible to depression. Garber et al (1979) suggest that experience with uncontrollable events leads to the following two primary deficits: reduced motivation to respond in new situations in which outcomes are controllable and impaired ability to learn about contingencies in new situations. Studies of animals and humans have shown that experience with uncontrollable aversive events is associated with a number of other factors including time, reduced aggression, weight loss, anorexia, deficits in social and sexual behavior, whole brain norepinephrine depletion, septal activation, as well as increased sadness, anxiety, and hostility. Close parallels exist between the behavioral science of learned helplessness and the signs and symptoms of depression.

The implications of the learned helplessness model for the etiology of depression in late life are apparent. Older persons are at greater risk than individuals at other stages of the life cycle (except children) for being placed in situations in which their own behavior has little effect on the behavior of other persons. This is especially true when the physical health or cognitive functioning of the older persons has been inaccurately assessed and therefore treatment interventions have been prescribed without consultation with the elder. An older patient being treated for chronic illness within a hospital who is transferred to a long-term care facility is especially vulnerable. Poor food, discomfort secondary to frequent venipuncture or intermuscular injections, and frequent transfers to diagnostic laboratories are virtually beyond the control of the patient. Lack of home care "necessitates" transfer to a long-term care facility that is equally uncomfortable. Many times older persons within these settings complain of the discomfort but are told, "It's for your own good." Therefore they feel unable to change the situation.

Any hypothesis that learning is a precipitant of depression must account for the effect of depression on learning. A study by Foster and Gallagher (1986) illustrates this effect. They evaluated the use of coping strategies in depressed versus normal adults, based on the theories of Billings et al (1983). The following five coping strategies were studied: logical analysis or efforts to understand the stressor and assess the consequences of the stressor; information seeking, such as obtaining guidance from others; problem-solving; affective regulation, such as direct efforts to control stressful emotions by suppressing impulsive acts; and emotional discharge, such as verbal expression of dysphoric emotions. In contrast to younger persons, who made more use of information-seeking and less use of problem-solving when depressed, older depressed adults did not differ from the nondepressed in the frequency of the use of these coping strategies, except that they did make significantly greater use of emotional discharge strategies. The perception by the depressed elderly, however, was that all types of coping strategies were less helpful when they were depressed compared with controls and the younger depressed. This may suggest a negative bias about learning strategies in the midst of a depression or the potential of these strategies to be effective in changing the situation.

■ PSYCHODYNAMICS

Psychoanalytic theories of depression have historically received more attention than all other theories of the etiology of depression except the biologic theories. Relatively little attention, however, has been directed to the changing psychodynamics of depression with increased age. Zetzel (1965) asserts that at the interpersonal and environmental levels, the elderly individual must adapt to loss or frustration (or both), consider a modified capacity for mobilizing adaptive and defensive reactions, and experience modifications in the instinctual pressures demanded in the psychic defenses during the postclimactic. Maturity, according to Zetzel, demands an essentially passive acceptance of painful and inevitable situations. Referring to Bibring's concept (1965) of depression as an ego state, she notes that anxiety stimulates the mobilization of active defenses appropriate to a wide range of threatened behaviors. These defense processes cannot be substituted for the more passive, depression-like affect, which is frequently more adaptive at late stages of the life cycle and which requires acceptance of reality. Late life demands the capacity to resign oneself to the inevitable without bitterness, self-reproach, or self-pity. This passive acceptance in turn facilitates the remobilization of available adaptive capacities in other areas. Zetzel's negative view of the consequences and necessary adaptations of aging is not shared by many clinicians today but was developed at a time when the cultural stereotype of aging was that of passive resignation to progressive loss.

Weissman (1965) contrasts despair with depression in late life. "Depression can occur as an instrument in the course of despair, but despair, a primary anxiety, is characteristic among the aged and particularly among dying patients." Despair, according to Weissman, includes apathy, absence of meaning, loss of aim, and deprivation. Sensory deprivation, deprivation of communication skills, and social deprivation all contribute to the psychic state of despair. The antithesis of despair is hope. The psychic state of the elderly may represent a return to an earlier state of psychic activity in that elders often feel more like they did when they were young than when they were middle-aged. Weissman noted four additional characteristics of psychic functioning in late life—disability, depletion, disappointment, and finally death. Disability is a state in which reality testing becomes less flexible and more restricted, whereas "psychologic sets" become fixed. Depletion is a state in which truths and fears are reduced, whereas old fantasies may recur and present conflicts are often relieved. Disappointments, on the other hand, are greater hazards in middle-age than during the more advanced years. Finally, death is the separation from important sources of love but also brings an end to extended frustration or delay in gratification. Weissman, like Zetzel, views the aging process as primarily negative and dominated by coping with loss.

The dynamics of depression are intimately interwoven with the psychologic reaction to loss of a significant object. Freud (1917-1950) determined that melancholia resembled mourning, occurring after the "loss of a loved person or the loss of some extraction which has taken the place of one, such as the fatherland, liberty and ideal." Unlike mourning, melancholia occurred only in individuals who are predisposed. The loss of a loved one may not occur in reality but only intrapsychically (i.e., emotional attachment to the person is withdrawn unconsciously because of hurt or disappointment). Spitz (1946) observed reactions of infants separated from their parents, which appeared similar to the adult reaction of depression. The extreme result of this anaclitic depression was death. Psychiatrists working with the elderly have noted similar reactions in their patients. The frequently noted phenomenon of death after entry into a long-term care facility has been equated with infant deaths after maternal separation. Failure to thrive may also be the result of late life equivalents of anaclitic depression (Blau, 1980).

Levine (1965), in discussing the disturbance in libido equilibrium that results from loss, suggests that, regardless of what type of object is lost, the same process occurs. Some events that can be thought of as loss are in fact loss equivalents. For example, someone else's gain might invoke feelings of envy and jealousy. The impact of loss also is determined by "rate of change," for a loss within a specific period of time significantly predicts the response of the individual to that loss. A high rate of change of an object of importance requires a major redistribution of libido in order for equilibrium to be reestablished. The sudden death of a spouse or other loved one is an example of a high rate of change. Yet one's own aging usually evolves slowly, since the resultant losses are typically gradual and partial, even though the self is highly affected.

Busse et al (1955), in their study of a longitudinal sample of elderly subjects, found that older adults were aware of more frequent and annoying depressive periods than they had experienced earlier in life. During such episodes, they felt so discouraged, worried, and frustrated that they often saw no reason to continue to live. About 85% of this group were able to trace the onset of most of these depressive episodes to specific losses. The authors concluded that these normal grief reactions may assume neurotic patterns by the following two possible pathways: (1) elderly persons blame themselves for the losses; or (2) they blame others, which leads to an overemphasis on neglect and rejection by other persons.

Abraham (1953) was the first psychoanalyst to document the presence of hostility and ambivalence in the psychopathology of depression. He postulates that the inherent self-reproach associated with depression and expostulated by Freud was in fact hostile feelings, which patients unconsciously had toward their loved objects and that, after these objects were lost or abandoned, were directed toward themselves. Cath (1965) did not find manifest guilt in older persons who were depressed as often as in younger persons. He suggests that the infrequency of guilt may be more apparent than real. Persons who suffer because of physical illness or emotional deprivation may balance these losses to satisfy a sense of guilt; thus compensation for anger and aggression occurred rather than guilt. Busse, et al (1954) suggest that, for the elderly, intrajection (the turning inward of unconscious hostile impulses) is seldom a mechanism for developing depression. Instead, depression is related to a loss of self-esteem that results from aged individuals' inability to supply needs and drives or to defend themselves against threats to security.

According to Gutheil (1959), external shocks are more likely to precipitate depression in elderly patients than in young individuals. One explanation is that the threshold for stress of the elderly is lowered with an added element of anxiety. Because these elders recognize they are at greater risk and are less capable of controlling the painful stimulus, they do not blame themselves for being bad, lazy, or unworthy. There is no objective evidence, however, that the elderly tolerate stressors better than do individuals at earlier stages of life. Levine (1965) notes that psychologic stressors include not only loss, but attacks, restraints, and threats as well. Attacks are external forces that lead to discomfort, pain, or injury. At the physical level an attack can vary in intensity from a mild pain to severe physical violence. Psychologically, an attack can vary in intensity from mild criticism to severe hostility. The elderly may be particularly susceptible to the physical attacks of illness and treatments associated with illness. They also are potentially susceptible to psychologic attacks that arise from common prejudices toward older persons (e.g., the older person perceives that he or she intrudes on the family of a child, perhaps after the spouse of the older person has died).

Restraints, according to Levine, refer to any external forces that restrict the actions necessary for satisfaction of instinctual drives. Any major restriction of activity can contribute to the development of a depression. Older persons are especially susceptible to restraints, given social isolation, decreased mobility, lack of access to transportation, and lack of a sexual partner. Threats are events that warn of possible future loss, attack, or restraint. The significance of a threat is not determined by external reality alone but by the individual's interpretation of that reality. Evidence of the significance of threats can be found in the manifest contents of dreams of elderly patients. Barad et al (1961) found that older persons, in their dreams, were preoccupied with loss of resources and threatening and aggressive environments and had a tendency to view themselves as unable to complete an action.

A thwarting of the basic drives is another proposed cause of depression. Abraham (1953) states that lack of sexual gratification leads to depression in many neurotics, and autoeroticism in the neurotic tends to prevent depression when it is threatened and to relieve it when it has occurred. As described previously, Levine (1965) emphasizes the role of restraint as an etiologic factor in depression. Sexual satisfaction continues to be important to the older person. Sexual drive, although persistent, may not readily be apparent, since it may not be apparent in the behavior of the elder. Although restriction of sexual drive results in part from repression, the cultural attitude that considers sexual outlets unimportant for the aged can appreciably reinforce repression. Continued sexual activity in late life is expected and provided for in many other cultures. Bibring (1965) also emphasizes the persistence of sexual impulses and fantasies in the elderly.

Wigdor (1980) notes that, in our achievement-oriented society, major reinforcers lead to the development of habit patterns and emphasize incentives for activity that may not be adaptive or appropriate to changing life situations with advanced age. With retirement, the mainstream of society, which reinforces the need for achievement, recognition, self-esteem, and confidence, is no longer available for many elders. Substitution of alternative social environments to meet these needs is not easy because our society does not have alternative formal roles for satisfying these needs. Erikson (1950), although establishing that the acquisition of integrity is the primary task of the older person (see Chapter 16), emphasizes that a continued striving toward the resolution of previous developmental crises persisted throughout the life cycle. Therefore striving for industry and generativity, the primary developmental tasks of earlier adulthood, continues to be important to the older adult.

Finichel (1945) was one of the first to describe the role of narcissism in the development of depression. "A person who is fixated on the state where his self-esteem is regulated by external supplies" has an inordinate need to be loved and places excessive demands on love objects. Severe depression results when these overly dependent individuals do not receive the vital supply of love and attention they seek. To the extent that their sense of well-being, safety, or security is dependent on love, money, social position, or power, the individuals are threatened by loss of these factors (Gaylin, 1968). In severe cases the persons despair of survival and give up. Chodoff (1972) carries this theme even further when he states that depression-prone individuals are inordinately and almost exclusively dependent on narcissistic needs derived directly or indirectly from other people for the maintenance of their self-esteem. Frustration tolerance is low, and the narcissistic person uses various techniques, including submission, manipulation, coercion, demands, and placation to maintain his or her desperately needed relationships with persons who provide these supplies.

According to Lazarus and Weinberg (1980), narcissistic pathology of the elderly patient may manifest itself in "recurring depressions or defensive grandiosity in response to minor slights or disappointments, self-consciousness, over-dependence on approval from others for maintenance of self-esteem, and the transitory periods of fragmentation in this cohesiveness of the self." The older person seeks a person to idealize and from whom approval, protection, and stabilization for a brittle sense of self and self-esteem can be acquired. "Self-centered and egocentric, he views others not as separate objects but as extensions of himself to be used for self-serving purposes, for enhancement and for stabilization of his self-esteem." Symptoms of the older narcissistic patient include hypochondriasis, an over-concern with physical appearance, possessions, and past accomplishments, seeking approval and assurance from others, and a special vulnerability to losses with aging. Meissner (1975) posits that narcissistic loss is the basic problem of aging. In turn the greatest test of narcissism is old age, with the inevitable depletion of energies, resources, and relationships.

Kernberg (1967) suggests that narcissistic injury is an expectable and unavoidable outcome for many as they grow older. In the vulnerable personality the impact of a narcissistic injury can be devastating. Depression will therefore result. For example, the retiree who worked very hard during his or her adult life may no longer be able to muster the usual defenses of rationalization, displacement, and sublimation that served him or her well in the workplace, thus leading to increased anxiety and depression.

Cath (1965b) suggests, as does Meissner, that the search for restitution secondary to the inevitable losses in late life is a major developmental task for aging individuals. The instinctual drive of older people, however, appears to be less intense. Biologic decline, according to Cath, the substrate of instinct, leads to a decline in drive. At the same time, the tyrannical demands of the superego and ego are reduced, which facilitates the ego's task of mediation, "especially since demand from the outside for achievement may be lessened." Unfortunately, this "ideal state of relative peace" may necessitate a renunciation of previous external activities and progressive interiority. If one lives for a sufficiently long time, the inevitable object loss, body change, and disease lead to a state of both internal and external depletion.

Depletion anxiety is the result of the recognition of these losses and is both qualitatively and quantitatively different from anxiety at other stages of the life cycle. Depletion anxiety is closely related to a threat of total emotional exile and eventual death. Cath goes so far as to consider depletion anxiety an epigenetic age-specific variant of the primary and secondary forms of anxiety. Progressive loss in late life leads to the need for a continuous countercathexis to maintain denial and to repress rage secondary to these losses. "One feels depleted when libido has been so consumed in maintaining countercathexis that the latter must be reinforced by drawing energy from other essential ego functions. However, one is depleted when, still later, energy is neither available nor evident as cathexis or countercathexis." Depletion anxiety may arise to such a magnitude as to call forth the most primitive defenses and therefore facilitate regression to much earlier modes of gratification. All available libido is required for self-preservative maintenance of the physical self, and psychic function is "in abeyance" because it is decathected. Cath considers the state of almost total depletion to be beyond the usual concepts of depression. Many take issue with Cath's formulation of depletion anxiety and its relation to depression in late life. The theories described previously associate late life depression with the frustration of drives rather than depletion.

Two investigators have departed from the traditional psychodynamic theories that view depression as a mood state characterized by loss of self-esteem. First, Bibring (1953), although acknowledging the importance of early childhood trauma and subsequent narcissistic injury, notes that self-esteem may be decreased in ways other than by frustration of the need for affection and love. Depression may result from frustration of other narcissistic aspirations, such as the desire to be good, the desire to be "clean," and the desire to not be resentful, hostile, or defiant. Bibring also theorizes that all depressions stem from conflict or tension within the ego itself rather than conflict between the ego and superego. Depression is a mood state that, in turn, is a state of the ego. Depression is "the emotional expression (indication) of a state of helplessness and powerlessness of the ego, irrespective of what may have caused the breakdown of mechanisms that establish self-esteem." Bibring's theory may be especially relevant to older adults, given that the sense of lack of control over the environment and a need to respond positively and accommodate environmental stimuli, especially what appear to be helpful gestures from the environment, may lead to the depressive state.

Second, Jacobson (1953) suggests that loss of self-esteem was the central psychologic problem of depression. The goals for development of self-esteem, superego, and ego ideal are the firm establishment of one's own identity, a differentiation of self from others, the maintenance of self-esteem, and the capacity to develop satisfactory object relationships (Beck, 1967). Self-esteem is the "degree of discrepancy or harmony between the self-representation and the wished-for concept of the self." Early disappointments in the first years of life lead to a premature devaluation of loved ones. This in turn interferes with normal establishment of self-esteem and leads to a fixation of ego and superego identifications at pre-Oedipal levels. In times of stress the superego and representations of object or self lose their distinctiveness and boundaries. Regression occurs, leading to an exaggerated dependency in these individuals. The object of this dependency may be persons, causes, or organizations. The patient's object representations are not sufficiently separated from the parental component of the ego ideal and therefore are unrealistically idealized. Exaggerated evaluation leads the patient to feel helpless and to be especially dependent on the loved one. Objects excessively idealized inevitably fail to live up to the patient's expectations. Psychotic depression results secondary to a regressive delusion of the identification with the loved object. Blan and Berezin (1975) note the significance of the loss of self-esteem that results from external losses in late life. Because of the experience of helplessness about life, the elderly become afraid of failure, which leads to further damage to their self-esteem.

Closely associated with Jacobson's theory is the epigenic theory of unresolved conflicts across the life cycle. Erikson (1950) suggests that the last of the eight stages of life requires the individual to resolve the conflict of "ego integrity versus despair." Erikson's description of ego integrity is similar to Jacobson's description of the development of self-esteem but incorporates a life-span perspective on the perceived meaning and value of one's life. When the older adult looks back through his or her life and views life as not having been worthwhile, self-esteem decreases and despair results. This despair will then take the form of depressive symptoms.

Regression to a more dependent state during the course of late life may at times be adaptive. Verwoerdt (1980) notes that dependent persons do not fare badly as aging progresses. Such individuals usually bring dependency features out in the open and are unambiguous to others in the social environment. These elders may welcome physical illness as a means to gratify dependency in late life. Depressive symptoms may serve a similar function. Bibring (1965) cautions that the term *regression* may be applied too liberally in the discussion of aging. It is assumed that psychic energy diminishes with the process of aging and the cathexis invested in others decreases. The resultant behavior is not identical with what is usually considered regression. The regression that follows a neurotic conflict leads to a withdrawal of cathexis but an increased libidinal pressure and subsequent displacement of instinctual wishes to less threatening yet potentially satisfying earlier goals. Displacement not only permits a discharge of libidinal tension but also decreases anxiety and guilt feelings. Rochlin (1965) states that, since the course of sexual life is not strongly affected by the aging process, regression may occur when sexual satisfaction is unavailable through usual modes. He notes that regressive phenomena inevitably reveal remarkably high and relatively unmodified sexual needs.

Psychodynamic theorists have paid special attention to those factors predisposing to depression throughout the life cycle. Bowlby (1952) provides abundant clinical evidence of pathologic effects on personality development of severe deprivations in early childhood, whereas more recent studies have documented the importance of stressful life events in the onset and the persistence of depression in early life and mid-life. The association of stressful events and depression are discussed in chapter 6. For the purposes of a psychodynamic orientation to depressive onset, such associations confirm the dynamic speculation that early loss serves as a predisposing factor to depression, regardless of age.

A somewhat variant approach to predisposing factors in depression can be found in the work of Klein (1948) and Balint (1952). According to Klein, intrajected aggression, which is closely associated with the death instinct, leads to a stage of development characterized by hostile and sadistic feelings as a reaction to frustration. She labeled this stage the *depressive position,* the point at which children can allegedly feel guilt and sorrow for the feared loss of loved object that they attribute to their own sadistic impulses. This depressive position thus becomes the prototype for all clinical depressions. Balint frees the depressive position from its aggressive ties. This developmental phase is characterized by a "deep, painful, narcissistic wounds which, as a rule, can be made conscious without serious difficulty somehow in this way; 'it is terrifying and dreadfully painful that I am not loved for what I am, time and time again I cannot avoid seeing that people are critical of me and it is an irrefutable fact that no one loves me as I want to be loved'." No known empirical studies have demonstrated that this view of a life-long pattern of the depressive position predisposes older people to develop depression. Nevertheless, many depressive symptoms experienced in late life, on historical inquiry, are found to have persisted for decades.

■ COGNITIVE THEORY

Beck (1967) proposes the most popular of the current theories regarding the psychologic etiology of depression—the cognitive theory. This theory has attracted clinicians primarily because of Beck's relatively simple and straightforward approach to psychotherapy (Beck et al, 1979). A number of investigators have adapted Beck's theories to the psychologic etiology of depression in the elderly. The work of Gallagher and Thompson (1983) is among the most extensive.

Adapting their model from Beck, Gallagher and Thompson suggest the following three specific concepts regarding depression: the negative triad, underlying beliefs or schemas, and cognitive errors. The negative triad consists of an interactive set of negative views of oneself, experience, and the future. For example, an older woman may be a caretaker for her husband whose health is progressively deteriorating. Because she is not able to reverse his deteriorating course through her caretaking efforts, she may view herself as not a good caretaker and therefore not a good wife to her husband. These views may expand in that she may see herself as always having been a "bad" person who has never been of help to other persons. She says to herself, "People are always becoming ill, and I cannot do anything to help those who are ill" despite the fact that she greatly comforts her husband through her caretaking efforts. Her views of the future change as well, in that she expects nothing to change, believes she will never be able to help anyone, and thinks no one will view her as a valuable or useful individual.

According to Beck, the second concept typical of the cognitive model of depression is an underlying belief or schema. For example, an older adult may say, "If I become a burden to my family, they will get in trouble and have all sorts of difficulties. The family depends on me. I am a failure if I do not make this family what it should be." This type of schema sets up unrealistic expectations for the individual based on a belief that can only lead to a sense of failure.

The third concept inherent in the cognitive model of depression is the development of cognitive errors (i.e., thinking that is typically distorted). Thinking may be distorted stylistically. For example, the individual can develop selective filtering, such as "I am a failure because I missed two items when I was tested for the renewal of my driver's license. Therefore I should no longer drive." Overgeneralization is another stylistic distortion. If a child does not follow some specific advice from the father, the father says, "No one in the family cares about my opinion anymore. They just feel like I'm a silly old man." A third stylistic distortion is catastrophizing for example, "When I discovered the lump in my shoulder, I knew it was cancer. I will be dead in about 3 months at the most."

Cognitive error may also be distorted semantically. Semantic errors are inexact labeling of events, such as overreaction and personalization. The individual who overreacts says, "My daughter disagrees with me about how to discipline her child. She hates the sound of my voice. I'll just keep my mouth shut from now on." An example of personalization is "My good friend did not come to visit me today. Therefore she must not care about me anymore. Because I'm getting older, she has found better friends."

Cognitive thinking can be distorted formally, too (i.e., the processes may tend to become automatic). Thought processes, take on a life of their own, leading to perseverating. Individuals who constantly worry about illness or finances exhibit formal cognitive distortion.

Once the individual develops the negative triad about the self, the world, and the future, develops schema that structure cognitive functioning into an enduring component, which in turn becomes formalized, then usual life events lead to depressive symptoms. This is because interpretation of those events are typically negative and idiosyncratic to the individual. In addition, autonomous depressive symptoms (e.g., sleep disturbance) can lead to negative interpretations of the environment and similar idiosyncratic contexts.

Evidence is beginning to accumulate that clarifies the relationship of depression in late life to cognitive distortion. Vezina and Bourgne (1984) studied 50 persons living in a home for the aged with the Dysfunctional Attitude Scale, the Beck Depression Inventory, and the Automatic Thought Questionnaire— instruments that attempt to establish thought distortions associated with depression. Depressed older adults reported significantly more dysfunctional attitudes and negative cognitions than nondepressed elderly. The strategies for coping with depression, such as help-seeking or emotional catharsis, did not vary between depressed elders and younger persons. The depressed viewed these strategies to overcome depression as less successful than the nondepressed, findings that are similar for those in younger subjects. Foster and Gallagher (1986) found that the depressed elderly, compared with the nondepressed elderly, expected a greater use of avoidance coping behavior and are more likely to use emotional discharge as a coping technique.

Lapointe and Crandell (1980) found depressed elders more likely to report irrational ideas and negative cognitions. Isaacs and Silver (1980), on the other hand, failed to find significant differences on the Dysfunctional Attitude Scale between depressed and nondepressed elderly. They therefore challenged the more consistent findings that depression in late life is associated with changes in cognitive structure. Lewinsohn and MacPhillamy (1974) found a decrease in activity to be related to depression and not to age. The depressed elderly had fewer activities than nondepressed elderly, and this in turn may have led to a more negative evaluation of the environment by the depressed elderly.

■ PERSONALITY AND DEPRESSIVE DISORDERS

Considerable literature has emerged examining the relationship between personality or personality disorders and depression. The specific association between personality problems and depression in late life has been relatively neglected, however. Nevertheless, personality has been studied in detail among older adults and this literature reflects on the well-documented association between personality disorders and the onset and duration of depressive symptoms. For example, Boyce et al (1990) studied a group of patients with remitted major depressed and found that nonmelancholic (versus melancholic) depressives had more vulnerable personality styles, specifically a more dependent personality. Much of the work has focused on the adaptation of stressors that is determined by personality and may result in depressive symptoms.

Dohrenwind (1961) proposes a paradigm of four main elements of the stress response. In addition to the nonspecific physical and chemical changes that occur in response to stress, a derailment of the mechanism of adaptation can occur. Disorders of adaptation may present in the form of psychiatric illness, specifically depression. Sociopsychologic adaptation syndromes must have affective components rooted in the arousal of fear and anger, behavioral components (e.g., changes in reemphasis of activities), and cognitive components (e.g., changes in orientation or the assimilation of new information and beliefs).

Thomae (1980) researched the ways in which a group of community elderly persons changed their patterns of reaction during a 17-year period. Although changes did occur in the ranked order of adjustment patterns to occupational problems, achievement-oriented behaviors continued to be the dominant pattern of adjustment. Maas and

Kuypers (1974) studied an elderly group aged 60 to 82 years who were the fathers and mothers of children being studied in the longitudinal panel. A full range of personality styles was found for each gender. Personality change was not shown to be related to significant life-cycle transitions, such as retirement and widowhood. These investigators (like many others but in contrast to Thomae) found that there is a large variability in personality styles among the elderly but with no single personality pattern being identified as characteristic of "the aged." In addition, Costa and McCrae (1980) have demonstrated the persistence of personality styles with the aging process.

Fiske (1980) describes a series of personality patterns in middle and late life that depended on stress and stress-response. Overwhelmed older adults are beset by many ostensibly stressful situations and dwell on them at length. They constantly discuss present and past ups and downs of their lives and appear at times to be reliving stressful experiences even though they occurred much earlier in life. Challenged adults appear to be besieged by many stresses but are not excessively preoccupied by them. They only briefly describe these stressful events, even when asked, and then quickly move on to other topics of discussion. Self-defeating personalities describe few stressful events but emphasize the weight of these events with life-event reviews dominated by scenes of loss and deprivation. The "lucky" are those individuals with few or mild stresses who rarely discuss these stresses in the description of their life experiences. According to Fiske, middle-aged men with a great deal of stress are more likely to be challenged, whereas middle-aged women typically are overwhelmed. These patterns are more likely related to the cohort in which these men and women were born than to inherent gender differences. Self-defeating individuals and the overwhelmed have a predisposition to developing depressive illness.

Fiske suggests that certain patterns of personality do change with aging, and some of these changes may protect older persons against the development of depression. Individual commitment, that patterning or configuration of the fundamental concerns harbored by an individual at a particular point in time, is an example of a personality trait that changes with time. Fiske writes of a maturing of commitment, a continuous process that evolves over time through adulthood. For example, secondary to the capacity of love for persons within the immediate social environment, individuals gradually develop concern for and a sense of unity with ever-widening circles of humanity. Occasionally, these altruistic commitments become the principal domain of an individual's life. Not only does the reflection of this commitment change during the life course, but the commitment is also influenced by those particular historical events that occur during the life of an elder. If an elder expands his or her horizons to these altruistic commitments, then individual failures during the life cycle on which the older adult may reflect and then develop despair may be mitigated (see previous discussion of Erikson [1950]).

The perception of time is another personality trait that has received attention in both the study of aging and the study of depression. Beck (1967) notes that depressed patients often feel time is passing more slowly than usual, although no objective evidence exists that actual judgment of time is impaired. For many depressed persons only the past matters, and painful memories dominate thinking and remind them of their unworthiness and inabilities. Verwoerdt (1980) suggests that, with advancing age, time's perspective is frequently altered. Some individuals believe time is running out and wish to make the most of the time that remains. Activities may be directed toward "catching up" with other individuals who have experienced more during their lives. The realization that life is finite often occurs in late middle life, the point at which an individual recognizes that less time remains to live than one has already lived (Jung, 1923). However, little evidence exists to support the idea that the subjective rate of time's passage increases with aging as it does with depression (Wigdor, 1980). More often, older persons value time because they view that there is less of it remaining.

A trait that has been explored with interest among the elderly is that of extroversion versus introversion. Cameron (1967) hypothesizes that there should be a continuous change with age from extroversion to introversion. This change parallels the physiologic changes from anabolism to catabolism, extroversion being survival by expansion and introversion being survival by controlled behavior and reduction of external activities. Thomae (1980) reviews the ambiguity in existing introversion with aging. For example, no age difference in the factor "reserve versus outgoingness" could be found by Angleitner et al (1971) in a study of residents aged 50 to 90 years in a home for the aged.

Rotter (1966) introduces the construct of locus of internal versus external control. This construct relates to the consistent expectation of individuals regarding their personal control of events or dependency on the social environment. A hypothesis has been proposed that a decrease in internal control accompanies the external loss of autonomy experienced by the elderly. Lao (1974) did not find this true of persons older than 60 years of age compared with younger persons, and the study previously described by Rodin (1986) suggests that control remains very important for older persons, even in long-term care facilities.

Personality style, even in late life, may be genetically determined. For example, Petersen et al (1989), in a study of how identical and fraternal twins react together and apart, report that 30% of the variance in a variety of locus of control measures were accounted for by genetic influences. Components of the contruct of locus of control, such as life direction and responsibility, were especially determined by genetic factors. Therefore the clinician working with the depressed elder must generally approach personality style as a given, and therefore determine to what extent personality style predisposes to depression either inherently (e.g., through excess dependency) or through increased vulnerability to stress.

Rigidity is another factor that has been thought to increase with age (Riegel, 1959). However, studies of rigidity are especially susceptible to the cohort effect. Schaie and Parham (1977), in a cross-sequential analysis, studied cohorts at three points in time and found that differences in rigidity between the cohorts was greater than differences within cohorts at different points in time. Rigidity (and therefore decreased adaptability to environmental change and increased susceptibility to depression) would therefore be the result of lifelong patterns in a particular group, with different cohorts showing different patterns as opposed to rigidity increasing with aging.

■ LIFE SATISFACTION AND DEPRESSION

Research of the elderly, especially the research that has its origins in sociologic theory, often includes the construct of life satisfaction. Life satisfaction is operationally defined as a "measure of mood that is not trait-oriented." According to Havighurst (1963), life satisfaction, morale, and adjustments or outcomes rather than conditions of adjust-ment represent a process-centered approach to the aging personality. Literature has shown a correlation of life satisfaction with a range of other variables, including health, socioeconomic status, social participation, income, and living arrangements (Thomae, 1980). Palmore and Kiuette (1977), in a 4-year longitudinal study, found that life sat-isfaction did not decline significantly in a cohort of older adults followed over time. This suggests that older persons are generally as satisfied with their lives as those per-sons at other stages of the life cycle.

Gillead et al (1981) compared elderly inpatient depressives with controls. They found satisfaction with past achievements differentiated depressives and controls both at ad-mission and at discharge (i.e., the depressed exhibited less life satisfaction). The oper-ationalized life satisfaction according to the model of Bigot (1974), which included (1) subject is as happy now as when younger; (2) subjects compared with others gets "down in the dumps" too often; (3) things done now by the subject are not as interesting as they once were; (4) looking back the subject did not get the most out of the important things that he or she wanted; (5) the current years are the best years of the subject's life; (6) compared with others of the same age, the subject has made many foolish de-cisions; (7) the subject would not change his or her life if he or she could; and (8) the subject's life could be happier than it is now. The study by Gillead is worth reviewing, since it demonstrates the difficulty in disentangling the constructs of personality and life satisfaction. According to this definition, life satisfaction very well could predispose to depression, for it appears to be more a personality trait than the state of an individual.

REFERENCES

Abraham K: Notes on the psychoanalytical investigation and treatment of manic-depressive insanity and al-lied conditions. In Abraham K (ed): *Selected Papers*. New York, Basic Books, 1953.

Angleitner A, Smitz-Schetzer R, Rudinger G: Altersab-Brangigkert der Personlichkeit in Sinne von RB Cat-tel, *Actuelle Gerontologie* 1:721, 1971.

Balint M: New beginning and the depressive syndromes, *International Journal of Psychoanalysis* 33:214, 1952.

Barad M, Altschuler KC, Goldfarb AI: A survey of dreams in aged persons, *Archives of General Psychiatry* 4:419-427, 1961.

Beck AT: *Depression: Causes and Treatment*. Philadelphia, University of Pennsylvania Press, 1967.

Beck AT, Rush AJ, Shaw BF, Emery G: *Cognitive Therapy of Depression*. New York, Guilford Press, 1979.

Benedict RF: *Patterns of Culture*. Boston, Houghton Mifflin, 1934.

Bibring E: Discussion notes. In Berezin MA, Cath S (eds): *Geriatric Psychiatry*. New York, International Uni-versities Press, 1965, pp. 188-201.

Bibring E: The mechanisms of depression. In Greenacre P (ed): *Affective Disorders*. New York, International Universities Press, 1953, pp. 13-48.

Billings A, Cronkite RC, Moose RH: Social environmental factors in unipolar depression: comparisons of depressed patients and non-depressed controls, *Journal of Abnormal Psychology* 92:119-133, 1983.

Blan D, Berezin MA: Neuroses and character disorders. In Howells JG (ed): *Modern Perspectives in the Psychi-atry of Old Age*. New York, Bruner/Mazel, 1975, p. 225.

Blau D: *Depression in Late Life: Psychodynamic Aspects*. Paper presented at a conference, "Depression in late life," Cleveland, Ohio, October, 1980.

Bowlby J: *National Care and Mental Health*. Geneva, World Health Organization, 1952.

Boyce P, Parker G, Hickie I, Wilhelm K, Grodaty H, et al: Personality differences between patients with remitted melancholic and non-melancholic depression, *American Journal of Psychiatry* 147: 1476-1483, 1990.

Buck R: *Human Motivation and Emotion*, New York, John Wiley and Sons, 1976.

Busse EW, Barnes RH, Silverman AJ: Studies of the processes of aging: factors that influence the psyche of elderly persons, *American Journal of Psychiatry* 110:897-903, 1954.

Busse EW, Barnes RH, Silverman AJ, Thaler M, Frost LL: Studies of the processes of aging: X. The strengths and weaknesses of psychic function in the aged, *American Journal of Psychiatry* 111:896-901, 1955.

Cameron N: Neuroses of later maturity. In Kaplan OJ (ed): *Mental Disorders in Later Life*. Stanford, California, Stanford University Press, 1956.

Cameron P: Introversion and egocentricity among the aged, *Journal of Gerontology* 22:199, 1967.

Cath S: Discussion notes. In Berezin NA, Cath S (eds): *Geriatric Psychiatry*. New York, International Universities Press, 1965, 128-129.

Chodoff P: The depressive personality: critical review, *International Journal of Psychiatric Medicine* 27:196, 1972.

Costa PT, McCrae RR: Still stable after all these years: personality as a key to some issues in adulthood and old age. In Baltes P, Brim O (eds): *Life Span Development and Behavior*. New York, Academic Press, 1980.

Dohrenwind BP: The social psychological nature of stress: a framework for causal inquiry, *Journal of Abnormal and Social Psychology* 62:294, 1961.

Eisdorfer C, Nowlin J, Wilkie F: Improvement of learning in the aged by modification of autonomic nervous system activity, *Science* 170:1327, 1970.

Erikson E: *Childhood and Society*. New York, WW Norton, 1950.

Fenichel O: *The Psychoanalytic Theory of Neurosis*. New York: WW Norton, 1945.

Fiske M: Task and crises of the second half of life: the interrelationship of commitment, coping, and adaptation. In Biren JE, Sloane RB (eds): *The Handbook of Aging and Mental Health*. Englewood Cliffs, New Jersey, Prentice-Hall, 1980, pp. 355-359.

Foster JM, Gallagher D: An exploratory study comparing depressed and non-depressed elders' coping strategies, *Journal of Gerontology* 41:91-93, 1986.

Freud S: Mourning and melancholia (originally published in 1917). In *Collected Papers (vol IV)*. London, Hogarth Press, 1950, pp. 152-172.

Freud S: On psychotherapy (originally published in 1924). In *Collected Papers (vol I)*. London: Hogarth Press, 1950.

Gallagher D, Thompson LW: Cognitive psychotherapy of late-life depression. In Breslau LD, Haug MR (eds): *Depression and Aging*. New York, Springer, 1983, pp. 168-192.

Garber J, Miller WR, Seaman SF: Learned helplessness, stress, and the depressive disorders. In Depue RA (ed): *The Psychobiology of Depressive Disorders*. New York, Academic Press, 1979. pp. 335-363.

Gaylin W: *The Meaning of Despair: Psychoanalytic Contributions to Understanding Depression*. New York, Science House, 1968.

Gilleard CJ, Willmott M, Vaddadi KS: Self-report measures of mood and morale in elderly depressives, *British Journal of Psychiatry* 138:230-235, 1981.

Gutheil E: Reactive depressions. In Arieti S (ed): *Anerican Handbook of Psychiatry*. New York, Basic Books, 1959, pp. 345-352.

Havighurst RJ: Successful aging. In Williams RH, Tibbets C, Donahue W (eds): *Processes in Aging. (Vol I)*. New York, Williams and Wilkins, 1963, pp. 299-320.

Hebb DO: Drives and the CNS (central nervous system), *Psychological Reviews* 62:243, 1955.

Isaacs K, Silver R: *Cognitive Structure in Depression*. Paper presented at the meeting of the Association for the Advancement of Behavior Therapy, New York, November, 1980.

Jacobson E: Contributions to the metapsychology of cyclothymic depression. In Greenacre P (ed): *Affective Disorders*. New York, International Universities Press, 1953, pp. 49-83.

Jung CG: *Psychological Types*. London, Routledge and Kegan Paul, 1923.

Kernberg OF: Borderline personality organization, *Journal of the American Psychoanalytic Association* 15:641-685, 1967.

Klein M. *Contributions to Psychoanalysis 1921-1945*. London, Hogarth Press, 1948.

Lao I: Developmental trend of the locus of control, *Personality and Social Psychology Bulletin* 1:348, 1974.

Lapointe HA, Crandell CJ: Relationship of irrational beliefs to self-reported depression, *Cognitive Therapy and Research* 4:247-250, 1980.

Lazarus LW, Weinberg J: Treatment in the ambulatory care setting. In Busse EW, Blazer DG (eds): *Handbook of Geriatric Psychiatry*. New York, Van Nostrand, Rheinhold, 1980, pp. 427-452.

Levin S: Depression in the aged. In Berezin MA, Cath S (eds): *Geriatric Psychiatry*. New York, International Universities Press, 1965, pp. 210-216.

Lewinsohn P, MacPhillamy DJ: The relationship between age and engagement in pleasant activities, *Journal of Gerontology* 29:290-294, 1974.

Lewinsohn TM, Weinstein M, Shaw D: Depression: a clinical research approach. In Rubin RD, Frank CM (eds): *Advances in Behavior Therapy.* New York, Academic Press, 1969.

Maas HS, Kuypers JA: *From 30 to 70.* San Francisco, Jossey-Bass, 1974.

Maddox GL: Persistence of life-style among the elderly: a longitudinal study of patterns of social activity in relation to life satisfaction. In Neugarten BL (ed): *Middle Age and Aging.* Chicago, University of Chicago Press, 1968, pp. 181-183.

Meissner WW: *Normal Psychology of the Aging Process Revisited. I.* Discussion presented at the fifth anniversary of the annual scientific meeting of the Boston Society of Gerontologic Psychiatry. Boston, November 1, 1975.

Mendelsohn M. *Psychoanalytic Concepts of Depression.* Springfield, Illinois, Charles C. Thomas, 1960.

Palmore EB, Kivett VR: Changes in life satisfaction, *Journal of Gerontology* 32:311-316, 1977.

Pedersen NL, Gatz M, Plomin R, Nesselroade JR, McClearn GE: Individual differences in locus of control during the second half of the life span for identical and fraternal twins reared apart and together, *Journal of Gerontology* 44:100-105, 1989.

Pfeiffer E, Verwoerdt A, Wang HS: The natural history of social behavior in a biologically advantaged group of aging individuals, *Journal of Gerontology* 24:193, 1969.

Riegel KF: Personality theory and aging. In Biren JE (ed): *Handbook of Aging and the Individual.* Chicago, University of Chicago Press, 1959, pp. 797-851.

Rochlin G: Discussion notes. In Berezin MA, Cath S (eds): *Geriatric Psychiatry.* New York, International Universities Press, 1965, pp. 226-227.

Rodin J: Aging and health: effects of the sense of control, *Science* 233:1271-1276, 1986.

Rotter J: Generalized expectations for internal *versus* external control of reinforcement, *Psychological Monographs* 80:(609), 1966.

Schaie KW, Parham IA: Cohort/sequential analysis of adult intellectual development, *Developmental Psychology* 13:649, 1977.

Schiffman S: Food recognition by the elderly, *Journal of Gerontology* 32:586-592, 1977.

Schmale AH: Relationship of separation and depression to disease. I. Report in a hospitalized medical population, *Psychosomatic Medicine* 20:259, 1958.

Seligman MEP: Depression and learned helplessness. In Friedman RJ, Katz NM (eds): *The Psychology of Depression: Contemporary Theory and Research.* Washington, DC, VH Winston, 1974.

Seligman MEP, Maier SF: Failure to escape traumatic shock, *Journal of Experimental Psychology* 74:1, 1967.

Spitz R: Anaclitic depression. *Psychoanalytic Study of the Child* 2:313, 1946.

Strelau J: Nervous system type and extroversion-introversion: a comparison of Eusench's theory with Pavlov typology, *POL Psychological Bulletin* 1:17, 1970.

Thomae H: Personality and adjustment to aging. In Biren J, Sloane RB (eds): *The Handbook of Aging and Mental Health.* Englewood Cliffs, New Jersey, Prentice-Hall, 1980, pp. 283-309.

Verwoerdt A: Anxiety, dissociation and personality disorders in the elderly. In Busse EW, Blazer DG (eds): *Handbook of Geriatric Psychiatry.* New York, Van Nostrand, Rheinhold, 1980, pp. 368-380.

Vezina J, Bourque P: The relationship between cognitive structure and symptoms of depression of the elderly, *Cognitive Therapy and Research* 8:29-36, 1984.

Weissman AD: Discussion notes. In Berezin MA, Cath S (eds): *Geriatric Psychiatry.* New York, International Universities Press, 1965, pp. 233-234.

Wigdor DT: Drives and motivation with aging. In Biren JE, Sloane RB (eds): *Handbook of Mental Health and Aging.* Englewood Cliffs, New Jersey, Prentice-Hall, 1980, pp. 245-261.

Zetzel E: Metapsychology of aging. In Berezin MA and Cath S (eds): *Geriatric Psychiatry.* New York, International Universities Press, 1965, pp. 109-118.

CHAPTER

6

SOCIAL ORIGINS

Most psychiatric disorders are caused by multiple factors, and social factors are recognized as important contributors to these disorders without denying the existence of biologic factors. The hypothesis that increased social stressors and decreased social support in late life contribute to depressive disorders is not new. Unlike many biologically based etiologic studies (characterized by the exploration of new relationships, associations, and pathways) the most valued studies of the social origins of late life depression have been based on refinement of the methodology used to test extant hypotheses.

As demonstrated in Figure 1-6, the web of causation for depressive disorders in late life includes many social factors. Loss and response to loss of significant objects within the environment have for many years been hypothesized to be associated with the depressive disorders (Freud, 1917; Gaylin, 1968; Spitz, 1942). Depression has been the prototype syndrome for testing the relationship between environmental stressors and psychiatric illness (Fieve et al, 1977; Ilfield, 1977; Jacobs et al, 1974; Paykel, 1974).

Focus on social stressors as etiologic factors in the onset of late life depression stems from at least three factors. First, many depressive episodes in late life are first-time events following an identifiable social stressor (Post, 1968; Slater and Roth, 1969). Persons with late onset depressive disorders also are less likely to report a family history of mood disorderss than persons with early onset mood disorders, suggesting that age-related neuropathologic changes and social factors predominate as causitive (Chessea, 1965; Hopkinson, 1954). The elderly face unique social and economic pressures secondary to transitions experienced in late life, such as ageism, declining incomes, and impaired physical health, which may place them at risk for depression (Bengtson and Haber, 1975; Palmore, 1969). Third, older people may be more susceptible to the adverse effects of social stress (Caudill, 1958; Lazarus, 1966).

This chapter first reviews the possible mechanisms by which social factors influence the onset and the outcome of late life depressive disorders and describes a social model of late life depression. Next, the literature on social factors and depression in late life is

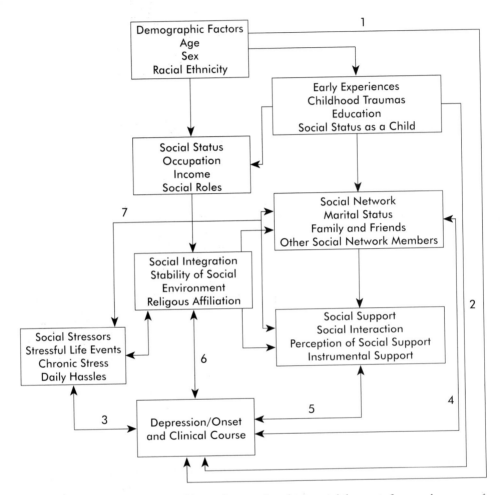

Figure 6-1. A model of the possible mechanisms by which social factors influence the onset of depression disorders, disaggregated by specific hypothesis.

reviewed with particular emphasis on the major hypotheses that make up the model of social factors and the onset of and outcome of late life depression (Figure 6-1).

■ SOCIAL ENVIRONMENT AS A CONTRIBUTOR TO DEPRESSIVE DISORDERS IN LATE LIFE

Interest in the relationship of the social environment to illness onset and outcome has blossomed during the past 20 years (MacMahon and Pugh, 1970; Nuckolls et al, 1972; Rahe et al, 1973). Not only do social conditions determine preferences, availability, and distribution of tangibles—such as food, services, and medical care—the social environment may directly alter function in the older adult (MacMahon and Pugh, 1970).

The association of the social environment with disease can be studied by applying the analogy of the infectious disease model (Cassel, 1976). The elements of this model are: (1) the disease agent (i.e., a pathologic organism); (2) the host; (3) the onset and outcome of the disease or disorder; and (4) the factors that modify the relationship between the disease agent and host, such as exposure and host resistance. Unlike the acute infectious disease model, however, most disease agents are ever present in the environment, yet most individuals are protected from these agents (Dubos, 1965). Cassel (1976) notes that "a full understanding of the distribution and determinants of the disease requires that we know both the prevalence and toxicity of these agents and the determinants of those factors which change the relationship between the host and these agents, thus transforming an innocuous, possibly symbiotic relationship to one in which clinical disease is the outcome."

The prime social contributor to chronic disease, such as late life depression, has been hypothesized to be stress (Cannon, 1935; Seyle, 1956; Wolff, 1950). Stress replaces the disease agent or pathologic organism in the disease model. As Cassel (1976) points out, however, semantic and methodologic problems surround the use of the word *stress* and therefore the concept. Wolff originally used the term to indicate "that state within a living creature which results from the interaction of the organism with noxious stimuli or circumstances, i.e., it is the dynamic state within the organism; it is not a stimulus, assault, load symbol, burden, or any aspect of environment, internal, external, social or otherwise" (Selye and Wolff, 1973). Over time, however, *stress* became associated with the noxious stimuli in the environment, although the term *stressor* is more accurate. According to Wolff (1973), the nature of psychosocial stressors is different from that of physicochemical disease agents. Physicochemical disease agents have a direct pathogenic effect on the organism by damaging and distorting structure and function (usually predictably), whereas psychosocial stressors effect the organism indirectly. The indirect action of psychosocial stressors may be secondary to their capacity to act as signals or symbols.

Although debate about the nature and characteristics of stressors continues, research in this area received great impetus after the operationalization of the construct of environmental stressors by Holmes and Rahe (1967). Following the tradition of Adolf Meyer (Leif, 1948), they documented a series of events that were uniformly recognized as requiring adaptation by members of the population, and therefore considered stressful. The simplicity of the concept of stressful life events coupled with an operational definition that was translated into a measurable variable resulted in many studies relating the onset and progression of illnesses, both physical and psychiatric, to these environmental events. (Hudgens et al, 1967; Paykel et al, 1974; Paykel et al, 1970; Thompson and Hendrie, 1972).

Harrell and Noelken (1978) note that the relationship of individuals to the social environment varies throughout the life cycle. Therefore results from studies of children and young adults cannot easily be applied to the elderly. The transitions of life, such as adolescence, the involutional period, and retirement, have been of great interest to investigators and clinicians in terms of the adaptation of individuals to these transitions. Adaptation to adolescence, however, is not the same as adaptation to retirement. Are the elderly more susceptible to role transitions than younger adults? Are older persons more capable of adapting to the impact of social environment stressors, given a lifetime of experience with adaptation? What are the events in late life to which elders have the most difficulty adapting?

As noted, many late life depressive episodes are first-time events. Can we assume, however, that depressive symptoms are secondary to environmental stressors? As noted in Chapter 4, the relative decrease of a genetic predisposition to late onset depression does not imply that biologic factors do not contribute significantly to the cause of late life depression.

The elderly are considered by some to be a greater risk for environmental stressors. Butler (1974) proposes that the elderly experience predictable stressful events that force them into a preconceived cultural definition as dependent, querulous, forgetful, fretful, and irritable. *Ageism* describes this prejudice toward the elderly. Loss of status and prestige also accompanies the absence of roles in late life. Loss of social roles results because of retirement from formally productive positions in the workplace and the absence of many socially prescribed roles, such as community leadership. Accompanying the loss of employment and roles is the parallel loss of economic status. Economic adversity secondary to a fixed retirement income and rising expenses (especially health care expenses) is common in late life. The elderly are also a greater risk for loss of spouse, siblings, friends, and even children.

Others argue that the elderly are more susceptible to the deleterious effects of the social environment (Caudill, 1958; Lazarus, 1966). Decline in perceptual abilities and other adaptative capacities render the older person particularly susceptible to social influences. Declining physical health may necessitate the availability of instrumental resources to carry on the usual activities of daily living. Increased dependence on the social environment may necessitate improved communication with that environment, thus placing particular responsibility on clinicians working with older persons (Blazer, 1978).

Dowd and Brooks (1978) suggest that the elderly are more anomic (i.e., they are more disconnected socially and emotionally from society). Lowenthal and Berkman (1967) found that many older persons are socially isolated, often by choice, and this limits their ability to participate in social activities. Because of a fixed income and the need to be within walking distance of needed services, such as a grocery store, older persons often persist in living in less desirable neighborhoods within the inner city. Geographic isolation decreases ties with families. Concern for security decreases social interaction with neighbors and friends (i.e., the elderly become prisoners in their own homes).

Shanas (1979), however, maintains that the family continues personal and effective ties with the older adult. She suggests geographic displacement does not interfere with emotional ties and, when necessary, instrumental resources are available from family to the older adult. A reciprocal relationship of instrumental and emotional support between generations is a special emphasis of Shanas' argument. Cumming and Henry (1961), in their discourse on the disengagement theory of aging, suggest that decreased social interaction is a mutual process. Society and the aging person withdraw from one another, with the aging individual accepting, perhaps even desiring decreased interaction. The aging individual's withdrawal has developmental and responsive qualities in that it is accompanied or preceded by an increased preoccupation with the self and a decreased emotional investment in persons and objects in the environment. Disengagement is therefore a natural rather than an imposed process. Maddox (1964), however, argues against the disengagement theory, stating that activity and the persistence of socially engaged life-style are the most adaptable means of achieving life satisfaction in later years. Examination of life-styles and life satisfaction of most older persons would confirm Maddox's conclusion.

■ A MODEL OF THE SOCIAL ORIGINS OF LATE LIFE DEPRESSION

A model of the possible mechanisms by which social factors, specifically social stressors and social support, influence the onset of depressive disorders is presented in Figure 6-1. Although it appears complicated, this model is oversimplified in that the social stressors are considered as only one variable and social support is considered across only two parameters—social network and actual social support. Seven potential hypotheses are diagrammed. They are as follows:

Hypothesis 1: Demographic factors, such as age, gender, and race, may contribute to the onset of depression in late life. Prejudice related to age, such as loss of social roles, is included in this hypothesis. In addition, the differences in depression by race, not explained by confounding factors, such as socioeconomic status, are included.

Hypothesis 2: Early experiences, especially childhood traumas and impoverishment, may increase the risk for the onset of late life depression. Childhood deprivation may effect the onset of depression, regardless of age. In addition, childhood deprivation determines in part adult social relations, which in turn may indirectly contribute to late life depression. Demographic factors often interact with early childhood experiences.

Hypothesis 3: Recent social stressors may precipitate a depressive disorder in older adults. In addition, social stressors may aggravate the outcome of a depressive disorder in late life. Most of the studies associating stressful life events and depression are based on this hypothesis.

Hypothesis 4: An impaired social network, such as the absence of a spouse, few family, and few friends, increases the risk for depression in late life. Most studies relating marital status to depressive disorders are based on this hypothesis. In contrast to hypothesis seven, this hypothesis relates to the main effects of impaired social support.

Hypothesis 5: A decline in social interaction, perception of social support, and tangible (or instrumental) support leads to depression in late life. An impaired social network, impaired social status, and poor social integration in the community may all contribute to a decline in social interaction and impaired perceived personal support (i.e., interactive effects).

Hypothesis 6: Poor social integration may lead directly to the onset and persistence of late life depression, (i.e., social disintegration is a main effect). The absence of strong religious affiliations and an unstable environment may contribute directly to the onset and outcome of late life depression.

Hypothesis 7: The causal relationship between social stressors and late life depression may be buffered by both the social network and social support. When social network and support are impaired, the impact of social stress is enhanced. So called buffering hypotheses related to late life depression are based on this hypothesis.

The literature that addresses the social origins of late life depression will be reviewed within the context of these seven hypotheses. These hypotheses do not, however, exhaust the possible complex interactions of social factors that may contribute to late life depression. These hypotheses do not specifically address the relationship between social stressors and the biologic origins of depression. Nevertheless, the empiric clarification of the relative strength of these different pathways to depression enhance the ability of clinical investigators and clinicians to identify those social factors within the web of causation that contribute directly or indirectly to the onset and outcome of late life depression.

■ DEMOGRAPHIC RISK FACTORS FOR LATE LIFE DEPRESSION

Although older persons may be more predisposed to depression biologically (see Chapter 4), the frequency of major depression in late life is lower than at other stages of the life cycle and the frequency of depressive symptoms does not appear to be higher in late life than at earlier ages (see Chapter 1). These findings suggest that older persons may be less exposed to or protected from psychosocial risk factors compared with persons at an earlier age. This protection may derive from improved coping mechanisms and adaptation to psychosocial risk factors for depression. Despite the increased physical health problems that accompany advancing age, even the oldest old do not consistently experience a higher prevalence of either major depression or depressive symptoms. (Blazer et al, 1991; Warheit et al, 1975).

Female gender is a risk factor for depression throughout the adult life cycle (Myers et al, 1984; Weissman and Boyd, 1985). Gender differences in the prevalence of major depression, however, appear to narrow as age increases (Blazer et al, 1987; George et al, 1989). To date, no one has adequately identified those factors related to gender that may place women at increased risk for depression, regardless of age. If such factors exist (bias in case identification may contribute significantly to the reported gender differences), those risk factors appear to decrease in late life. Some presumed vulnerability in younger women, such as multiple roles (e.g., worker and homemaker), social isolation, and childrearing responsibilities, disappear with increasing age. Yet older women often face unique social stressors with greater frequency than older men, such as caretaking responsibility and widowhood.

Race and ethnic differences in the risk for depression are virtually nonexistent, regardless of age when appropriate control variables are included in the analysis—especially education and socioeconomic status (Blazer et al, 1985). Warheit (1975) found race differences in depressive symptoms in a community sample. Blacks were found to experience higher prevalence of depressive symptoms than whites, but this difference was explained by socioeconomic differences. As the socioeconomic status of blacks and whites tend toward equalization with advancing age, even the crude rates of depressive symptoms and major depression tend not to vary in later life by race.

■ EARLY EXPERIENCES AS RISK FOR DEPRESSION IN LATE LIFE

Studies of the risk factors for depression in mid-life have substantiate that adverse early childhood experiences increase the risk for depression in mid-life. For example, lower levels of education have been associated with a higher risk for depression (Holzer et al, 1986). The relationship between depression and education, however, may be more complex (George, 1991). For example, the relationship may be curvilinear, with both very low and very high levels of education associated with greater risk of depression than with moderate levels of schooling (Blazer et al, 1985). In addition, the relationship between education and depression may be weaker among older adults than among young and middle-aged persons (George, in press).

Brown and Harris (1978), in their influential book *Social Origins of Depression*, established that events occurring earlier in life with severe, long-term threatening implications, most of which involved some major loss, played a major role in predisposing to depressive disorders, both among patients in psychiatric treatment and among women in the community (Brown and Harris, 1978; Murphy, 1982). In these studies, however, there were significant social class differences in the prevalence of depression among working class, middle-aged women. Not only were the women predisposed to developing depression secondary to the early experience of childhood deprivation (a predisposing factor), they were much more likely to have experienced a severe stressful life event in the year before developing the depressive disorder (a provoking factor). Those long-term social difficulties, identified as vulnerability factors, included loss of the mother before the age of 11.

Other childhood traumas that have been associated with overall mental health during adulthood include childhood poverty and sexual assault (O'Neil et al, 1987; Tennant, 1982). Exposure to parents with alcohol problems also appears to increase the risk for depression in adult life (Mathew et al, unpublished manuscript). George (1991), in analysis based on epidemiologic catchment area data from North Carolina, found the relationships between childhood traumas and psychiatric disorders in the elderly to be as strong for persons aged 60 and older as for those aged 18 to 59. She notes that epidemiologic studies examining this relationships are complemented by findings from clinical studies, some of which focus specifically on older persons (Kaminsky, 1978; McMordie and Blom, 1979).

The elderly are more anomic according to Dowd and Brooks (1978) (i.e., they lose ties to their culture because they are conscious of recent trends in social policy and values away from traditional values). Older persons may believe that society is under the control of a group of influential, higher-income, college-educated "bureaucrats" (i.e., the new middle class). This anomie is accompanied by a conscious estrangement from dominant societal institutions. Since Dowd and Brooks reported these observations, factors have changed. For one, older persons have improved in both their educational and income status as younger cohorts have matured. In addition, older persons have recognized that they are powerful (although not necessarily united) political force and have asserted their influence in many areas.

Neugarten (1970) noted that older persons experience frequent life events, such as the death of a spouse or a sibling, and postulates that they may be better prepared to accept and adapt to these events than persons at earlier stages of life. Adaptation to these events is facilitated if the events are anticipated, expected, or "on time" during the life cycle (see Chapter 5). Unanticipated events are more likely to be traumatic. The debate will continue about whether older persons experience more social stress than younger persons in our society. Older persons do experience unique stressful events that disrupt the social network, and an understanding of the relationship of these events to both physical and mental health is essential for intervention and management.

The elderly are considered by some to be at greater risk for impaired social relations and support (Butler, 1974; Lowenthal and Berkman, 1967). Lloyd (1980) in her review of the literature on stressful life events and depression, divided these events into predisposing and precipitating etiologic factors. Early adverse experiences are predisposing factors, and recent losses are precipitating factors. Most studies of early loss, unfortunately, do not include individuals in late life but rather focus on the onset of depression between the ages of 20 and 45 years. Kay et al (1964), however, found that the prevalence of mental disorder in a community population of the elderly was increased in individuals who had experienced some type of childhood trauma. However, this study has not been replicated, and the results have therefore not been verified. No known clinical report to date suggests that early loss contributes to first onset depressive disorders in late life.

■ SOCIAL STRESSORS AS A RISK FOR LATE LIFE DEPRESSION

Proximal stressors in the social environment that may contribute to the onset and continuance of depression in older adults have been divided into life events, chronic stress, and daily hassles (George, 1991). Life events are those identifiable, discrete changes in life patterns that disrupt the elder's usual behavior and threaten or challenge his or her well being, such as the death of a sibling. Chronic stress includes those long-term conditions that challenge or threaten the elder's well-being, such as ongoing financial deprivation, interpersonal difficulties, or living in a dangerous neighborhood (Krause, 1987; Pearlin and Schooler, 1978). Daily hassles are the ordinary but stressful events and transactions between the person and the physical or social environment (Lazarus and Folkman, 1984). Examples of daily hassles include household responsibility, managing household finances, home maintenance, and unpleasant interactions with neighbors. These hassles tend to be long-term but are of lower intensity than chronic stress.

Much attention has been given to the loss of a spouse as a precipitant of depression (Briscoe and Smith, 1975). The symptoms of a major depressive episode are similar to those of an uncomplicated bereavement (see Chapter 12), but most investigators and clinicians have observed a case where the death of a spouse precipitated depression in a depression-prone elder and in which symptoms exceeded the symptoms of normal bereavement. Birtchnell (1970) found an increased prevalence of recent parental death among 500 inpatients with depression. Since the young old often experience the loss of parents, as well as siblings and friends, these findings apply to the elderly and the young.

Others who investigate the origins of depression have not concentrated on specific events, such as loss of a spouse, but instead on the occurrence of accumulated stressors. For example, Paykel et al (1970) found that depressed patients had an increased frequency of eight life events during the 6 months before the onset of depressive symptoms. These events included marital arguments, marital separations, starting a new type of work, change in work conditions, serious personal illness, death of an immediate family member, serious illness of family members, and family members leaving home. Murphy (1982), when comparing the depressed elderly with normal elderly in the general population, found an association between the accumulation of severe life events, especially in the presence of poor health, and the onset of depression.

As noted, a debate persists about whether stressful life events are more or less frequent in older adults compared with young adults. Hughes et al (1988) found that life event differences using a standard scale did vary between young and old, but the differences were not as great as might be expected. For example, the experience of someone close to the informant suffering a serious illness was no more frequent among the elderly than in younger persons. Murrell and Norris (1984) found that, although overall life events decrease with aging, specific types of events occur more frequently (e.g., events related to physical functioning and health). Investigators also debate the relevance of traditional scales that assess stressful events in older adults, such as the Schedule of Recent Events (Holmes and Rahe, 1967). For example, retirement may be a positive event among the elderly but a negative event at earlier ages. In addition, most studies do not account for the positive influence of certain events. Rewards and recognition to older persons are generally not considered in the stressful life event literature. A move to a retirement community may represent the reward of a lifetime of difficult work as opposed to a stressful event. Thoitis (1981) found that, when health-related events are removed from the measures of life events, the relationship between life events and psychophysiologic distress decreases significantly.

Stressful events contribute not only to the onset of depressive disorders but also to the persistence of these disorders as well. Tennant et al (1981) found that the report of adverse life events 3 months before evaluation were associated with remission of neurotic disorders in 800 subjects between the ages of 18 and 64 years of age. Neutralizing events were associated with remission as well. A neutralizing event, according to Tennant and colleagues, was an event that neutralized the impact of an earlier threatening event or difficulty. For example, if an older man loses a position as a volunteer that he valued, that event would be neutralized if he obtains another equally satisfying volunteer position.

According to George (1991), many investigators find that chronic stress has a stronger effect on the onset and outcome of depression than life events. These findings are based on samples of all ages (Billings and Moos, 1984; Krause, 1986). Arling (1987) suggests that older persons may be able to adapt to specific changes in their lives but have more difficulty with ongoing sources of strain, such as chronic physical health problems, economic deprivation, and social isolation. Pearlin et al (1981) was the first to suggest the concept of *life strain* (here described as chronic stress and daily hassles). Life strain is a set of enduring and basic problems that discrete life events may exacerbate, create, or bring into focus.

George (1991) suggests that some chronic stressors may be more closely related to depression than others. She provides the example of the study by Krause (1986). In this study, chronic financial deprivation was more strongly related to depression for older women than chronic health problems (Willis Recent Life Events). Ezquiaga (1987) found that stressful events were more likely to occur associated with the first two episodes of major depression than with later such episodes of major depression. There was no difference, however, in the prevalence of chronic stress across the different depressive episodes. There are few studies of the relationship between daily hassles and depression.

■ SOCIAL SUPPORT AND THE ORIGIN OF LATE LIFE DEPRESSION

The complexity of conceptualizing and measuring stressors has lead researchers and clinicians to consider the importance of factors in the social environment that modify the adverse consequences of environmental stressors (Berkman and Syme, 1979; Cassel,

1976; Cobb, 1976; Durkheim, 1950; Kaplan et al, 1977; Leighton, 1959; Lowenthal, 1965). Most of these investigators have investigated the support function of the social environment. Social support is the provision of meaningful, appropriate, and protective feedback from the social environment to the person that enables the person to negotiate intermittent or continual environmental stressors. Social support is an attractive concept because it is more amenable to interventions than environmental stressors.

Although a number of studies suggest a relationship between social support and depression, conceptual and methodologic advances are necessary to firmly establish the nature of that relationship (Krause, 1987; Holihan and Holihan, 1987; Norris and Murrell, 1984; Kaplan et al, 1983; Lin et al, 1979). As noted by Cassel (1976), one of the most important requirements of future social environmental studies is improvement of the conceptual framework. Meaningful and relevant models of social support that are adaptable to measurement must be developed. Before hypotheses can be tested, a series of pathways that may lead to expected outcomes should be developed. Given the nature of social support as a variable, longitudinal research design is essential for studies. Of special importance is the potential contamination of perceptions of the social environment by physical and psychiatric disorders. In a recent study, however, Blazer and Hughes (1991) found that depressive symptoms, although highly correlated with perceived social support, was a separate construct. This longitudinal study illustrates the value of disaggregating potential confounding effects of variables explored in social psychiatric investigation.

The roots of the construct "social support" go back to the early twentieth century. Durkheim (1950) proposes that persons who are not integrated into society (i.e., anomie) are at greater risk for suicide. Mead (1934) closely connects human development with social support. Through language individuals take on, or internalize, the attitudes of others toward both the environment and themselves (i.e., the human acquires a social self). This social self, or the "me," is an organization of the internalized attitudes of others, the conventional as opposed to the active part of the self, and therefore depends for its existence on the social environment, especially supportive and informative aspects of that environment.

Parsons (1951) reflects on the importance of social support as follows:

The first element of any social control mechanism . . . may be called "support" . . . its primary significance is . . . to give a basis for reassurance such that the need to resort to aggressive/ destructive and/or defensive reactions is lessened. Support may be of various kinds, but the common element is that somewhere there is the incorporation or retention of ego in a solitary relationship so that he is a basis of security. (The therapist) readiness to "help" and his "understanding" of the patient . . . (function to) localize the focus of strain, making it possible for the ego to feel that his insecurity is not "total" but can be focused on a limited problem area.

The epigenetic theory of childhood development, postulated by Erikson (1950) and described in Chapter 5, illustrates the importance of the social environment to proper psychologic functioning throughout the life cycle. According to Erikson, "The human personality, in principle, develops according to steps predetermined and the growing persons readiness to be driven, to be aware of, and to interact with, a widening social radius and society, and in principle, tends to be so constituted as to meet and invite the succession of interactions in attempts to safeguard and to encourage the proper weight and proper sequence of the unfolding."

Developing an operational definition and measuring social support may be even more problematic than defining and measuring social stressors. The supportive functions of the social environment continuously influence the individual through time, albeit change and supportive functioning can occur over time, and reflect the effectiveness of the individual's interaction with the social environment. An adequate understanding of social support necessitates an understanding of the nature of the social environment itself.

The supportive aspects of the social environment can be considered from many different viewpoints. For example, the overall ecology of a given environment can be contrasted with the factors within the environment that directly affect individuals, or structural and transactional aspects of the social environment can be contrasted. Social structure is the multidimensional space of social positions among which the persons are distributed and reflects and effects role relations and social associations (Blau, 1977). Social structure, for the most part, can be directly observed and measured and includes concepts such as status, role, stratification, and differentiation. In the model presented in Figure 6-1, social status is operationalized by variables such as occupation, income, and social roles.

Social transactions are the interactions between the social environment and the individual, as well as interactions among social organizations. Social transactions are less easily measured, yet can be defined in terms of durability, intensity, frequency, and flexibility. The quality of social transactions between social organizations directly influences and defines in large part social integration (see Figure 6-1) (i.e., the stability of the social environment). The quality and frequency of interactions between individuals is captured by the construct of social support in Figure 6-1.

Social support in the model is operationally defined as (Blazer, 1980):

1. Social network, or roles and available attachments—the individuals and groups of individuals within the social network available to the subject, such as spouse, children, and group membership.
2. Social interactions—the frequency of interactions between social network members and the subject.
3. Perceived social support—the subjective evaluation by the individual of his or her sense of a dependable social network, ease of interaction with the network, sense of belonging to the network, and a sense of intimacy with network members.
4. Instrumental support—concrete and observable services provided to the subject from the social network.

This operational definition of social support is directly impacted by social status, social integration, and social stressors (especially those stressors that remove individuals from the social network or change interaction within the network).

In what ways is social support operative? The most frequent explanation of social support to the individual is that it provides feedback, information, and guidance. According to Cassel (1976):

Failure of various forms of behavior to elicit predictable responses leads to one of three types of responses on the part of the animals involved, the most common of which is repetition of the behavioral acts. Some acts are always accompanied by profound neuroendocrine changes and presumably chronic repetitions lead eventually to permanent alterations in the levels of hormones to the degree of autonomic nervous system arousal reported on the conditions of animal crowding.

Increased levels and disruption of the circadian output of hormones from the hypothalamic pituitary adrenal axis are associated with depressive disorders (see Chapter 4), and therefore the lack of social support may contribute to the onset of a mood disorder through the mechanisms described by Cassell.

Other authorities postulate that social support is operative through an integration at the emotional level, namely, the perception of attachment and bonding. Mead (1934) claims that messages from the social environment are essential for the definition of the personality. Bowlby (1969) suggests that biologic factors in mother and child help establish an attachment between the parent and child from the early stages of life. A number of behaviors called *attachment behaviors*, such as smiling, touch, and feeding, bond mother and child in a way analogous to *imprinting*, the phenomenon noted in ground-nesting birds (Scott, 1962).

Still others have suggested that social support is of value to an individual in that it provides nuturance or support at the physical level. Bovard (1959, 1962) notes that stressful psychologic stimuli are mediated cerebrally through the posterior and medial hypothalamus. Stressful stimuli cause a release of neurotransmitter to the anterior pituitary, which in turn produces a general protein catabolic effect. A second center located in the anterior lateral hypothalamus produces a "competing response" that inhibits, masks, or screens the stress stimulus when appropriate social stimuli are produced. Hofer and Weiner (1971) show that behavioral and physiologic changes occur when young rat pups are denied physical nuturance and body contact with their mother. This lack of nuturance, which is only partially nutritional, predisposes the rat to altered physiologic responses to stress in later life. Early childhood deprivation may therefore predispose to depression physiologically and psychologically.

Caplan (1974) and Moss (1973) note that one value of a supportive network to an individual is the provision of task-oriented assistance. Families and other members of the network provide supervision or checking services to the older adult, educational services that help develop or improve skills, and training in the instrumental functions of living and personal care, such as aiding the individual in bathing, dressing, and feeding. These activities are measurable and undoubtedly contribute to the emotional well-being of the individual. Closely associated with this personal assistance is the provision of material goods to the person (i.e., food, clothing, and shelter) (Caplan, 1974). These provisions are the more basic expectations of persons in society.

Moss (1973) speculates that support may operate by protecting participants from encounters with "information incongruities." According to this theory, support in some way deflects stress from the individual. This theory can be appreciated in the phenomenon of herd immunity. The individual organism is sometimes protected from an environmental stressors, such as poverty or war, secondary to membership in the group. In other words, immunity possessed by most members of the group protects persons within the group who are not immune.

As noted by George (1991), however, social support is not always an unqualified benefit. Dissatisfying and conflictual transactions may affect the older adult more adversely than the absence of transactions (Rook, 1984). Excessive support, even if it is welcomed, may lead to a loss of autonomy, self-reliance, and feelings of personal control (Lee, 1985). Elders may also vary in their desire for a need of supportive transactions (Henderson et al, 1981).

Most studies of social support do not substantiate significant differences in either the support network or perceived support by age. Most older persons are embedded in an extensive social network and are generally satisfied with that network (Shanas, 1979; Markides et al, 1986). Network size also does not appear to be significantly different for the young-old compared with the old-old (Cantor, 1975). It is well known that isolation is associated with loneliness and therefore increases the risk for depression. Dean et al (1992) found that, among older persons living alone, depressive symptoms were more frequent, and this relationship was independent of the expressive support from friends, face-to-face interaction with friends, undesirable life events, disability, and financial strain. Antonucci (1985), in a large study based on a national sample of noninstitutionalized adults 50 years of age and older, found that age was negatively related to the amount of support provided by nonfamily members and that older persons tended to be more satisfied with their support networks than younger members of the sample.

■ SOCIAL DISINTEGRATION AS A RISK FOR LATE LIFE DEPRESSION

Leighton (1974) has championed the hypothesis that overall social disintegration contributes to significant psychopathology, regardless of age. An integrated society is "a system in that it has patterns of interpersonal behavior that are essential to the survival and welfare of the whole." These patterns enable the group to obtain what is needed for subsistence, protection against weather and disease, control of hostility and other forms of disruption, the creation of new members and their education, disposal of the dead, networks of communication, storage of information, ways for arriving at decisions and taking united action, and much else. Such collective, patterned activities have been called *the functional prerequisites of society.* A society is disintegrated if there is no system to permit individuals within society attaining these goals, but rather a "collection of human beings whose precuring of food, shelter, defense against attacks and so on are purely individual matters." Leighton tested his model and found that, at all ages, when the frequency of mental illness (such as depression) was compared between integrated and disintegrated communities, the rates were higher in disintegrated communities (Leighton et al, 1963).

Studies of social integration are ecologic in that there is no direct attempt to associate the environmental stressor with a given individual in a society, but rather the overall level of societal disruption is associated with the overall level of psychopathology. As can be imagined, such studies are most difficult to implement and therefore have received little attention since Leighton attempted to test his hypothesis in Nova Scotia.

A specific indicator of social integration that has been the focus of recent epidemiologic studies is urban versus rural residence. A number of studies document that both depressive symptoms and major depression are more prevalent in urban when compared with rural residence (Blazer et al, 1985; Prudo et al, 1981; Comstock and Helsing, 1976). These differences are greater among younger adults than among older adults (Crowell et al, 1986; Blazer et al, 1986).

George (1991) has adapted the construct of social integration to the individual level, concentrating on religious activities and participation in voluteer organizations as evidence of integration. She quotes evidence that both formal religious participation (i.e., church attendance) and personal religions devotions (e.g., prayer, Bible reading) are related to decreased risk of psychiatric disorders in general and depression in particular (Bergin, 1983; Ellison, 1991). Participation in volunteer organizations appear to have similar benefits (Grusky et al, 1985).

■ SOCIAL SUPPORT AS A BUFFER OF SOCIAL STRESSORS

The interaction of social factors in causing depression in older persons is complex. A review of Figure 6-1 reveals a number of potential interactions. For example, early life experiences not only may directly affect the onset and outcome of clinical depression, they may also impact the social network and the social status of an elder. The most frequent interaction studied by investigators is the so-called stress-buffering hypothesis (Kessler and McCloud, 1985). This interaction is based on the hypothesis that the effects of social stressors on depression will be greater when social support is impaired. Landerman et al (1989) compared a main effects model (a model that does not consider interaction) for predicting the onset of depression across the life cycle in a community sample with a stress buffering model. In the main effects model, high levels of support promoted decreased depression, regardless of stress and stress leads to increased depression regardless of support. He found that the interaction of life events and social support were "model dependent" (i.e., when a linear probability model was used, significant life event by support interactions were observed for both depressive symptoms and major depression). When a logisitic regression model was used, however, no significant event by support interactions were observed. Krause (1986), as well as Murrell and Norris (1984), suggests that a combination of weak social resources and a high number of stressors results in higher levels of depression, thus confirming an interaction model when depressive symptoms are the outcome variable. They studied middle-aged and elderly in community samples. Weinberger et al (1987), however, failed to find either a direct or a buffering effect for social support.

A number of investigators have studied the stress-buffering hypothesis with a focus on more specific stressors and support. For example, Krause (1986), when focusing on bereavement, crime, and crisis in the social network, found that specific types of social support served to buffer the impact of specific types of stressors. Health-related events, on the other hand, required more instrumental support, such as someone to take the older adult to a doctor. The stress of a non–health-related event, such as death of a spouse, may be buffered by the presence of a confidant.

Arling (1987), in a community sample of older adults, found women, whites, those living alone, and those with little education had greater sources of strain. Individuals with greater sources of strain were also more likely to receive social support, although they tended to have a smaller social networks and less social contact. Social support had a moderating influence on the relationship between impairment in activities of daily living and psychosomatic symptoms of distress. A major life strain may therefore cause a constriction of the social network and reduce contact with others, thus contributing to the interaction of social support and social stressors.

The degree of social support necessary to buffer against stress is not known. McFarlane et al (1983) found that individuals with a small core of intimates were better able to buffer themselves against stressful events than persons with wider networks who lacked the intimate sources of support.

REFERENCES

Antonucci TC: Personal characteristics, social support and social behavior. In Benstock RH, Shanas E (eds): *Handbook of Aging and the Social Sciences.* New York, Van Nostrand Reinhold, 1985, pp. 94-128.

Arling G: Strain, social support and distress in old age, *Journal of Gerontology* 42:107-113, 1987.

Bengston VL, Haber DA: Sociological approaches to aging. In Woodruff DS, Birren JE (eds): *Aging: Scientific Perspectives and Social Issues.* New York, Van Nostrand Reinhold, 1975.

Bergin AE: Religiousity and mental health: a critical re-evaluation and meta-analysis, *Professional Psychology: Research and Practice* 14:170-184, 1983.

Berkman LF, Syme SL: Social networks, host resistance, and mortality: a nine-year follow-up study of Almeda County residents, *American Journal of Epidemiology* 109:186, 1979.

Billings AG, Moos RH: Coping, stress and social resources among adults and unipolar depression, *Journal of Personality and Social Psychology* 46:877-891, 1984.

Birtchnell J: Depression in relation to early and recent parent death, *British Journal of Psychiatry* 116:299, 1970.

Blau P: *Inequality and Heterogeneity.* New York, Free Press, 1977.

Blazer DG: Life events, mental health functioning, and use of health care services by the elderly, *American Journal of Public Health* 70:1174, 1980.

Blazer DG: Social support and mortality in an elderly community population, *American Journal of Epidemiology* 115:684-694, 1982.

Blazer DG: Techniques for communicating with your elderly patient, *Geriatrics* 33:79, 1978.

Blazer DG, Burchette B, Service C, George LK: The association of age and depression among the elderly: an epidemiologic exploration, *Journal of Gerontology: Medical Sciences* 46:M210-M215, 1991.

Blazer DG, Crowell BA, George LK, Landerman R: Urban-rural differences in depressive disorders: does age make a difference? In Barrett JE, Rose RM (eds): *Mental Disorders in the Community: Progress and Challenge.* New York, Guilford Press, 1986, pp. 32-46.

Blazer DG, George LK, Landerman R, Pennybacker M, Melville ML, et al: Psychiatric disorders: a rural/urban comparison, *Archives of General Psychiatry* 42:651-656, 1985.

Blazer DG, Hughes DC, George LK: The epidemiology of depression in an elderly community, *The Gerontologist* 27:281-287, 1987.

Blazer DG, Hughes D: Subjective social support and depressive symptoms: Separate phenomena or epiphenomena, *Journal of Psychiatric Research* 25:199-203, 1991.

Bovard EW: The balance between negative and positive brain system activity, *Perspectives in Biological Medicine* 6:116, 1962.

Bovard EW: The effects of social stimuli on the response to stress, *Psychological Research* 66:267, 1959.

Bowlby J: *Attachment and Loss: Attachment,* (vol 1). New York, Basic Books, 1969.

Briscoe CW, Smith JB: Depression and bereavement and divorce, *Archives of General Psychiatry* 32:439, 1975.

Brown GW, Harris TO: *Social Origins of Depression.* London, Tavistock, 1978.

Butler R: Old age. In Arieti S (ed): *American Handbook of Psychiatry* (vol 1, ed 2). New York, Basic Books, 1974, pp. 646-661.

Cannon WB: Stresses and strains of homeostasis, *American Journal of Medical Science* 189:1, 1935.

Cantor MH: Life space and the social support system of the inner city elderly of New York, *The Gerontologist* 15:23-27, 1975.

Caplan G: *Support Systems and Community Mental Health.* New York, Behavioral Publications, 1974.

Cassel J: The contribution of the social environment to host resistence, *American Journal of Epidemiology* 104:107, 1976.

Caudill W: *Effects of Social and Cultural Systems in Reaction to Stress.* Pamphlet #14, New York, Social Services Council, 1958.

Chessea ES: *A Study of Some Etiologic Factors in the Affective Disorders of Old Age.* Unpublished PhD dissertation. Institute of Psychiatry, University of London, 1965.

Cobb S: Social support as a moderator of life stress, *Psychosomatic Medicine* 38:300, 1976.

Comstock G, Helsing K: Symptoms of depression in two communities, *Psychological Medicine* 6:551-563, 1976.

Crowell BA, George LK, Blazer D: Psychosocial risk factors and urban/rural differences in the prevalence of major depression, *British Journal of Psychiatry* 149:307-314, 1986.

Cumming E, Henry WH: *Growing Old: The Process of Disengagement.* New York, Basic Books, 1961.

Dean A, Kolody B, Wood P, Matt GE: The influence of living alone on depression in elderly persons, *Journal of Aging and Health* 4:3-18, 1992.

Dowd JJ, Brooks FP: *Anomie and Aging: Normalessness of Class Consciousness.* Paper presented at the 31st Annual Scientific Meeting of the Gerontological Society, Dallas, Texas, November, 1978.

Dubos R: *Man Adapting.* New Haven, Yale University Press, 1965.

Durkheim E: *Suicide.* New York, Free Press, 1950.

Ellison CG: Religious involvement and subjective well-being, *Journal of Health and Social Behavior* 32:80-99, 1991.

Erikson E: *Childhood and Society.* New York, WW Norton, 1950.

Ezquiaga E, Gutierrez JLA, Lopez AG: Psychosocial factors and episode number and depression, *Journal of Affective Disorders* 12:135-138, 1987.

Freud S: Mourning and melancholia. (Originally published in 1917). In *Collected Papers,* (vol 4). London, Hogarth Press, 1950.

Gaylin W: *The Meaning of Despair: Psychoanalytic Contributions to Understanding Depression.* New York, Science House, 1968.

George LK: *Social Factors and Depression in Late Life.* Paper prepared for the National Institute on Health Consensus Development Conference on the Diagnosis and Treatment of Depression in Late Life. November 4-6, 1991, Bethesda, MD.

George LK: Social factors and the onset and outcome of depression. In Schie W, House J, Blazer DG (eds): *Aging, Health Behaviors and Health Outcomes.* Hillsdale, New Jersey, Erlbaum Associates, 1992.

George LK: Stress, social support, and depression over the life-course. In Markides KS (ed): *Aging, Stress, Social Support and Health.* Chichester, England, John Wiley and Sons, (in press).

George LK, Blazer DG, Hughes DC, Fowler N: Social support and the outcome of major depression, *British Journal of Psychiatry* 154:478-45, 1989.

Grusky O, Tierney K, Manderscheid RW: Social bonding and community adjustment of chronically-mentally-ill adults, *Journal of Health and Social Behavior* 26:49-63, 1985.

Hall KS, Dunner DL, Zeller G, Fievre RR: Bipolar illness: a prospective study of life events, *Comprehensive Psychiatry* 18:497, 1977.

Harel Z, Noelken L: *The Impact of Social Integration on the Well-being and Survival of Institutionalized Aged.* Paper presented at the 31st Annual Meeting of the Gerontological Society of America, Dallas, November, 1978.

Henderson S, Bryne DG, Duncan-Jones P: *Neurosis and the Social Environment.* New York, Academic Press, 1981.

Hofer MA, Weiner H: Physiological and behavioral regulation by nutritional intake during early development of the laboratory rat, *Psychosomatic Medicine* 33:468, 1971.

Holihan CK, Holihan CJ: Self-efficacy, social support, and depression and aging: a longitudinal analysis, *Journal of Gerontology* 42:65-68, 1987.

Holmes TH, Rahe RH: *Schedule of Recent Events.* Seattle, University of Washington, 1967.

Hopkinson G, Ley P: A genetic study of affective disorder, *British Journal of Psychiatry* 115:917, 1969.

Hudgens R, Morrison J, Barchha R: Life events and onset of primary affective disorders, *Archives of General Psychiatry* 16:134, 1967.

Hughes DC, George LK, Blazer DG: Age differences in life events: a multi-variant controlled analysis, *International Journal of Aging and Human Development* 27:207-220, 1988.

Ilfield FW: Current social stressors and symptoms of depression, *American Journal of Psychiatry* 134:161, 1977.

Jacobs S, Prusoff BA, Paykel ES: Recent life events in schizophrenia and depression, *Psychological Medicine* 4:444, 1974.

Kaminsky M: Pictures from the past: the use of reminiscence in case work with the elderly, *Journal of Gerontological Social Work* 1:19-31, 1978.

Kaplan BH, Cassel JC, Gore S: Social support and health, *Medical Care* 15:47, 1977.

Kaplan HB, Robins C, Martin SS: Antecedents of psychological distress in young adults: Self-rejection, deprivation of social support and life events, *Journal of Health and Social Behavior* 24:230-243, 1983.

Kay DWK, Beamish P, Roth M: Old age mental disorders in Newcastle-Apon-Tyne. I. A study of prevalence, *British Journal of Psychiatry* 110:146, 1964.

Kessler RC, McLoed JD: Social support and mental health in community samples. In Cohen S, Symes L (eds): *Social Support and Health.* New York, Academic Press, 1985, pp. 219-240.

Krause N: Chronic financial strain, social support and depressive symptoms among older adults, *Psychology and Aging* 2:185-192, 1987.

Krause N: Chronic strain, locus of control and distress in older adults, *Psychology and Aging*, 2:375-382, 1987.

Krause N: Social support, stress and well being among older adults, *Journal of Gerontology* 41:512-519, 1986.

Krause N: Stress and coping: reconceptualizing the role of locus of control beliefs, *Journal of Gerontology* 41:617-622, 1986.

Landerman R, George LK, Campbell RT, Blazer DG: Alternative models of the stress buffering hypothesis, *American Journal of Community Psychology* 17:625-642, 1989.

Lazarus RS: *Psychological Stress and the Coping Process.* New York, McGraw-Hill, 1966.

Lazarus RS, Folkman S: *Stress, Appraisal and Coping.* New York, Springer, 1984.

Lee GR: Kinship and social support of the elderly: the case of the United States, *Aging and Society* 5:19-38, 1985.

Leaf PJ, Meyers JK, George L, Bednarski P: The increased risk for specific psychiatric disorders among persons of low socioeconomic status, *American Journal of Social Psychiatry* 6:259-271, 1986.

Leif A: *The Common Sense of Psychiatry of Dr. Adolpf Meyer.* New York, McGraw-Hill, 1948.

Leighton AH: *My Name is Legion.* New York, Basic Books, 1959.

Leighton AH: Social disintegration and mental disorder. In Caplan G (ed): *American Handbook of Psychiatry* (vol 2, ed 2). New York, Basic Books, 1974, pp. 411-423, 1974.

Leighton DC, Harding JS, Macklin DB, MacMillan AM, Leighton AH: *The Character of Danger.* New York, Basic Books, 1963.

Lin N, Simone RS, Ensel WM, Kuo W: Social support, stressful life events, and illness: a model and empirical tests, *Journal of Health and Social Behavior* 20:108-119, 1979.

Lloyd C: Life events and depressive disorders reviewed. I. Events as predisposing factors, *Archives of General Psychiatry* 37:529, 1980.

Lowenthal MF: Antecedents of isolation in mental illness in old age, *Archives of General Psychiatry* 12:245, 1965.

Lowenthal MF, Berkman PL: *Aging and Mental Disorder in San Francisco: A Social Psychiatric Study.* San Francisco, Jossey-Bass, 1967.

MacMahon B, Pugh TF: *Epidemiology: Principles and Methods.* Little, Brown and Company, 1970.

Maddox GL: Disengagement theory: a critical evaluation. *The Gerontologist* 4:80, 1964.

Markides KS, Boldt JS, Ray LA: Sources of helping an intergenerational solidItary: a three generation study of Mexican Americans, *Journal of Gerontology* 41:506-511, 1986.

Mathew R, Wilson W, Blazer DG, George LK: Psychiatric disorders in individuals with alcoholic parents, an epidemiologic inquiry, *American Journal of Psychiatry* (in press).

McFarlane AH, Norman GR, Streiner DL, Roy RG: The process of social stress: stable, reciprocal, and mediating relationships, *Journal of Health and Social Behavior* 24:160-173, 1983.

McMordie WR, Blom S: Life-review therapy: psychotherapy for the elderly, *Perspectives in Psychiatric Care* 4:162-166, 1979.

Mead GH: *Mind, Self, and Society.* Chicago, University of Chicago Press, 1934.

Meyers JK, Weissman MM, Tischler JL, Holzer CE, Leaf PJ, et al: Six-month prevalence of psychiatric disorders in three communities, *Archives of General Psychiatry* 41:959-970, 1984.

Moss GE: *Illness, Immunity and Social Interaction,* New York, John Wiley and Sons, 1973.

Murphy E: Social origins of depression and old age, *British Journal of Psychiatry* 141:135-142, 1982.

Murrell S, Norris FH: Resources, life events and changes in positive effect and depression in older adults, *American Journal of Community Psychology* 12:445-464, 1984.

Newgarten BL: Adaptation and the life cycle, *Journal of Geriatric Psychology* 4:71, 1970.

Norris FH, Murrell SA: Protective function of sources related to life events, global stress and depression in older adults, *Journal of Health and Social Behavior* 25:424-437, 1984.

Nuckolls KB, Cassel JC, Kaplan BH: Psychological assets, life crisis and prognosis of pregnancy, *American Journal of Epidemiology* 95:431, 1972.

O'Neil MK, Lancee WJ, Freeman SJ: Loss and depression: a controversial link, *Journal of Nervous and Mental Diseases* 175:354-257, 1987.

Palmore E: Physical, mental, and social factors in predicting longevity, *Gerontologist* 9:103, 1969.

Parsons T: *The Social System.* New York, Free Press, 1951.

Paykel ES: Recent life events and clinical depression. In Gunderson EK, Rahe RH (eds): *Life Stress and Illness.* Springfield, IL, Charles C. Thomas, 1974.

Paykel ES, Myers JK, Diene H, Klerman GL, Lindenthal JJ, et al: Life events and depression, *Archives of General Psychiatry* 21:753, 1970.

Pearlin LI, Menaghan EG, Lieberman MA, Mullan JT: The stress process, *Journal of Health and Social Behavior* 22:337-356, 1981.

Pearlin LI, Schooller C: The structure of coping, *Journal of Health and Social Behavior* 19:2-21, 1978.

Post F: The factor of aging in affective illness. In Oppen A, Walsh A (eds): *Recent Developments of Affective Disorders*, *British Journal of Psychiatry* (special publication #2, 1968).

Prudo R, Brown GW, Harris T, Dowland J: Psychiatric disorder in a rural and an urban population: I. Etiology of depression, *Psychological Medicine* 11:581-599, 1981.

Rahe RH, Bennett L, Romo M, Siltanen P, Arthur RJ: Subjects' recent life changes and coronary heart disease in Finland, *American Journal of Psychiatry* 130:1222, 1973.

Rook KS: The negative side of social interaction: impact on psychological well-being, *Journal of Personality and Social Psychology* 46:1097-1108, 1984.

Scott JP: Criticial periods in behavior development, *Science* 138:949, 1962.

Selye H: *The Stress of Life*. New York, McGraw-Hill, 1956.

Selye H, Wolff HG (quoted in Hinkle LE): The concept of "stress" in the biological and social sciences, *Science of Medicine and Man* 1:31, 1973.

Shanas E: Social myth as hypothesis: the case of the family relations of older people, *The Gerontologist* 19:3, 1979.

Slater E, Roth M: *Clinical Psychiatry* (ed 3). Baltimore, Williams & Wilkins, 1969.

Spitz R: Anaclitic depression: an inquiry into the genesis of psychiatric conditions in early childhood, *Psychoanalytic Study of the Child* 2:313, 1942.

Tennant C, Bebbington P, Hurry J: The short-term outcome of neurotic disorders in the community: the relation of remission to clinical factors to "neutralizing" life events, *British Journal of Psychiatry* 139:213-220, 1981.

Tennant C, Hurry J, Bebbington P: The relation of childhood separation experiences to early adult depressive and anxiety states, *British Journal of Psychiatry* 141:475-482, 1982.

Thoitis PA: Undesirable life events and psychophysiological distress: a problem of operational confounding, *American Sociological Review* 46:97-109, 1981.

Thompson KC, Hendrie HC: Environmental stress in primary depressive illness, *Archives of General Psychiatry* 26:130, 1972.

Warheit GH, Holzer CE, Arez SA: Race and mental illness: an epidemiologic update, *Journal Health and Social Behavior* 16:243-256, 1975.

Weinberger M, Heiner SL, Turney WM: Assessing social support in elderly adults, *Social Science and Medicine* 25:1049-1055, 1987.

Weissman MM, Boyd J: Affective disorders: epidemiology. In Kaplan HI, Sadork BJ (eds): *Comprehensive Textbook of Psychiatry*. (vol I) Baltimore, Williams & Wilkins, 1985, pp. 212-241.

Wolff HG, Wolf SG, Hare CC: *Life Stress and Bodily Disease*. Baltimore, Williams & Wilkins, 1950.

CHAPTER 7

Existential Depression

This chapter is an exception to others in this book, yet an essential chapter nevertheless. The science of clinical investigation and interpersonal interactions has served clinicians well in assessing and treating late life depression. To acquire the art of treating late life depression, the clinician must become aware of the existential aspects of late life depression. Perhaps the starting point for any exploration of existential depression is empathy. Clinicians tend to diagnosis diseases and conceptualize etiologies in terms of empirically observed biologic, psychologic, and social processes interacting in a web of causation, the final pathway being the depression syndrome. Patients, however, experience illnesses, and in the case of depression, experience a challenge to the very meaning and purpose of their lives. Regardless of the etiology of depression in late life, the older adult is likely to view the structure and purpose of his or her life in negative ways when depressed, which significantly impacts the clinical management of the depressed elder.

Yalom (1980) identified four essential themes relevant to existential illness and psychotherapy–death, freedom, isolation, and meaninglessness. Meaninglessness is especially important in the manifestation of late life depression and therefore is the focus of this chapter. Death is discussed in Chapter 13 on bereavement, and isolation is discussed in Chapter 6 on the social origins of depression. Although not necessarily expressed, meaninglessness often takes the form of questions, such as "What is the meaning of life?" "What is the meaning of my life?" "Why do we live?" "Why were we put here?" "What have I accomplished in my life?" "If I must die, if nothing endures, then what is the sense of doing anything?" Camus (1970) said, "I have seen many people die because life for them was not worth living. From this I conclude that the question of life's meaning is the most urgent question of all." Frankl (1965) believes 20% of the neuroses he encountered in his clinical practice evolved from a lack of meaning.

The work of Erikson (1950), however, may provide the best approach to understanding meaninglessness in late life. In Erikson's discussion of the eight stages of man, the conflict of integrity (i.e., integration) versus despair is the unique psychologic challenge faced by older adults (see Chapter 5). Resolution of this conflict leads to the trait of wisdom. Erikson et al later expanded on his view of integration (Erikson et al, 1986). They found that during this last stage of life, the life cycle "weaves back on itself" leading to integration of hope, will, purpose, competence, fidelity, love, and care. To confront the existential dread of "not being," which looms ever closer as one ages, the older person continually integrates previous actions and restraints, choices and rejections, and strengths and weaknesses of the present and past. In summary, integration is "the acceptance of one's one and only life cycle and of the people who have become significant to it as something that had to be and that, by necessity, permitted no substitutions" (Erikson, 1986).

The following case example illustrates the importance of meaninglessness in the care and management of a depressed older adult. This older man is not unlike those elders who are treated daily by geriatric psychiatrists, psychologists, nurses, and social workers. The symptoms may easily be ascribed to cognitive distortions and biologic dysregulation, yet, to this man, his despair was closely interwoven with the lack of fulfillment in his past life.

■ CASE REPORT

Dr. Smithfield practiced surgery in a small community until he was 44 years of age. His practice flourished, he did well financially and he was respected as a community leader. Nevertheless, the long hours and demands on a single practitioner in a community finally convinced Dr. Smithfield that he should seek different employment.

He learned that a position as a staff surgeon in a Veterans Administration Hospital had opened in a larger city and he took the position. He was placed on a straight salary and therefore made less money (although job security and benefits were better). He actually performed more surgical procedures in his new position and worked a much easier call schedule. He enjoyed his work but was less active in community life in the larger city than in the small town.

When Dr. Smithfield was 67 years of age (he planned to retire when he was 70), he suffered a severe myocardial infarction. Congestive heart failure persisted after the heart attack, and he was forced to relinquish his surgical practice immediately. His health remained severely impaired for 2 years, and he was barely able to leave the house. Exacerbation of his illness led to frequent hospitalizations. After 2 years, his health improved, he could leave the house when he chose, and the emergency hospitalizations were no longer necessary. By this time, however, his social life had virtually disappeared, and the opportunity to return to practice had disappeared. His physician advised him not to return to any type of medical practice. Although he was secure financially, he was not "well off." For this reason his wife (who was some years younger) continued to work.

Dr. Smithfield became very depressed. He experienced classic symptoms of major depression, including poor appetite, weight loss, sleep difficulties, and a profound anhedonia. In addition, he expressed extreme guilt that he had made a serious mistake early in his life by not remaining in the small community where he had been such a popular surgeon. He believed that the latter portion of his life (the time after his move to the Veterans Administration Hospital) had been wasted. His dream of a comfortable and successful retirement was shattered.

Dr. Smithfield responded well to a tricyclic antidepressant, nortriptyline. His sleep improved, weight loss was reversed, and he was able to enjoy many activities on a day-to-day basis. Nevertheless, he could not reintegrate himself into his previous social activities. Although he participated in volunteer activities with the Veterans Hospital and a number of civic groups, he could never "give of himself" to these activities. He described these volunteer activities as basically "a way to pass time."

At times, Dr. Smithfield would become so discouraged that he would discontinue his medication, only to experience a significant return of the symptoms of major depression. He then would return to the medication. His health, after the depressive illness, deteriorated slightly (he became more short of breath). Nevertheless, his physical problems did not significantly interfere with his usual daily activities.

In psychotherapy the therapist working with Dr. Smithfield initially encouraged him to find more and more enjoyable activities. Dr. Smithfield would duly comply by adding yet another volunteer activity but never experienced a return of his former enthusiasm. The therapist interpreted that Dr. Smithfield had displaced his affect from his physical problems over which he had no control, to a decision that he had made many years prior over which he did had control. He controlled the decision to move from private practice to the Veterans Hospital. Dr. Smithfield recognized that control was a major issue for him and accepted that he probably had overstated the importance of the job change many years prior in terms of his current depressive mood. This interpretation, however, was ineffective in reversing Dr. Smithfield's depressed mood.

Finally, Dr. Smithfield approached his therapist and said that he was seriously considering giving up therapy and the medication (yet again), for he could find nothing that would enable him to overcome the depressive symptoms that he faced. He felt that he just "couldn't stand" the continued depression, although he denied any suicidal thoughts. He related an incident where he had spoken with a prisoner of war from Vietnam during his days as a surgeon at the veterans hospital. The young pilot, whom he was treating, described the year during which he was held captive by the North Vietnamese. The conditions were terrible yet this young pilot had clearly been a survivor and had been able to withstand the deprived conditions and the psychologic torture of wartime captivity. Dr. Smithfield noted that he, himself, was not a survivor and probably would not have lived through the captivity. He had no fear of death, but he had great fear of being in a situation where he was out of control.

The therapist interpreted that Dr. Smithfield was not as he believed himself to be. Actually, Dr. Smithfield was a survivor. He had survived the stresses of a difficult surgical practice in a small community (the only surgeon within a 75-mile radius) for 15 years, longer than any surgeon in the history of this community. Dr. Smithfield had made a mid-life job transition successfully, having relinquished many friends and securities to make new friends and to develop new important factors in his life. Dr. Smithfield had survived the health problems that he had suffered later in his life. Although not in control of these conditions, they had not defeated him. The therapist worked with Dr. Smithfield and helped him recognize his survival skills. Dr. Smithfield was able to incorporate survival as a meaning of his life and his depression began to lift.

■ THE IDENTIFICATION OF MEANINGLESSNESS

How can the therapist establish that the depressed older adult is suffering from a sense of meaninglessness? Asking global questions is usually not the best means of establishing meaninglessness. In fact, such questions may be threatening. Rather, the clinician must carefully listen to the theme woven by the depressed elder and throughout interaction with the elder attempt to expand that theme. For example, in the case presented previously, the therapist inquired, after Dr. Smithfield's suggestion that he had made a terrible mistake at the age of 46, "Do you feel that this means that you haven't achieved your life goals?"

Meaning in life may be correlated with life satisfaction, but it is not necessarily the same. An older adult may have been chronically dissatisfied through most of his adult life and into late life yet find significant meaning in life and a sense of purpose. A useful life may not be a meaningful life. Many persons find that they have served their spouses, children, and grandchildren, yet question the meaning of their lives. Did they spend too much time helping others, only to neglect themselves?

Clinicians must take care not to confuse meaning with current affect. An individual in the depths of depression may profess no meaning to live. When the elder is depressed, he or she views not only the present but their past lives through grey-colored glasses. In general, however, meaning does not correlate highly with mood. Listening over many days and weeks enables the clinician to determine if a theme of meaninglessness challenges the psychologic integrity of the elder.

The clinician must also recognize that meaninglessness not only manifests itself in depressive symptoms but in other symptoms that may mask the existential despair of the older adult. One expression of meaninglessness is through compulsive activity. Continued activity and subsequent dissipation of the elder's energy drains the elder of the discomfort experienced when he or she reflects upon life. Unfortunately, if this activity has no true meaning or sense of "rightness," sooner or later it fails the older adult. Pike (1953) refers to this phenomenon as *false centering* of life.

Yet another expression of meaninglessness is a sense of helplessness. Yalom (1980) suggests that if the older person believes that he or she has found meaning, this simultaneously brings a sense of mastery. Older persons crave meaning and are uncomfortable in its absence. They not only cling to causes or purposes periodically throughout their lives, they also cling to individuals when they feel a lack of meaning or purpose.

What is meaning? There is no definition that will apply to each older adult. The question is one for philosophers to ponder and discuss rather than clinicians. Nevertheless, the clinician must develop the ability to search in the right areas to determine if meaninglessness is a major component of the depressive syndrome. Yalom (1980) suggests that *meaning* can take on several meanings. *Meaning* usually refers to a sense of coherence. Terms that are related to meaning are *purpose, intention, aim, function,* and *significance.*

Clinicians should explore different aspects of the older person's life and thoughts during therapeutic interaction over time. The older person may directly question the overall meaning of life. Yalom describes this as *cosmic meaning* (i.e., whether life in general or at least human life fits into some overhaul coherent pattern). Cosmic meaning by definition implies a design outside of and probably superior to an individual and usually includes some spiritual order of the universe as part of its purpose. The Jewish, Christian, and Muslim religions offer a comprehensive meaning or schema regarding the world and human life for most older adults in western society. Jung (1961), for example, believed that no one could find meaning in life unless he or she regained a religious outlook on life. "Among all my patients in the second half of life—that is to say, over thirty-five—there has not been one whose problems in the last resort was not that of finding a religious outlook on life. It is safe to say that every one of them fell ill because he had lost what the living religions of every age have given to their followers, and none of them has been really healed who did not regain his religious outlook. This of course has nothing whatever to do with a particular creed of membership of a church" (Jung, 1933). Most elders, in the midst of a depressive episode, do not ask these larger questions regarding life nor do they lose their religion. At times, however, older persons facing crises do experience a concomitant crisis in their religious life and/or their understanding of the cosmic meaning of life. Clinicians would do well in these circumstances to refer the older person to the clergy and to work closely with clergy to assist the elder in addressing these existential questions. Most questions regarding meaning, however, are, according to Yalom (1980), terrestrial (i.e., "What's the meaning of my life?"). The individual who has a terrestrial sense of meaning tends to experience his or her life as having some purpose or function to be fulfilled, some goal or goals to which to apply one self, and some accomplishments on which to rely. Persons who have attained a sense of cosmic meaning usually incorporate into that cosmic meaning a terrestrial meaning as well. Terrestrial meaning may take many forms.

First, terrestrial meaning may be found in suffering and survival. Even the most fatalistic of individuals can find meaning in the acquisition of a true understanding of the plight of the individual within this world. The existential philosophers provide excellent examples of finding meaning in the pain of meaninglessness. Camus (1946), in his novel *The Stranger*, uses the word *absurd* to refer to the human being's position in the world. We are absorbed in that we are meaning-seeking beings forced to live in a world that has no meaning (Yalom, 1980). Camus believed that humans could only gain meaning in life by living with dignity in the face of absurdity. Sartre (1965) attempted to overcome his despair at finding no meaning in the world by generating a system of personal meaning (i.e., a system that included self-developed values and guidelines for conduct, such as courage, a willingness to rebel, love, suffering, and loneliness).

Another terrestrial meaning, according to Yalom (1980), is dedication to a cause. Frankl quotes Jaspers, "What man is he has become through that cause he has made his own." The older person who finds cause in this life may not find a large, cosmic changing purpose but rather purpose in even the smallest of activities. For example, an older man may find meaning in visiting with a lonely young boy for only a few minutes out of every day. An older woman may find meaning in helping her husband through a terminal illness.

The clinician working with the depressed elder often faces a crisis in meaning when the elder perceives that he or she must abandon a cause. For example, older persons may despair that they have been forced to borrow money or use part of the family savings for a severe illness. Others may have promised that they would never spend time in a long-term care facility. The clinician must work with the older person to enable that older person to adjust their causes to the realities of the world in which they live and to seek the more general causes that are beyond the specific promises made to spouses, parents, and children.

Still others, according to Yalom (1980), find meaning in creativity. The teacher, the craftsman, the automobile mechanic, as well as the physician, the scientist, and the rabbi can find creativity in their activities. As individuals age, the opportunities for creativity may decrease. The older person who was creative in administrative activities may lack an outlet for a talent once he or she retires. Creativity in late life can find its outlets in many activities, such as cooking, gardening, writing, sewing, and painting. When physical disabilities hamper former outlets of creativity, the individual may turn to other outlets. An often cited example is Grandma Moses, who in late life was forced to relinquish her previous creative outlet in knitting, was able to take up painting, and painted some of those popular works in the twentieth century (Comfort, 1976).

Meaning in life often takes the form of generativity, the stage in Erikson's eight stages of the man that precedes that of integration versus despair (Erikson, 1950). Most older persons continue to look to the future and expect to continue living for the forseeable future. At the same time, they recognize that the life cycle nears completion and that they have lived more years than they will live. Therefore elders often look to the next generation as a means by which they can achieve some sense of immortality. Erikson et al (1986) suggest that older persons not only look to what they have taught their children and grandchildren but to the physical features of their children and grandchildren. They may identify with particular grandchildren for reasons as diverse as eye color, facial expression, occupation, and special interests.

At times elders are frustrated with today's world (even when they are not depressed) and can find little in life that provides a sense of generativity. Reactions to these feelings include statements such as "I'm glad you are the one that's going to face the world in the future and it's not me." "I'm certainly pleased that I will not have to live in the world that our children are inheriting, for I worry about the future of this planet." The sensitive therapist, in such cases, must explore the disappointments that these elders often feel in not having left a better world than the one they inherited. For example, the therapist may need to assist the elder to recognize that he or she did, through most of his or her life, live by certain principles that rendered the world a better place to live, even though, overall, the world may appear more difficult. An older person might say, "I can only do the best I can. I have tried to live my life in a way that would make this world a better place for everyone."

Yet another way that meaning acrues to an individual is through self-transcendence. Buber (1961) suggests that as individuals search for meaning within themselves they find that there is something beyond themselves. Excessive concern with self (through self-expression and self-actualization) leads to a decrease in life satisfaction. The older person, through self-exploration, should find that he or she focuses less on self and more on others. Erikson's generativity could be viewed as self-transcendence. Yet Buber was concerned with a much larger sense of the other, the thou, which circles back to cosmic meaning.

■ APPROACHES TO FINDING MEANING IN LATE LIFE

What are the approaches that elders can take so they may find meaning in their lives? Erikson et al (1986) suggest the following four steps toward the integration of one's life and finding meaning: role models, looking at both sides of an issue, togetherness, and involvement or activity. Since elders cannot escape the finitude of the past and they face physical limitations and a finite future, integrating one's life can present a challenge to an older adult who has experienced a difficult life, regardless of mood. Integration is not a task confined to late life alone, however. Each stage of life requires the individual to integrate old experiences with new experiences. Finding a resolution for conflicts, such as generativity versus stagnation and intimacy versus isolation, is not confined to late life. Yet late life presents unique opportunities to solidify a sense of meaning in life. The therapist should take advantage of these unique opportunities.

Role models can provide an excellent means by which the older person can move to integrate his or her life and establish meaning for one's life. As described below, the therapist himself or herself often becomes a role model through continued activity and care for the elderly patient. Parents may also serve as role models as the elder recalls how his or her parents aged successfully. A changing social milieu, however, renders the application of role models from the past more difficult. Therefore elders may seek contemporaries whom they admire (e.g., entertainers, such as George Burns; political leaders, such as Ronald Reagan; and even sports figures who continue their athletic pursuits, such as George Forman the boxer). If the role model is approximately the same age and has reflected publicly on his or her own life experiences (similar as those of the elder), the role model takes on added meaning. Older celebrities are popular speakers at gatherings of older adults.

Erikson et al (1986) suggest that a second aspect of integration is the ability to observe both sides of an issue. They suggest the example of the lifelong liberal activist who has developed the ability to see both sides of her liberal political ideas and has modified those ideas towards conservatism. Conservatives, in contrast, express a more tolerant view toward persons of a more liberal persuasion. Many elders take pride in their newfound acceptance and ability not to become overly disturbed when confronted by extremes in society.

Yet another approach to finding meaning and integration is through a sense of togetherness. Most elders have developed formal and informal support networks within which they feel great comfort. A disturbance in that social network can be most threatening to the older person, and investigators of psychiatric illness in elders usually concentrate on deficits in the social milieu, such as stressful life events and impairment of the social network. Perhaps more attention should be directed to the positive aspects of social support, especially the perception of belonging. Many senior citizens groups, such as local chapters of the American Association of Retired Persons (AARP), as well as local senior centers, render elders a sense that they are not alone. Other elders, who remain in a particular neighborhood for a half century or more take comfort that many of their neighbors have lived in the neighborhood equally as long. Meaning is found in the neighborhood growing old together. Still others experience a sense of belonging through church or synagogue. Some elders explore their family or cultural history to establish a sense of belonging through traditions.

Yet another means of finding meaning in life is through involvement or activity. The so-called activity theory (in contrast with the disengagement theory) of aging highlights the importance of remaining actively involved as a means of successfully adapting to late life (Erikson et al, 1986). Thoughts about dying, feeling ill, and grief over the loss of loved ones are integral to old age. Those elders who age successfully, however, usually struggle to counterbalance these pessimistic perceptions with more optimistic, "life-affirming" involvement. Life takes on meaning when the elder is meaningfully involved.

Finally, elders find meaning in their lives when they confront and come to grips with death. (Erikson et al, 1986). Most elders do not fear death itself. Rather, they fear the pain and suffering that precedes death. The loss of control associated with a chronic illness is often a more threatening thought than death for most elders. Therefore approaching older persons with proposals for living wills and advanced directives is not as disturbing as many younger persons may believe. Having a role in deciding their fate if afflicted with terminal illness is most important to older persons.

■ PSYCHOTHERAPY FOR EXISTENTIAL DEPRESSION IN OLDER ADULTS

Yalom (1980) outlines an approach to psychotherapy with individuals who have experienced the existential challenge of meaninglessness. Many components of this approach are applicable to psychotherapy with older adults experiencing depression. The first component of Yalom's approach is engagement. Elders who find life meaningless are likely to have removed themselves from an active involvement in life, seeing current experiences as irrelevant and of no value. The therapist can break into this self-developed isolation by engaging actively with the older adult. Two aspects of engagement are useful in breaking through the isolation. First, the therapist engages the patient by therapeutic relationship itself. The interest shown by the therapist in the patient and commitment of the therapist to the relationship help the older adult to engage in at least one relationship—the therapeutic relationship.

Second, the therapist should encourage the older person to become involved in activities and with people. Although simply participating in a relationship (e.g., joining a discussion group in a retirement community) does not lead to a sense of involvement in the depressed elder, experiences derived from the relationship provide material that can be used by the therapist. Initially, the depressed elder may only express curiosity regarding other persons with whom he or she comes in contact. The therapist explores these curious reflections and encourages the depressed elder to question his or her own isolation compared with the activities and interest of other elders.

Next, the therapist can often challenge the pessimistic and nihilistic view of life of the elder through logical inconsistencies in his or her world view (Yalom, 1980). For example, if the older person professes that "nothing matters," then it should not matter that nothing matters. Of more importance, however, is that current doubts, isolation, and pessimism cannot eliminate the reality of past concern and involvement with life. The therapist should help older persons to look back to times in their lives when things did matter and enable the elder to explore how he or she dealt with these situations.

Yalom (1980) suggests that yet another means of effecting improvement in existential depression is to confront the "hedonistic paradox." The clinician does no service to the elder by simply suggesting that searching for pleasure and excitement in this life will lead to life satisfaction. Pleasure is a by-product of meaning instead of the reverse. When the elder becomes engaged (e.g., enjoying the visit of grandchildren or a game of cards with good friends), such enjoyment does not refute the pessimism and troublesome questions that emerge from existential depression. Yet the more the older becomes engaged in the day-to-day activities of life, the less these questions are dwelt on and the less they matter. Wittgenstein said, "the solution of the problem of life is seen in the vanishing of the problem."

Yet another means by which the therapist may enhance the therapeutic process with the existentially depressed elder is through modeling (Yalom, 1980). Many young therapists doubt that older adults look to them as models (given the many years of life experience that the older adult appears to possess by virtue of advanced age). Nevertheless, the existentially depressed elder is often looking for a model for reawakening feelings that were present when the elder was the age of the therapist. Therefore the elder identifies with the care the therapist expresses about his or her professional mission, the growth of other persons, and the desire to help other persons achieve these goals.

Finally, the therapist assists the elder in clarification of his or her values. A value may be defined as "a conception, explicit or implicit, distinctive of an individual or characteristic of a group, of the 'desirable' which influences the selection of available modes, means and ends of action" (Kluckholm, 1951). Therapists cannot develop values for their patients yet they can assist the older person in identifying values that may be implicit but have not been explicitly stated. The ability of elders to state their values and to review their lives within the context that the elder was consistent in those values through life is a major step in confronting existential depression in older persons. An integral component of values is the interim spiritual resources of the elder. Inquiring should not only be directed to current spiritual resources but should review what spiritual resources were called on in the past during difficult situations.

Existential depression does not fall within our usual diagnostic nomenclature but rather cuts across many different depressive syndromes. The skills acquired in the training of most modern psychiatrists is not usually in existential psychotherapy. Nevertheless, the clinician working with an older adult who experiences an existential depression cannot serve that older adult adequately unless he or she recognizes and confronts existential issues faced by the elder. Existential concerns are not mere epiphenomena of biologic or psychologic disorders. They are part and parcel of life.

REFERENCES

Buber M: The Way of Man According to the Techniquies of Hasidicm. In Kauffman W (ed): *Religion from Toscoloy to Camus*. New York, Harper Torch Books, 1961, pp. 425-441.

Camus A: *The Stranger*. New York, Alfred Knopf, 1946.

Camus A, Cide D, Jaffe A: *The Myth of the Meaning in the Work of CJ Jong*. London, Hodden and Stroughton, 1970, title page.

Comfort A: *A Good Age*. New York, Crown, 1976, p. 74-75.

Erikson E: *Childhood in Society* (ed 2). New York, Norton, 1950, pp. 268-269.

Erikson EH, Erikson JM, Kivnick HQ: *Vital Involvement in Old Age*. New York, Norton, 1986.

Frankl V: *The Doctor and the Soul*. New York, Alfred Knopf, 1965.

Jaspers C, Cide D, Frankl V: *Will to Meaning*. New York, World Publishing, 1969 p. 38.

Jung C: *Memories, Dreams and Reflections*. New York, Penthom Books, 1961, pp. 255-256.

Jung C: *Modern Man in Search of a Soul*. New York, Basic Books, 1933, p. 229.

Kluckholm C: Values and Value-Orientation in the Theory of Action. In Parsons T, Shils E (eds): *Toward a General Theory of Action*. Cambridge, Massachusetts, Harvard University Press, 1951, p. 396 (as quoted in Yalom, 1980).

Pike J: *Beyond Anxiety*. New York, Charles Scribner, 1953.

Sartre JP, Cide D, Hepburn R: Questions about the Meaning of Life, *Religious Studies* 1:125-140, 1965.

Wittgenstein L: *Tractatous Logico-Philosophicous*, translated by Pears D, McGinnis B. London, Henly, Rutledge and Kagan-Paul, 1961, p. 73 (as quoted by Yalom, 1980).

Yalom I: *Existential Psychotherapy*. New York, Basic Books, 1980.

PART THREE

The Diagnosis and Differential Diagnosis of Late Life Depression

8

Diagnostic Workup of the Elderly Depressed Patient

The foundation of the diagnostic workup of the elderly depressed patient is the diagnostic interview. In this chapter, attention is first directed to techniques for communicating with the older patient. Next, identification of the common symptoms of depression is emphasized. Finally, routine and experimental laboratory tests that can assist the clinician in the diagnosis and differential diagnosis of late life depression are reviewed.

■ COMMUNICATING WITH THE ELDERLY DEPRESSED PATIENT

Communicating is an important aspect of human behavior (Hine et al, 1972). The personality is largely shaped through interactions with the social environment. Orderly communication between two people or among individuals within a group is a prerequisite to adaptive behavior by each individual. Disordered communication may result in disordered or maladaptive behavior. For example, a misunderstanding between a clinician and a depressed older adult may lead to behavior patterns that are not adaptive for the patient and are antitherapeutic for the clinician. Many malpractice problems in the United States probably result more from poor communication than from incompetent medical care.

In every human interaction, each participant makes a contribution that influences the outcome. The clinician and the patient must be considered as individuals before the interaction can be understood. Factors influencing each person may inhibit effective communication (Blazer, 1978). Patient factors and physician factors are described next.

■ PATIENT FACTORS

- **Anxiety.** Many older patients function with a high level of anxiety. The increased stress of a new situation, such as visiting the clinician's office or being interviewed in the hospital setting, may lead to intense anxiety, impairing the older person's ability to communicate effectively (Eisdorfer, 1968). However, anxiety may not be easily appreciated by the clinician. Tension and agitation may be manifested directly, or they may be diverted into symptoms of withdrawal, shame, fear, or uncooperativeness.

- **Sensory problems.** Hearing loss is usually the most difficult sensory problem for the elderly. It affects men more often than women and occurs in 30% of older persons (Butler and Lewis, 1977). The most common auditory problem that older persons experience is understanding speech (Marsh, 1980). Specific auditory deficits contribute to this lack of comprehension. These deficits include loss of sensitivity to frequencies above 1000 Hz, decreased pitch discrimination, and decreased sound localization.

  Although 80% of older persons have fair-to-adequate vision, visual problems may interfere with effective communication. For example, poor orientation, decreased ability to read, and an occasional frightening visual stimuli may complicate communication in the clinician's office. Visual acuity decreases with decreased light input, increased scattering of light from the various ocular structures, aging of the crystalline lens, and loss of retinal elements in the macula.

- **Cautiousness.** Older persons tend to make fewer errors of commission than errors of omission (Botwinick, 1966). When a clinician is obtaining a history from the older adult, he or she must be aware that elders may omit important aspects of their history. Older people also take longer to respond to inquiries. The clinician who rushes through the history interview may overlook valuable information.

- **Transference.** The older patient may develop an unrealistic view of the clinician based on previous experiences. This process has been called *transference* in psychoanalysis. Older persons may view the clinician as a parent, leading to marked dependence, or as a child, leading to inquires about the clinician's health and behavior (see Chapter 17 on Psychotherapy). The parental transference reaction is likely to occur when the therapist is of similar age to the patient's children (Lazarrus and Weinberg, 1980). Patients may idealize the therapist because of belief in the therapist's healing powers, projection onto the therapist of the patient's own grandiosity, or an overevaluation of the therapist secondary to feelings of emptiness and despair.

  Negative transference reactions occur fairly often. If a depressed older person is forced to go to the clinician's office by family members or other health care professionals, the first reaction may be suspiciousness and lack of cooperation. Frequently, the patient fears that the therapist will reject him or her. Therefore the patient tests the sincerity of the therapist with initial hostility. More often, however, the transference reaction will be positive (Goldfarb and Turner, 1953). If handled properly, a positive transference can be beneficial in the management of the patient.

- **Frequent themes.** Regardless of the psychiatric state of the older adult, certain topics are often prominent in the initial diagnostic interview. These topics include somatic concerns, loss reactions, life review, fear of losing control, and death. These topics are reviewed in more detail in Chapters 5 and 17.

■ PHYSICIAN FACTORS

- **Attitudes towards the elderly.** Fears of aging and death are frequent in our youth-oriented society (Bunzel, 1973). This "gerontophobia" may severely limit the clinician's ability to establish a therapeutic relationship with the patient. Recognizing these fears is of utmost importance in establishing effective communication with the older adult.

- **Countertransference.** Psychotherapy with older adults may rekindle the clinician's unresolved conflicts with parents and grandparents. Omission of a sexual history from the interview of older patients may represent an unconscious prohibition against discussing sexual matters with one's elders (i.e., one's parents) (Lazarrus and Weinberg, 1980). Unfortunately, therapists often concentrate on countertransference issues that are most applicable to the patients of their own age and neglect countertransference toward older adults. Therefore the potential for a damaging countertransference with the older patient is increased because of the lack of training and experience in working with older adults.

- **Lack of understanding.** The clinician must constantly separate the myths about aging from reality. A persistent myth is the assumption that people become grouchy, cranky, and depressed as they age. Stereotyping the older person is a significant barrier to communication. The elderly are especially sensitive to being labeled "cranky," "hypochondriacal," or "crazy." The clinician should empathize with older persons, but this skill is not easily learned from textbook and can only be learned through experience with healthy elders.

■ TECHNIQUES OF EFFECTIVE COMMUNICATION*

- **Approach the older patient with respect.** If the depressed older adult is seen in the office, the clinician should leave the inner office and greet the patient in the outer office and escort the patient into the inner office. If the patient is hospitalized, the clinician should knock before entering the hospital room, approach the patient from the front if possible, and greet the patient by surname (Mr. Jones, Mrs. Smith) rather than by given name unless the patient wishes to be addressed by the given name.

- **Assume a position near the older patient.** The clinician should make every attempt to place himself or herself close enough to reach and touch the patient if desired. The most comfortable arrangement is usually for parties to be seated at a 45-degree angle to each other. If possible, chairs should be of the same height, and the clinician should avoid standing or walking during the interview.

- **Speak clearly and slowly.** The older person may have auditory difficulties and may not be able to distinguish the clinician's speech. Clarity of speech and the use of simple sentences are most effective in communicating with the elderly, especially for those who have hearing loss and/or organic mental syndromes.

  Telephone interviews are frequently used in the follow-up of older adults. Many persons who hesitate to come to the clinician's office and who are quiet and withdrawn on arriving will be loquacious over the telephone. One reason is that the

---

*Modified from Blazer DG: Techniques for communicating with your elderly patient, *Geriatrics* 33:79, 1978.

telephone enables the older patient to take advantage of preserved bone conduction in the presence of mild-to-moderate hearing loss. In addition, older persons may feel less pressure or stimulation over the phone than in person and thus may be better able to process information.

- **Inquire actively and systematically about problems presented.** Older persons do not reveal many of their symptoms spontaneously, as previously noted. Clinicians should actively inquire about common physical and psychologic symptoms of late life depression, such as hearing deficits, memory loss, weight loss, feelings of hopelessness about the death of friends or loved ones, recent retirement, and financial setbacks.
- **Pace the interview.** Older patients must be given enough time to respond to the clinician's questions. In contrast with most younger persons the elderly are not, as a rule, uncomfortable with silence. Pauses in the interview give them the opportunity to formulate answers to questions and to elaborate on certain points. A slow, relaxed pace in the interview will do much to decrease anxiety.
- **Pay attention to nonverbal communication.** The clinician must be alert for changes in facial expressions, gestures, posture, and touch as auxiliary methods of communication by the elderly. Some of these nonverbal expressions are described in Chapter 2.

Touch is frequently an effective way to make contact with the elderly patient. As a rule, older persons are less inhibited about physical touch than younger persons. Many of the sexual connotations of touch that complicate psychotherapy at earlier stages of the life cycle do not apply in late life. Holding the patient's hand or resting a hand on the patient's arm may be very reassuring, especially in the hospital or in long-term care settings.

■ DIAGNOSTIC WORKUP

History

The components of the diagnostic workup for an elderly patient with depressed symptoms are presented in the box on p. 143. Although it is occasionally difficult to elicit a history from the patient, a combination interview with the patient and family can aid the clinician in obtaining information necessary to make the correct diagnosis and to institute therapy. Symptoms of depressive disorders in late life are frequently different from symptoms at other stages of the life cycle because of comorbid physical illness or cognitive impairment (as outlined in Chapters 13 and 15). Therefore the clinician must be alert to the common symptoms of depression in the elderly, such as confusion, memory disturbance, somatic complaints, agitation, sleep disturbance, and constipation. Nevertheless, as noted in Chapter 2, the older patient, on inquiry, will usually report either a depressed mood or a loss of interest in usual activities.

One of the major difficulties in diagnosing late life depressive disorders is making the distinction between depression and organic mental disorders. For this purpose, it is valuable to obtain an accurate chronologic history of onset, duration, and fluctuation of symptoms over time. The depressed patient frequently loses a sense of time, and therefore the clinician must engage family members or friends in the diagnostic workup. It is essential to collect data on possible precipitating events, acuteness of onset, the con-

Office Diagnostic Workup of the Elderly Patient with Depressive Symptoms

History
Symptoms

Present history, including onset, duration, and change in symptoms over time.

Past history of depressive or manic episodes and other psychiatric and medical disorders.

Presence or absence of symptoms of a thought disorder, such as schizophrenia, organic brain disease, or significant physical illness.

Medication History

Family history of depression, other psychoses, or alcoholism.

Physical Examination

Special attention should be paid to the evaluation of possible endocrine disorders, occult infection, neurologic deficits, cardiac function, and evidence of occult malignancy.

Mental Status Examination

Disturbances of consciousness
Disturbances of mood and affect
Disturbances of motor behavior
Disturbances of perception
Presence or absence of hallucinations
Disturbances of thinking (delusions)
Self-esteem and guilt
Suicidal ideation
Disturbances of memory and intelligence (usually should be tested on at least two or three occasions)
Memory (e.g., "Do you know the date today?")
Ability to abstract (e.g., "In what way are a pear and a banana alike?")
Ability to perform simple calculations (e.g., "Subtract 3 from 20 and keep subtracting 3 from each number you get until you reach 0.")
Knowledge of important current events (e.g., "Who is the President of the United States?")

trast between the patient's present symptom state and previous personality style, and the presence of significant remissions, especially for the chronically depressed patient. Regardless of chronicity, most clinicians encounter patients with recent onset or recently exacerbated depressive episodes. Careful inquiry into the nature of the recent episode often places the episode properly within the context of the patient's overall history of psychiatric and physical disturbance.

Although approximately one half of the those persons with depressive episodes in late life experience the initial episode after the age of 65 years, a significant number of depressive episodes evaluated by clinicians, either unipolar or bipolar, are recurrences. Recurrences of depressive episodes with initial onset in late life is frequent. Unfortunately, older adults do not spontaneously associate present symptoms with past problems. Many patients ignore or even forget past psychiatric difficulties and become irritated or angry when clinicians seek information about the past. They wish to concentrate on their present suffering, and, given the frequent occurrence of somatic symptoms in late life depressions, they make no connection between emotional problems at earlier stages of life and depressive symptoms in late life. To further complicate the problem, early significant mood swings may have been disguised as periods of decreased productive activity, episodes of excessive alcohol intake, or vague physical problems. Many elders had the onset of their first depressive episodes before modern constructs of recurrent depressive disorders were formulated and antidepressant medications were available. Clinicians may therefore have labeled the symptom pattern as a problem other than a depressive episode.

Recent studies of the natural history of depressive disorder, regardless of age, solidify the clinical impression that recurrent depressive disorders "breed true." For example, if an older person initially experiences a depressive disorder with psychotic features, then a recurrent episode is likely to be psychotic. The collateral history from family members and a review of past medical records can assist the clinician in characterizing the current depressive episode within the context of previous depressive episodes.

The high probability that older persons with depressive disorders will experience a concurrent medical problem or history of medical difficulties makes the distinction of depressive symptoms in the medically ill difficult for the clinician. Schwab et al (1965) note that all medical patients express some of the usual symptoms of depression, many of which may seem to a result from their medical illness. Symptoms, such as guilt, crying, loneliness, and anorexia, in addition to the generalized somatic problems encountered by the medically ill, were particularly characteristic of depressed medical inpatients. Schwab et al found depressive symptoms among all age groups in a hospital sample, and approximately 20% of the patients in the hospital ward were clinically depressed. They suggested that clinicians question patients about recent losses and chronicity of symptoms and carefully evaluate the patients reaction to his or her recent illness. Disaggregating the depressive symptoms from the direct reaction to the acute medical problems frequently enables the clinician to determine the nature of the depression associated with the physical illness (see Chapter 14). Butler and Lewis (1977) found that 86% of depressed patients have chronic health problems of some type. In addition, sensory losses, especially losses of hearing and visual impairment, may exacerbate the depressive symptoms by contributing to a sense of isolation and loss of control.

Essential for the evaluation of every older psychiatric patient suffering depressive illness is an accurate medication history. The physician, trained nurse, social worker, or paraprofessional should carefully determine present and past medication use. Mechanisms for obtaining this history are described in Chapter 19. Many medications prescribed for older persons can either exacerbate or produce depressive symptoms, especially centrally acting beta blockers (e.g., propranolol), sedative hypnotic agents, and corticosteroids.

A careful family history should be taken to elicit evidence of depressive symptoms in relatives, especially first-degree relatives (siblings, children, and parents). A history of depression or mood disorder may be disguised as alcoholism, work-related difficulties, or undiagnosed physical illness. If possible, the clinician should interview one member of the family from each generation, such as the patient's spouse or sibling, the patient's child, and a grandchild. These interviews should be directed toward eliciting the presence of affective symptoms in the family member being interviewed, and a careful questioning of the family member concerning symptoms in other family members.

Physical Examination

Physical examination of the patient with depression is essential. Although most psychiatrists do not routinely perform physical examinations, such an examination often helps the clinician establish a therapeutic relationship with the patient and show concern about the physical complaints that are frequently expressed by depressed elders. Given that medications are often prescribed by psychiatrists to depressed elders, the physician should at least check sitting and standing blood pressure, as well as pulse. Since physical problems often accompany depressive symptoms, a careful physical examination may also reveal the presence of an illness not previously noted. Careful evaluation of the endocrine system (especially the thyroid gland), neurologic deficits (especially frontal lobe signs and other soft signs that may assist the clinician in the diagnosis of cerebral pathology), cardiac dysfunction, and signs of an occult malignancy is essential. The clinician must determine whether an examination of the rectum and genitalia is necessary. Depressed patients with paranoid ideation frequently become frightened or upset during such an examination. Nevertheless, some forms of cancer (e.g., prostatic and uterine cancer) can only be diagnosed via rectal and genital examination. If the treating clinician is uncomfortable in performing such an examination (or feels incompetent to perform the examination), then referral to an appropriate specialist is indicated.

Depression in the elderly may lead to problems that can only be diagnosed on physical examination, such as peroneal palsy (Massey and Bullock, 1979). Older and active patients with weight loss are particularly prone to this condition. The diagnosis of peroneal neuropathy is important for the following reasons: (1) it may be subacute and therefore not apparent to the physician or patient until it leads to stumbling or severe falls; (2) although it is not rare, it is frequently missed because it is not specifically looked for during the physical examination; and (3) it is frequently correctable. Patients with peroneal palsy may complain of numbness of the lower anterolateral part of the leg and the dorsum of the foot. The foot may "flop" on examination. Sensation in this area is supplied by the peroneal nerve as well. Weakness can be elicited in dorsiflexion of the foot and toes. Loss of weight leads to a lack of protection by fatty tissue of the peroneal nerve during extended periods of leg crossing in the inactive depressed patient and contributes significantly to the condition. Treatment is straightforward, namely instructing patients not to cross their legs.

Mental Status Examination

Although physicians and other health care personnel may frequently omit a formal mental status examination, either to save time or to avoid insulting or irritating the patient, the mental status examination of the depressed patient, especially the elderly patient, is central to the diagnostic workup. A clinician can determine the patient's mood and affect by observing the patient during the interview. Affect is the feeling tone, pleasurable or unpleasurable, that accompanies the patient's cognitive output (Linn, 1975). Affect may vary considerably during the interview; however, fluctuation of affect is generally less extensive with the elderly depressed patients than with younger persons. Mood is the feeling state that underlies affect and is sustained over a period of time. Although the affect of the depressed patient may not reach the degree of dysphoria seen in younger persons, mood is usually depressed and is sustained during successive interviews in depressed elders.

Next, the clinician must determine if disturbances in the motor aspects of behavior are present. Psychomotor retardation or underactivity is characteristic of a depressive disorder, yet older depressed patients commonly exhibit hyperactivity or agitation as well. Severely depressed elders frequently ring their hands and complain of extreme suffering and an inability to remain still. Pacing is often observed when the elder is admitted to a hospital ward. Occasionally, increased activity will take the form of compulsive acts, such as frequent excursions to the toilet, hand washing, adjusting bed covers, and so on. On the other hand, the severely depressed elder may become so retarded in his or her activity as to simulate catatonic stupor. Unlike the schizophrenic patient with catatonic stupor, the depressed patient often has a grimaced face with eyes closed and may actively resist any attempts to move the extremities. On questioning, an elderly patient with depressive retardation may respond with statements such as, "I just can't do anything. I'm going to die."

Next, the clinician should evaluate the perceptions of the patient. Perception is the awareness of objects in relations that follow stimulation of peripheral sense organs (Linn, 1975). Typical disturbances in perception that accompany depression are the presence of hallucinations or false sensory perceptions not associated with real external or internal stimuli. Severe depressive disorders in the elderly are usually not associated with hallucinations. However, if hallucinations are present, they often take the form of false auditory perceptions, false perceptions of movement or body sensation, and false perceptions of smell, taste, and touch. The propensity of older persons to manifest psychic distress as body function symptoms is apparent.

A thorough evaluation of the content and process of cognition is essential in the diagnosis of the depressed elder. Thinking is the goal-directed flow of ideas, symbols, and associations that is initiated in response to a problem or task and that leads to a reality-oriented conclusion (Linn, 1975). Disturbances of thinking may present as problems with the structure of associations, the speed of associations, and the content of thought. The agitated depressed older person may pathologically repeat the same word or idea in response to a variety of probes. Some depressed elders demonstrate circumstantiality, or the introduction into conversation of many details only distantly related or entirely unrelated to the main subject. Such interviews can proceed at a frustratingly slow rate for the clinician. On rare occasions, depressed elders appear incoherent, with no logical connection to their thoughts, or they produce irrelevant answers when questioned. Most often, however, depressed patients demonstrate no disturbance of the structure of associations.

The agitated depressed elder may produce rapid verbalizations, shifting from one idea to another. In the retarded depressed patient the speed of thought is slowed significantly with an occasional blocking or interruption in the train of thinking. Disturbances in thought content, however, are the most common disturbances of cognition noted in depression. The depressed patient often has beliefs that are inconsistent with objective information obtained from family members about the patient's abilities and social resources. These beliefs, which generally cannot be corrected by reasoning, include delu-

sions of bodily dysfunction, such as the belief that cancer or some other incurable illness is present. Depressed patients may state, "I've lost my mind."

Patients who complain about their memory are often depressed. When the family
members complain of the memory problems the patient is more likely to have a real
memory loss. This problem is discussed in detail in Chapter 16. Older persons are less
likely to suffer from delusions of self-remorse, guilt, or persecution, yet they often believe they are no longer of use to others, especially family members. It is difficult to
classify this belief as a delusion, because it is frequently associated with events that have
progressively removed the patients from productive roles in society. Preoccupation, or
centering of thoughts on a particular idea, is not uncommon in depressed older adults.
Preoccupation is closely associated with obsessional thinking or irresistible intrusion of
thoughts into the conscious mind. Patients frequently act on these thoughts compul-
sively. Unlike thoughts of younger depressed patients, these obsessive thoughts are less
commonly guilt-provoking or self-accusing. It is more common for such obsessive preoccupied thinking to center around an unfinished domestic task or physical discomforts.

Spontaneous revelation of suicidal thoughts is not common among depressed elders.
A stepwise probe is the best means of assessing the presence of suicidal ideation. First,
the clinician should ask the patient if he or she has ever thought life not worth living.
If so, has he or she considered doing anything about it? How would the patient attempt
to harm himself or herself? If definite plans are presented, it should be determined
whether the implements for the attempt are readily available. For example, if the patient reveals a plan to take an overdose of sleeping pills, the clinician should ask, "Do
you have sleeping pills at home?" Next, the interviewer should question whether the
patient has activated the plan (e.g., actually taking the pills out of the medicine cabi-
net) or has actually attempted suicide. Clinicians should become progressively concerned
when the patient has done the following: (1) seriously considered suicide and the implements are available, (2) activated a plan, and (3) made a suicide attempt. Unfortunately, negative responses do not guarantee that the patient is not a risk for suicide (see
Chapter 1).

Disturbances of memory and intelligence are commonly elicited during the mental
status examination of the depressed older individual (see Chapter 16). However, these
disturbances may not reflect mental retardation or dementia but may reflect instead the
psychic distress or cognitive dysfunction experienced by the depressed older person.
Therefore memory and intelligence testing should be performed on two or three occasions and generally should be complemented by psychologic testing (see section on psychologic testing at the end of this chapter). During the acute-depressive episode, however, only simple cognitive testing should be performed. Most clinicians base their examination of memory on the following three essential processes: (1) registration—the
ability to record an experience in the central nervous system; (2) retention—the persistence and permanence of a registered experience; (3) recall—the ability to consciously
summon the registered experience and report it (Linn, 1975). The impairment in memory noted in tests of these essential processes of the patient with organic mental disorder are beyond the scope of this chapter. Therefore the specific deficits that might be
encountered in depressed patients with minimum or no cognitive impairment are emphasized. Registration generally depends on the level of consciousness of the individual
being tested. Barring the presence of a sensory deficits, such as hearing and visual losses,

or the presence of a delirium/stupor, the older depressed patient rarely has difficulty registering environmental events. Although elders may appear uninterested and may claim lack of interest in their surroundings, examination after the resolution of a depressive episode reveals that most experiences perceived are registered. Registration can only be tested indirectly through assessment of the individual's ability to recall events or through techniques for eliciting events seemingly not observed. These techniques include hypnosis, narcoanalysis, and psychoanalysis.

Retention of experience, on the other hand, may be impaired in the depressed elder. When psychic distress is expressed, especially in the agitated patient, memories may be registered but not retained. This is especially true of the unimportant data frequently asked for on the mental status examination. For example, asking the depressed older adult to remember three things for 5 minutes frequently reveals a deficit. This deficit is not persistent, however, as with the primary dementia of senile onset. Retention, as with registration, can only be tested indirectly through questioning or through techniques previously mentioned.

Disturbances of recall can be tested directly. The most common test of recall involves typical questions relating to orientation to time, place, person, and situation. However, clinicians must take care, for questions of orientation assume that individuals have registered the oriented experience. Most persons are constantly orienting themselves by reading newspapers, listening to the radio, reading signs, conversing with others, or looking at a time piece. There are various reasons older adults may not be exposed to these experiences. For example, an elderly person living alone may have difficulty seeing (which may prevent him or her from reading the newspaper or watching television), may have lost interest in media, or may be socially isolated. Poor orientation to time or current events should be expected. This lack of orientation does not reflect a memory disturbance but social and asymmetric isolation.

Recall is generally tested by asking the individual to repeat a series of digits spoken by the examiner, usually beginning with three and working up to six or seven digits. The patient may also be asked to repeat the digits in reverse order, but this task requires cognitive operations other than registration, retention, and recall. Older persons of average intelligence can usually recall five to six digits forward and three to four digits backward.

Recent memory may be assessed by asking the patient to recall certain events during the past 12 to 24 hours, such as what he or she ate during the most recent meal. As suggested previously, recent memory can also be tested by asking the patient to remember three things for 5 minutes. The distinction can usually be made between experiences that are registered and recalled, although they never are stored in unconscious memory and experiences that are registered and retained unconsciously and then are returned to the conscience mind when remote memory is tested. Immediate registration, retention, and recall versus recent memory is a valid distinction. Memory for remote events can be evaluated by asking the patient about important dates in the past, such as date of birth, date of marriage, or date of children's births. The clinician must take care to avoid culture bias, because in some subcultures memory for such dates is less important. Although many authorities have suggested that remote memory is maintained in primary dementia senile onset, objective testing suggests that there is little qualitative difference between deficits in recently remote memory.

Depressed older adults, especially patients who are severely agitated or retarded, will have trouble with digit-span testing. Such patients may or may not attend to the task at hand, which generally can be determined by the patient's ability to repeat digits in the order given by the examiner. Other patients will attend to the task but have difficulty concentrating because of psychic distress. Distress is more often reflected by the patient's inability to recall digits in reverse order. Memory for recent and remote events is generally intact given the significance of the event and the life-style of the patient. Depressed elderly patients with high psychic distress may have difficulty recalling something after 5 minutes because of the seeming unimportance of this particular cognitive exercise within the context of his or her distress. On the other hand, some depressed elders have trouble remembering seemingly important information, such as past presidents of the United States, which probably reflects the life-style and previous interest of the patient. Therefore test of recent memory must be as free of culture bias as possible. For example, the elderly homemaker who cannot recall past presidents of the United States may be able to recall other relevant information, such as the ingredients of a favorite recipe.

Amnesia, the partial or total inability to recall certain past experiences, usually within a circumscribed time period, occasionally occurs in depressed older persons. These amnestic episodes may be associated with an organic brain syndrome, but in the absence of good evidence for such a syndrome the most likely cause is the excessive psychic distress of the depressive episode leading to psychogenic amnesia. Older persons who have previous major depressive episodes treated with electroconvulsive therapy may experience both anterograde and retrograde amnesia around the period of the electroconvulsive therapy (see Chapter 20). These patients even complain that they have little if any memory of the hospital in which such treatments were administered.

Intelligence is the ability to constructively understand, recall, mobilize, and integrate previous learning when meeting new situations (Linn, 1975). Intelligence testing and the mental status examination includes tests of the ability to abstract, the ability to perform simple arithmetic calculations, the fund of knowledge, and tests unrelated to previous experience. The capacity of abstract thinking is usually tested by asking the patient to interpret a well-known proverb, such as "People who live in glass houses should not throw stones." A better means of testing abstraction is to ask the patient to classify objects into a common category. For example, the patient is asked, "In what way are an apple and a pear similar?" Elderly depressed patients have little difficulty in performing abstraction.

The usual test for calculation is to ask the patient to subtract 7 from 100 and to repeat this operation until 0 is reached (or until five or six subtractions have been completed). For the older adult, a more practical test may be to ask the patient to subtract 3 from 20 and to continue to repeat this operation until 0 is reached. The examiner must not rush the patient nor penalize the patient for lack of speed when scoring the test. Mistakes that are subsequently corrected should not be counted as wrong. Tests of calculation require not only calculating ability but also memory and the ability to concentrate on a particular task. The individual with acute psychic distress may be unable to perform this task. These patients will frequently do well when given a common arithmetic problem set in the context of their everyday lives, such as "If you go to the store and buy a loaf of bread that cost $1.26 and give the grocer $2.00, how much change should the grocer return to you?"

The general fund of knowledge may be determined by asking the patient to recall as many items as possible from one or two common categories, such as animals, vegetables, and states of the United States. The patient should be able to recall at least eight to ten items from each category. This task also involves memory and attention.

Fluid intelligence, which consists in the manipulation of new information or complex problem solving—solving capacity and speed, appears to decline linearly with age, peaking in the early twenties. A more rapid decline can be seen in individuals with primary degenerative dementia of senile onset (Siegler, 1980). Fluid intelligence can be tested during the mental status examination by asking the patient to perform a complex but short task, such as arranging a group of four to eight matches in a geometric pattern that has previously been demonstrated by the examiner and then disassembled. Since this task requires very little time and is emotionally sterile, it may prove to be a useful adjunct to the mental status examination.

Laboratory Tests

The elderly patient suffering from a major depressive episode secondary to the unipolar or bipolar mood disorder demonstrates no unusual findings on routine laboratory diagnostic tests. Nevertheless, the extensive differential diagnosis of depression in the elderly, as outlined in Chapter 9, necessitates certain routine tests (see box below). A complete blood count and urinalysis will not always reveal physical disorders that lead to depressive symptoms (see Chapter 14). Nevertheless, anemia or urinary tract infections are not uncommon findings among chronically depressed older adults.

A clinical chemistry screen is routine for almost all older persons admitted to the hospital and for most elders evaluated in outpatient clinics. Although the yield of positive results on these screens is usually low, the low cost and potential for treatment of undetected medical illness has rendered them of value in psychiatric diagnosis. The Council of Scientific Affairs for the American Medical Association (1986) provided a

---

Laboratory Workup of the Depressed Older Adult

Routine

Complete blood cell count
Urinalysis
T3, T4, FTI, TSH
VDRL
Vitamin B12 and folate assays
Chemistry screen (Na, Cl, K, BUN, Ca, Glucose, Creatinine)
Electrocardiogram

Elective

Dexamethasone suppression test
Polysomnography
Magnetic resonance imaging (or computed tomography)
Cerebrospinal fluid assays
TRH stimulation test

consensus report on those laboratory tests that should be included in the diagnosis workup for dementia patients routinely (AMA, 1986). These tests are equally applicable for the depressed older adult. They include complete blood count, electrolytes, blood sugar, blood urea nitrogen, creatinine, liver function tests, thyroid function tests, serologic test for syphilis, toxicology screen, B12 and folate concentrations, sedimentation rate, and urinanalysis.

Abnormal sodium and chloride levels suggest dehydration that may contribute to symptoms of delirium and lethargy. Overhydration can also precipitate delirium and lethargy, as well as weakness and muscle twitching. Respiratory or metabolic acidosis (revealed by an increased CO_2 level) may precipitate symptoms of drowsiness and weakness, often mistaken for a chronic depression. Respiratory alkalosis secondary to hyperventilation during episodes of anxiety may contribute to symptoms of unreality and paresthesias.

Although disorders in potassium are rare (and most often result from laboratory error secondary to hemolysis), they are nevertheless critical to identify. The muscle paralysis and paresthesias accompanying a low potassium level should alert the clinician to the possible onset of severe erythema and cardiac failure. An increased level of calcium secondary to hyperparathyroidism can precipitate paranoid ideation and other mental changes, including depressive symptoms. Psychiatric symptoms secondary to hypoparathyroidism include agitation and psychosis. Hyperinsulinism, secondary to increased insulin intake in a diabetic, may cause hypoglycemia and be manifested by anxiety, perspiration, weakness, and shortness of breath. Hyperglycemia, secondary to adult-onset diabetes in older persons, initially leads to lethargy but later may progress to diabetic coma and ketoacidosis.

Monitoring thyroid function is especially important in diagnostic workup on the depressed older adult. The three tests used in most laboratories for screening the psychiatric patient include a direct assay of thyroxine (T4) by radioimmunoassay, a triiodothyronine (T3) uptake, and a calculation of a free thyroxine index. These tests should be augmented by an estimate of thyroid stimulating hormone (TSH). Frequently, in the midst of a severe depressive episode, thyroid function will be increased and will return to normal with usual treatment. Subclinical hypothyroidism is not an uncommon depressive symptom in older adults.

More specialized tests can be used selectively. For example, the thyrotrophin releasing hormone (TRH) stimulation test is the most sensitive of clinical tests available for a thyroid disorder. The test is described in Chapter 4 during the discussion of the psychobiology of late life depression. After a drug-free period of 7 days, subjects fast overnight. The test begins at 9:00 in the morning, and subjects retain a supine position. TRH, in a dose of 0.5 mg, is injected and TSH is recorded at intervals of 30 minutes for 3 hours. A blunted TSH response TRH is seen not only in depressive disorders but also in patients with toxic goiters and occasionally in patients with pituitary hyperthyroidism. Poor nutrition may also contribute to an abnormal response. An elevated serum cortisol (see Chapter 4) also appears to reduce the TSH response in most patients with endocrine disorders. The TSH response is often blunted in older persons who are medically ill.

The dexamethasone suppression test is discussed in greater detail in Chapter 4. Although this test has been used to diagnose Cushing's syndrome for many years, only recently has it been applied to the diagnosis of psychiatric disorders, especially depression. The test was adapted by Carroll et al (1981) to the diagnosis of depression by lowering the dose of dexamethasone administered. The usual procedure is to administer 1 mg of dexamethasone orally at 11:00 PM the night before the test. The next day, venous blood samples are obtained for cortisol at 3:00 PM and (optionally) at 10:00 PM. Although laboratories differ, an abnormal test is usually defined as a postdexamethasone cortisol of greater than 5 μg/dl.

Many factors may lead to a false-positive DST, although sensitivity of this test is relatively good (Carroll et al, 1981). Some factors that may create false-positive results include medications (e.g., phenytoin, barbiturates, and carbamazepine), endocrine disorders (especially Cushing's syndrome or pregnancy), medical problems (especially a severe infection), metabolic problems (e.g., recent withdrawal from alcohol or rapid weight loss and malnutrition), and neurologic problems (e.g., multi-infarct dementia). A false-negative result can occur when synthetic corticosteroids are used.

The dexamethasone suppression test probably adds little to the ability to make the diagnosis of major depression in older persons versus another psychiatric disorder. Nevertheless, a positive dexamethasone suppression test provides a useful marker for response to biologic therapies. If the test remains positive, even after the administration of an adequate trial of antidepressant medications or electroconvulsive therapy, then the likelihood of relapse (even if symptoms improve) is greatly increased. On the other hand, if the test reverts to negative during biologic intervention, the likelihood that the individual will improve symptomatically and will retain his or her improvement is increased. As noted in Chapter 4, the sensitivity of the test is increased in older persons compared with younger persons, but the specificity is decreased.

Magnetic resonance imaging (MRI) has become a relatively common diagnostic test in the workup of the depressed older adult. The abnormalities found on MRI screening of depressed older adults are described in detail in Chapters 4 and 15. In general, MRI scanning is not recommended for routine evaluation of depressed older adults, however. The test is expensive and, at this time, the yield of results that would change treatment orientation is limited. Nevertheless, in those older persons with combined depression and significant cognitive and/or neurologic deficits, MRI screening is indicated.

Routine electroencephalographic (EEG) studies do not assist the clinician in diagnosing depressive disorder in the elderly nor do the studies enable the clinician to differentiate between depression and Alzheimer's disease. Nevertheless, EEG changes do occur with normal aging and also with dementing disorders.

Polysomnographic studies, on the other hand, are among the more specific tests available for diagnosing major depression, regardless of age. Reynolds et al (1988) have demonstrated, despite the fact that the changes on polysomnographic EEG studies found in normal aging are similar to those findings in depression, that quantative evaluation permits the clinician to differentiate aging from depression. Nevertheless, polysomnographic studies in older persons are not easy studies to perform. First, the older person must be drug free for 7 to 14 days. In a severely depressed older person the struggle to withdraw the older person from medications and maintain them in a withdrawn state may be more damaging to therapy than the value of obtaining the polysomnographic study. The recent advent of mobile procedures for polysomnographic tracings, permitting the older person to return home for the usual 2 nights of study required improves the availability of polysomnographic studies. Nevertheless, polysomnographic studies remain expensive studies to perform in the diagnostic workup on the depressed elder.

Polysomnographic studies are not routine and therefore should be limited to those older persons in whom significant sleep problems predominate and there is some significant question regarding the degree to which the older person is suffering from sleep abnormalities. For example, if the older person complains excessively of sleep problems but, by report of family, sleeps relatively well, then polysomnographic evidence may assist in differentiating subjective complaints versus objective time in sleep. If it is found on polysomnographic studies that the older person is sleeping poorly, then more aggressive biologic treatment of the depressive disorder might be indicated.

The electrocardiogram is not a test to screen for depressive disorder per se but is an integral part of the workup of the depressed older adult. In some cases, however, cardiovascular disease can present with psychiatric manifestations. Congestive heart failure and pulmonary edema may lead to confusion and agitation in older persons. Lethargy is also a symptom of these disorders. In the diagnostic workup of the older person, screening for cardiovascular disease that would preclude the use of antidepressant medications or electroconvulsive therapy and monitoring the effects of these therapies on cardiovascular function is essential.

As described in Chapter 19, the cardiotoxic effects of the tricyclic antidepressants are a concern, but usually these drugs are safe, even in patients with documented cardiovascular disease. Ventricular rhythms may actually improve with therapy using tricyclic antidepressants. These drugs to lead to a prolonged T-R intervals and prolongation of the QRS complex. Although not intrinsically dangerous, these changes should be monitored by repeated ECGs during drug therapy and after therapy is discontinued. If the older person experiences a preexisting heart block, then the potential for this block to increase must be determined.

Routine blood pressure monitoring, both sitting and standing, is essential in following the older person taking antidepressant medications in both hospital and office settings. Postural hypotension can be easily monitored through sitting and standing blood pressure.

Psychologic Testing

The use of psychologic tests for cognitive impairment in the evaluation of depressed older persons is commonplace. Not only are such tests useful in making the distinction between transient and permanent cognitive impairment, they may also reveal the nature and the extent of the depressive cognitive dysfunction. Some caution must be taken in interpreting cognitive tests with the elderly, however, because the test scores must be adjusted for age and the state of the older person during testing will greatly affect the results of the test.

Neuropsychologic testing for cognitive function is best postponed until after the older person has recovered from the severe symptoms of the depressive episode, since the lack of motivation and actual cognitive dysfunction that may accompany a depressive episode will undoubtedly bias the results of psychologic testing (see Chapter 16). If the older person is suffering from mild-to-moderate depressive symptoms or has recovered fully from a more severe depressive episode, then the clinician may proceed with testing. Most tests administered in the routine mental status examination, such as the Mini Mental State Examination, are not sensitive to mild neurologic impairment. The clinician may then wish to supplement the examination by the administration of additional neuropsychologic tests such as the Wechsler Adult Intelligence Scale-Revised (WAIS-R) or the Stanford-Binet Intelligence Scale (Lezak, 1983; Terman and Merrill, 1973). The WAIS-R is composed of 11 subtests, divided into verbal and performance categories. These subtests, which may be used independently, include information, comprehension, arithmetic, similarities, digit span, and vocabulary (the verbal test), and performance tests of digit symbol, picture completion, block design, picture arrangement, and object assembly. Memory can be evaluated by the revised Wechsler memory scale (Russell, 1975). Other neuropsychologic tests that may be administered include the Trail-Making Test and the Halstead-Reitan Battery.

In general the use of the WAIS-R, supplemented by a few memory and performance tests, such as the Trail-Making Test and the Wechsler Memory Scale, are sufficient for the evaluation of cognitive function. Repeated use of these tests over time is necessary if scores are to be interpreted effectively in older persons.

The Minnesota Multiphasic Personality Inventory (MMPI) is the most frequently used individual psychologic test for personality assessment. This test has recently undergone extensive revisions with the development of more appropriate norms across the life cycle. It provides scores on a number of clinical scales that correspond to Axis I diagnoses, such as depression. It also includes various scales to correct for biases resulting from nonresponse or "faking." The interpretation of the MMPI must be within the context of clinical judgment, and the results should not supersede the clinical evaluation. In addition, some of these scales have low reliabilities. Aaronson (1958) notes that older persons have higher scores on the hysterical, hypochondrical, and social introversions scales than do younger adults. Older individuals tend to appear more neurotic than the young on the MMPI as well. Bernal et al (1977) pointed out that the MMPI is a long and tedious test for older adults, especially if the attention span is short and visual problems are present. It is also particularly difficult for seriously ill or seriously agitated individuals to complete the test in a self-administered form. The use of a keyboard, however, may render the test more easily administered to older persons than in its typical pencil and paper form. Subscale scores and profiles *do not* substitute for either Axis I or Axis II DSM-III-R diagnoses.

Another psychologic test used in the evaluation of older adults in clinical practice is the Thematic Apperception Test (TAT). Neugarten (1964) found that older persons, through their responses to this test, appear to take a different orientation to the outer world. They consider the world complex and dangerous. It cannot be reformed according to the personal wishes of an individual, but instead the individual must conform and accommodate to the demands of the environment. Ego function is turned inward, yet the ego appears to be less in contact with and less perceptive in controlling and channelling internal impulses. These findings may also be confounded with a typical findings from the response of depressed individuals Neugarten presented in the TAT. The test is not useful for distinguishing between depression and dementia.

Of the projective tests, however, the Rorschach is the most extensively used (Crombach, 1984). Many of the responses typically found in younger depressed persons are noted as general trends in the older population. Klopfer (1946) suggests that the trend for older individuals is one of constriction, decrease in the number of responses, decrease in the number of human figures and movement, increase in animal responses, and decrease in the form of level ratings. Brink (1978) notes that responses to the ten standard Rorschach Ink Blocks by depressed elders showed tendencies toward restriction of attention to detailed responses, shading responses, inaminate movement responses, anatomic responses (especially in hypochondrasis), marked delay in response to card seven, and a unique response to card ten. The Rorschach test is of no value in distinguishing depression and dementia.

In general, personality and projective tests are not of great value in diagnosing depressive disorders in late life. Nevertheless, characteristics of late life depression that might be useful in the psychotherapeutic and milieu management of the patient may emerge from such testing. Therefore the selection of appropriate tests and expections from these tests must be determined during the diagnostic workup. Psychologic tests are expensive to administer and clinicians must select patients carefully from whom they chose to test.

REFERENCES

Aaronson BS: Age and sex differences on MMPI profile peak distributions in an abnormal population, *Journal of Consulting Psychology* 22:203, 1958.

Bernal, GA, et al: Psychodiagnostics of the elderly. In Gentry WD (ed): *Geropsychology: A Model of Training and Clinical Service.* Cambridge, Massachusetts, Ballinger, 1977, pp. 43-77.

Blazer DG: Techniques for communicating with your elderly patient, *Geriatrics* 33:79-83, 1978.

Botwinick J: Cautiousness in advanced age, *Journal of Gerontology* 21:347, 1966.

Brink TL: Geriatric rigidity and its psychotherapeutic implications, *Journal of the American Geriatric Society* 26:274, 1978.

Bunzel JH: Recognition, relevant and the deactivation of gerontophobia, *Journal of American Geriatric Psychiatry* 21:77, 1973.

Butler RN, Lewis MI: *Aging and Mental Health: Positive Psychosocial Approaches,* (ed 2). St. Louis, Mosby, 1977.

Carr AC: Psychological testing of personality. In Caplan HI, Sadock BJ (eds): *Comprehensive Textbook of Psychiatry/IV.* Baltimore, Williams and Wilkins, 1985, pp. 514-535.

Carroll BJ, Feinberg M, Greden JF, Tarika J, Abala AA, et al: A specific laboratory test for the diagnosis of melancholia: standardization, validity, and clinical utility, *Archives of General Psychiatry* 38:15-22, 1981.

Council on scientific affairs of the American Medical Association: Dementia, *Journal of the American Medical Association* 256:2234-2238, 1986.

Eisdorfer C: Arousal and performance: experiments in verbal learning and a tentative theory. In Falland GA (ed): *Human Aging and Behavior.* New York, Academic Press, 1968.

Goldfarb AI, Turner H: Psychotherapy of aged persons: utilization and effectiveness of brief therapy, *American Journal of Psychiatry* 109:916, 1953.

Hine FR, Friedel RO, Maddox GL, Henn RH: *Behavioral Science: A Selective View.* Boston, Little, Brown and Company, 1972.

Klopfer WG: Personality patterns of old age, *Rorschach Research Exchange* 10:145, 1946.

Lazarrus LW, Weinberg J: Treatment in the ambulatory care setting. In Busse EW, Blazer DG (eds): *Handbook of Geriatric Psychiatry.* New York, Van Nostrand Reinhold 1980, pp. 427-452.

Lezak MD: *Neuropsychological Assessment* (ed 2). New York, Oxford University Press, 1983.

Linn L: Clinical manifestations of psychiatric disorders. In Friedman AN, Kaplan HI, Sadock BJ (eds): *Comprehensive Textbooks of Psychiatry.* Baltimore, Williams and Wilkins, 1975, pp. 783-825.

Marsh GR: Perceptual changes with aging. In Busse EW, Blazer DG (eds): *Handbook of Geriatric Psychiatry.* New York, Van Nostrand Reinhold, 1980, pp. 147-168.

Massey EW, Bullock R: Perineal palsy in depression, *Psychiatry Digest,* January, 1979, p. 41 (abstract).

Neugarten BL, et al: *Personality in Middle and Late Life.* New York, Atherton, 1964.

Reynolds CF, Kupfer DJ, Hauch PR, Hauch CC, Stack JA, et al: Reliable discrimination of elderly depressed and demented patients by electroencephagraphic sleep data, *Archives of General Psychiatry* 45:258-264, 1988.

Russell EW: A multiple screening method for the assessment of complex memory functions, *Journal of Consulting and Clinical Psychology* 43:800-809, 1975.

Siegler IC: The psychological of adult development in aging. In Busse EW, Blazer DG (eds): *Handbook of Geriatric Psychiatry*. New York, Van Nostrand Reinhold, 1980, pp. 169-221.

Terman LM, Merrill MA: The Stanford-Binet intelligence scale. *Manual for Third Revision*. Form L-M. Boston, Houghton Mifflin, 1973.

9

Differential Diagnosis of Late Life Depression

The clinician's first diagnostic task is to distinguish clinical depression (i.e., syndromes that arise without preexisting mood disorders and are grossly out of proportion to any life events that may have preceded them) from normal fluctuations in mood, situational depression, or depressive symptoms secondary to an underlying physical or psychiatric disorder (Akiskal, 1979). Next, mood disorders should be subclassified into one of the diagnostic categories from an existing classification scheme, such as the Third Edition (revised) of the Diagnostic and Statistical Manual (DSM-III-R) or the Tenth Edition of the International Classification of Diseases (ICD-10) (APA, 1987; The International Classification of Diseases, Tenth Edition). A new edition of the Diagnostic and Statistical Manual will be available within the next few years. The classification of mood disorders in DSM-IV will not vary greatly from the current revised edition.

First, the diagnostic categories in DSM-III-R applicable to late life mood disorders are reviewed in this chapter (see box on p. 158). Some of these diagnoses are discussed in more detail in other chapters (e.g., bipolar disorders, major depression, bereavement, minor depression, and depressive disorders secondary to alcohol abuse). Then, the differential diagnosis of depression from three common syndromes—dementia, hypochondriasis, and sleep disorders—are discussed.

■ DIAGNOSES OF DEPRESSION IN THE ELDERLY

Dementing Disorders

Dementing disorders are frequently associated with depression (see Chapter 16). The most common of the dementing disorders is primary degenerative dementia, where the prevalence of depressive symptoms meeting criteria for a major depressive episode reaches 20%. The comorbidity of major depression with multiinfarct dementia may be even higher.

Differential Diagonsis of Depression in the Elderly

I. Organic mental disorders
   A. Dementias arising in the senium
      1. Primary degenerative dementia of the Alzheimer's type (with depression) 290.2
      2. Multiinfarct dementia (with depression) 290.43
   B. Substance-induced organic mental disorders associated with depression
      1. Sedative, hypnotic, or anxiolytic intoxication 305.40
      2. Caffeine intoxication 305.90
      3. Antihypertensive agents, such as guanethedine and reseperine 305.90
      4. Antiarrhythmic agents, such as propranolol 305.90
   C. Alcohol abuse (305.00) and dependence (303.90) with depression
   D. Organic mood syndrome (293.83) with depression secondary to
      1. Hypothyroidism
      2. Cushing's syndrome
      3. Occult malignancy, such as carcinoma of the pancreas
      4. Vitamin deficiency syndromes, especially a deficiency in the B complex vitamins and folic acid
      5. Mass lesions of the brain, especially slowly growing lesions affecting the frontal lobe, such as meningioma
      6. Parkinson's disease
      7. Stroke
II. Schizophrenia, paranoid 295.3x (with intermixed depressive symptoms)
III. Schizoaffective disorder (uncommon in late life) 295.70
IV. Mood disorders
   A. Bipolar disorder
      1. Mixed 296.6x
      2. Depressed 296.5x
      3. Manic 296.4x
   B. Major depression
      1. Single episode 296.2x
      2. Recurrent 296.3x
   C. Cyclothymic disorder 301.13
   D. Dysthymic disorder (or depressive neurosis) 300.40
   E. Depressive disorder not otherwise specified 311.00
V. Anxiety disorders
   A. Generalized anxiety 300.02 (often comorbid with depression)
   B. Posttraumatic stress disorder 309.89
VI. Somatoform disorder
   A. Somatoform pain disorder 307.80 (often accompanied by depressive symptoms)
   B. Hypochondriasis (or hypochondriac neurosis) 300.70
VII. Adjustment disorder with depressed mood 309.00
VIII. Personality disorders: A depressed affect frequently accompanies narcissistic (301.81) and dependent (301.60) personality disorders in the elderly.
IX. Sleep disorders
   A. Primary insomnia 307.42
   B. Sleep-wake schedule disorder 307.45
X. Other (301.60)
   A. Uncomplicated bereavement V62.82
   B. Marital problems V61.10
   C. Phase of life problem or other life circumstance problem V62.89

Adapted from the *Diagnostic and Statisical Manual of Mental Disorders* (ed 3), revised, Washington, DC: American Psychiatric Association, 1987.

Drug Dependence and Intoxication

Depressive disorders are often associated with medications, especially medications used to treat other psychiatric symptoms, such as sleep problems. These medications are reviewed in Chapter 13 in more detail. Older persons who have recently used a sedative, hypnotic, or anxiolytic may exhibit maladaptive behavior changes, including disinhibition, aggressive impulses, impaired adjustment, and impaired social or occupational functioning (APA, 1987). Slurred speech, incoordination, unsteady gait, and impairment of attention or memory also accompany abuse of sedative, hypnotic, or anxiolytic medications. Mood lability or even a chronic depressed mood is a common symptom of use of these medications, especially in the elderly. Older persons may respond adversely to these medications even when the doses fall within a therapeutic range. Caffeine intoxication can lead to restlessness, nervousness, excitement, insomnia, flushed face, diuresis, and gastrointestinal complaints (APA, 1987). The agitation, insomnia, and irritability may mimic an agitated depression in older adults. A careful history of caffeine use should reveal caffeine intoxication, but the reviewer should not only inquire about beverages containing caffeine but also analgesics and over-the-counter stimulants.

Medications used to treat cardiovascular disease are especially likely to cause depressive symptoms in older persons. Even the relatively benign diuretics, such as hydrochlorothiazide, may lead to significant weakness, lethargy, and secondary depression. Guanethidine and reserpine are especially prone to precipitate depressive episodes. The more commonly used beta-blocking agents also may precipitate a significant depressed mood. Not only can these agents lead to a depressed mood directly, the lethargy that is common with their use has been associated with a significant decline in life satisfaction (leading some to question the risks versus the benefits of using these agents).

Alcohol Abuse and Dependence

Both alcohol abuse and chronic alcohol use can lead to significant depressive symptoms. Alcohol is known to be a risk factor not only for depression but also for suicide (see Chapter 1). Older persons may hide their drinking habits from the clinician and family. More commonly, the older person begins to experience problems with unchanging alcohol intake over months or even years. Therefore neither the elder nor family members associate alcohol intake with problems in mood and performance. The elder suffering alcohol problems frequently becomes suspicious, withdraws socially, and may even exhibit paranoid symptoms, as well as depression. Amnesia for events is frequent during more acute episodes of intoxication, and memory problems, in turn, suggest the diagnosis of a dementing disorder. Alcohol use over many years often contributes to significant memory impairment that can be stalled but not reversed on cessation of alcohol use. Intoxication itself may lead to acute medical problems, even death. More commonly, the older adult becomes intoxicated and then experiences some type of trauma (e.g., a fall or an automobile accident). Alcohol occasionally precipitates physical aggression in older adults, but it is more likely to precipitate attempts to harm oneself. The association of a depressed mood and alcohol is not difficult to identify if the clinician is aware of the increased association of alcohol use and depression in late life.

Organic Mood Disorder

The essential feature of an organic mood syndrome is a prominent and persistent depressed (or elevated) mood resulting from a specific organic factor. Clinical presentation of the syndrome is similar to manic episodes or major depressive episodes and organic mood disorders may range from the mild to the severe (APA, 1987).

Cognitive impairment is a common accompaniment of organic mood disorder, especially in older adults. Typical accompanying features of an organic depressed syndrome are agitation, irritability, excessive somatic concerns, suspiciousness, and occasional delusions of worthlessness. The organic manic syndrome is usually accompanied by irritability and aggressiveness.

Organic mood syndrome in late life is most often secondary to structural disease of the brain, such as stroke, Parkinson's disease, and dementing disorders. The dementing disorders with a depressed mood are assigned to a separate diagnostic category, however (see box on p. 158). The organic mood syndrome may also be caused by toxic or metabolic factors and medication. A common cause in late life is depressive or manic symptoms secondary to endocrine disorders, especially hyper/hypothyroidism and hyper/hypocortisolism. Carcinoma of the pancreas has been associated with depressive disorders as well. Organic mood disorders must be distinguished from depressions that are reactive to a disability and other life changes that a medical condition causes; this discrimination is frequently difficult to make (see Chapter 13).

Schizophrenia

Schizophrenic disorders, especially schizophrenic disorders of late onset, are often associated with depressive symptoms. In the Third Edition of the Diagnostic and Statistical Manual (APA, 1980), persons with the onset of schizophrenic-like symptoms after the age of 45 could not be diagnosed as suffering from a schizophrenic disorder. Although the onset of schizophrenia usually occurs during adolescence or young adulthood, onset in late life does occur. Schizophrenic symptoms with onset in late life are generally less severe than those at earlier stages of the life cycle and usually are of the paranoid variety. Cognitive function typically remains intact. In general the diagnosis of a mood disorder, as opposed to a schizophrenic disorder, will be based on the predominance of the depressed mood over the psychotic thinking and the presence of mood-congruent delusions and hallucinations. In other words the delusions and hallucinations can be explained by the severe mood disturbance. As noted in Chapter 10, psychoses associated with severe major depression are more common in late life than at other stages of the life cycle.

Schizoaffective Disorder

Schizoaffective disorder is a debated diagnosis, since many clinicians and clinical investigators suggest that these persons can be classified either as persons with a severe mood disorder accompanied by psychotic symptoms or as suffering from a schizophrenic disorder. There is virtually no literature on schizoaffective disorder in older adults, and detailed information on the prevalence, age of onset, and course of the disorder is virtually lacking. The diagnosis of schizoaffective disorder is made only when it cannot be established that the older adult cannot be classified with a mood disorder with psychotic features, schizophrenia, or an organic mental disorder with depressive or manic symptoms.

Mood Disorders

As reviewed in Chapter 2, older persons, without complicated physical or cognitive problems, can be diagnosed as easily with major depression when suffering from a severe depressive syndrome as people at other stages of the life cycle. Although many nosologists debate the validity of the DSM diagnosis of major depression (originally deriving from the Research Diagnostic Criteria category for major depression), there is no reason to believe the diagnosis is less valid in the elderly than at other stages of the life cycle (Spitzer et al, 1978). More severe depressive episodes that last for 2 weeks or longer qualify for the diagnosis of major depression. Major depressive episodes in late life, as during other stages of life, may be single or recurrent and mixed with intermittent manic episodes (bipolar disorder). Older persons are more likely to experience major depression with psychotic features (delusions or hallucinations) but are no more likely to experience melancholic major depression or major depression with a seasonal pattern. Seasonal mood disorder is probably less common in late life and the unique symptoms of seasonal mood disorder, such as excessive sleep or increased appetite during the depressed episode, are less frequent in late life. Melancholic depression is important to identify, for persons suffering from melancholic depression are more likely to respond to somatic therapies and less likely to respond to psychosocial therapies.

Bipolar disorder is less common in late life than at other stages of the life cycle yet the disorder can have its first onset in late life (see Chapter 10). Euphoria and an expansive mood are less common in late life, whereas irritability and agitation are more common. Sleep disturbance, confusion, pressure of speech, distractibility, decrease in goal-directed behavior, and a relatively acute onset are characteristics of manic episodes in older adults. In contrast to younger persons, older persons are more likely to complain of manic symptoms as being ego-dystonic.

Cyclothymia is a disorder that is not often diagnosed in clinical settings. The symptoms are less severe than in bipolar disorder and older adults who manifest such symptoms are more likely to be treated by primary care physicians than mental health specialists. The essential feature of cyclothymia is a chronic mood disturbance of at least 2 years' duration, involving numerous hypomanic episodes and numerous periods of depressed mood or loss of interest that are of insufficient severity or duration to meet criteria for major depression or manic episode. The category of "minor depression" (see Chapter 12) may include individuals who suffer cyclothymia. Angst (1990) describes a syndrome with recurrent brief but relatively severe episodes of mood disturbance that fit rather closely the criteria for cyclothymia. The major difference between Angst's recurrent brief mood disorder and cyclothymia is that the episodes, although less than 2 weeks (and often lasting only 2 or 3 days) are nevertheless severe enough to warrant a classification of major depression or mania.

Dysthymia (or depressive neurosis) is a common disorder in late life. Most dysthymic disorders presenting in late life have their onset earlier in life. The essential feature of dysthymic disorder is a chronic disturbance of mood, involving a depressed mood for most of the day more days than not for at least 2 years (APA, 1987). Typical symptoms of dysthymic disorder in older persons include poor appetite, chronic insomnia, chronic low energy or fatigue, difficulty concentrating, inability to make decisions, and persistent chronic expressions of hopelessness. Older persons may suffer from a "double depression," in that they may experience a dysthymic disorder all or most of the time and periodically experience an episode of major depression. As noted in Chapter 12, persons may be treated for the major depression and partially recover, yet their mood never becomes euthymic. If the initial onset of dysthymia immediately follows a major depressive episode, then the correct diagnosis would be major depression in partial remission (APA, 1987). According to DSM-III-R, the diagnosis of dysthymia can be made after major depression only if there has been a full remission of the major depressive episode lasting at least 6 months before the development of dysthymia.

One category of DSM-III-R of especial interest to clinicians working with older persons is the "wastebasket" category of depressive disorders not otherwise specified (NOS). The following two examples are provided that are directly relevant to older adults: (1) a recurrent, mild, depressive disturbance that does not meet criteria for dysthymia; (2) non–stress-related depressive episodes that do not meet criteria for a major depressive episode (APA, 1987). Considerable interest has emerged in the construct of minor depression (Broadhead et al, 1990; Blazer, 1991). Many persons with symptoms of depression that do not meet criteria for major depression or dysthymic disorder and are not associated with obvious stress (i.e., an adjustment disorder) may best be classified in the DMS-III-R nomenclature as depressive disorder NOS. Further studies are needed, however, to explore the construct of minor depression (see Chapter 12).

Generalized Anxiety Disorder

Generalized anxiety disorder (GAD) is one of the more common disorders across the life cycle, with about 4% of older persons in the community suffering the disorder (Blazer et al, 1991). The essential feature of GAD is unrealistic or excessive anxiety and worry (apprehensive expectations) about multiple life circumstances, such as finances, health, or social relations. Since anxiety is a symptom that is comorbid with many psychiatric disorders, especially mood disorders, the diagnosis should not be made when a mood disorder is prominent. The following three categories of symptoms contribute to the syndrome of generalized anxiety: motor tension (trembling, muscle tension, and aches); autonomic hyperactivity (shortness of breath, palpitations, and sweating); and symptoms of vigilance and scanning (feeling on edge, experiencing exaggerated startled response, and difficulty concentrating (APA, 1987). Symptoms of depression are common with generalized anxiety. To make the diagnosis, an individual must suffer the disorder at least 6 months and the anxiety symptoms should be predominant. In addition, no organic factor should be present as the cause of the disorder, such as hyperthyroidism or caffeine intoxication.

Posttraumatic Stress Disorder

Posttraumatic stress disorder (PTSD) is uncommon in the elderly, being much more common in young adulthood. In late life the symptoms do not usually result from traumatic war experiences but rather from distressing events outside the severity of general experience that occur during the usual daily activities of an individual. The trauma may be an accident, such as an automobile crash, head injury, or a frightful experience (e.g., a rape or an assault). The recurrent and intrusive recollections of the event lead to difficulties with sleep and episodes of panic that may resemble an agitated depression in older adults. Nevertheless, the event usually can be identified leading to PTSD. Persistent symptoms of hyperarousal also may resemble a mood disorder and include difficulty falling or remaining asleep, irritability, difficulty concentrating, and an exaggerated startle response. The person experiencing a PTSD may withdraw socially and restrict his or her affectional ties.

Somatoform Disorders

The somatoform pain disorder is a disorder that usually occurs in mid-life, and most commonly involves back pain. The essential feature is a preoccupation with pain in the absence of physical findings to account for the pain's intensity and location (APA, 1987). Although the person may experience actual structural damage to the back (or other body parts), the pain is inconsistent with the anatomic distribution and/or the severity of the pain is not consistent with the structural damage. Depressive symptoms are frequent, especially anhedonia and insomnia in individuals suffering from a somatoform pain disorder (APA, 1987). The diagnosis of a major depressive disorder can be made in conjunction with a somatoform pain disorder if the symptoms are severe enough to warrant the diagnosis. The depressive symptoms may be treated in the usual manner, and the pain accompanying the depressive disorder often improves with improvement in depressive symptoms.

One of the more important distinctions for the clinician to make is the distinction between depression in late life and hypochondriasis. This is discussed more fully in a later section.

Adjustment Disorder with Depressed Mood

The diagnosis of adjustment disorder is made when an elder develops a maladaptive reaction to an identifiable psychosocial stressor that occurs within 3 months after the onset of the stressor and persists for no longer than 6 months (APA, 1987). The maladaptive reaction may lead to occupational dysfunction, decline in usual social activities, and emotional pain. The stressors leading to an adjustment disorder may be single, such as retirement, or multiple, such as marital problems and chronic physical illness. When the predominant feelings are depressed mood, tearfulness, and hopelessness, the diagnosis of adjustment disorder with depressed mood is made. It is most difficult to distinguish an adjustment disorder with depressed mood from a major depressive episode, for frequently a major depressive episode follows a stressful event. In addition, depressive syndromes after a clearly identifiable stressor often last longer than the 6-month criterion necessary for a diagnosis of adjustment disorder. Usually, in such circumstances, the diagnosis of major depressive episode should be made if the symptoms meet criteria for major depression. When the symptoms are less severe, the diagnosis of adjustment disorder may be made. Nevertheless, the clear association of the depressive symptoms with the stressor is not easy to establish.

Personality Disorders

Personality traits are enduring patterns of perceiving, relating to, and thinking about the environment and oneself and therefore are ubiquitous with the human experience (APA, 1987). When these personality traits become inflexible and maladaptive and cause significant functional impairment, they constitute a personality disorder. Personality disorders begin early in life and persist throughout life. Personality disorders usually become less severe with aging. Nevertheless, stressors in late life may lead to an exacerbation of the symptoms of a personality disorder.

Two personality disorders are especially associated with depressive symptoms in late life—narcissistic personality disorder and dependent personality disorder. The essential feature of a narcissistic personality disorder is a pattern of grandiosity, hypersensitivity to evaluation of others, and lack of empathy. These elders tend to exaggerate their accomplishments and talents and expect to be noticed as special (APA, 1987). In late life the gratification of their sense of importance often decreases and therefore they become depressed when they feel neglected or are preoccupied with the change in physical appearance (especially when it is perceived that the youthful appearance has deteriorated). Persons with a narcissistic personality disorder in late life may be at greater risk for suicide because they cannot tolerate the losses associated with aging.

The dependent personality disorder is characterized by a pervasive pattern of dependence and submissive behavior that usually begins early in adulthood and persists throughout life. Dependent persons usually find roles in life that permit them to rely on others. Excessive dependence on others, however, may lead to difficulties in initiating and doing things on one's own (APA, 1980). Dependent elders feel uncomfortable or helpless when alone and go to great lengths to avoid being alone. Loss of a spouse can be devastating and severe depression is common. Persons with dependent personality disorder invariably lack self-confidence and tend to belittle their own abilities and assets. When faced with taking more independent roles in late life (e.g., after bereavement), they frequently believe themselves incapable of assuming the new roles. They become a burden to their families, which further complicates the depressed mood.

Sleep Disorders

Two sleep disorders commonly lead to depressive symptoms in older persons—primary insomnia and sleep-wake cycle disorder. Primary insomnia is characterized by a persistent inability to sleep not related to other known mental or physical problems (APA, 1987). The older person with primary insomnia worries excessively during the day about not being able to fall asleep and stay asleep, which may become the major preoccupation of his or her life. The elder insomniac makes intense efforts to fall asleep and goes through elaborate rituals at night, only to be frustrated that sleep does not ensue. Daytime napping may contribute to primary insomnia. To meet criteria for insomnia, the elder must have difficulty at least three times a week for at least a month, and the problem must be sufficiently severe to result in either a complaint of significant daytime fatigue or the observation by others of some symptom that is attributable to the sleep disturbance, such as irritability or impaired daytime functioning (APA, 1987).

Perhaps an even more common sleep problem among older persons is sleep-wake cycle disorder. In this disorder the older adult becomes uncoupled from the normal sleep-wake schedule, usually resulting in a complaint of insomnia. A life-style that is characterized by irregular sleep-wake patterns may predispose the disorder. Such a life-style is frequent in late life when the usual factors that orient sleep-wake cycle are lacking. For example, the older person no longer must arise at a given time in the morning to go to work and, because of loneliness, may either go to sleep early in the evening or watch television into the early hours of the morning. These irregular sleep cycles lead to a disruption in the sleep-wake pattern.

Sleep-wake schedule disorder may be either advanced or delayed. In advanced sleep-wake cycle disorder the elder goes to sleep early in the evening, only to awake early in the morning. In the delayed cycle the person goes to bed early in the morning only to awaken late in the morning. Advanced sleep-wake schedule disorder is much more common in older persons.

Other Disorders Associated with Mood Disturbance

There are a number of syndromes in late life that often lead to depressive symptoms but that are not classified as psychiatric disorders. These include uncomplicated bereavement (see Chapter 13), phase of life problems (e.g., retirement or a marriage in late life) and marital problems (which may arise for the first time in late life). These conditions should not be classified or conceptualized as psychiatric disorders. Nevertheless, they may contribute to depressive symptoms and deserve attention by the clinician.

■ DIFFERENTIAL DIAGNOSIS

Three syndromes have traditionally confounded clinicians in their attempts to distinguish a primary mood disorder from other psychiatric problems associated with a depressed mood. These conditions are pseudodementia, hypochondriasis, and sleep disorder disturbances.

Pseudodementia

Pseudodementia is a syndrome in which dementia is mimicked or characterized by functional psychiatric illness, most often depression (Wells, 1979). The comorbidity of depression and neurologic conditions is presented in Chapter 15. Patients with pseudodementia respond to the mental status examination in ways similar to those with true degenerative brain disease. Kiloh (1961) notes that pseudodementia "is descriptive and carries no diagnostic weight," yet he observed that patients with pseudodementia were in danger of inaccurate diagnosis and therapeutic neglect.

A number of investigators suggest that a frequent overlap of depressive symptoms and symptoms of organic mental disorders occurs in late life. Kahn et al (1975) studied 153 persons 50 years of age and older who had various degrees of depression that altered brain function. Depressed persons in this study tended to exaggerate their memory complaint, in contrast to individuals with altered brain functions but who were not depressed. Earlier, Lowenthal et al (1967) found that memory complaints were common in a community population of the elderly. These complaints corresponded to the typical stereotype that older persons lose their memory as they age. Grinker et al (1961) found impaired recent memory in 21% and poor remote memory in 14% of persons they studied with depressive disorders at all ages.

Findings from a series of cross-national studies suggest that diagnostic discrepancies exist between clinicians in Great Britain and the United States. Duckworth and Ross (1975) found, when comparing diagnoses assigned to older persons in New York, London and Toronto, that organic brain syndromes were diagnosed 50% more frequently in

New York than in London or Toronto. Wells (1979) concluded that clinicians in New York quite likely were incorrectly labelling individuals with depression as demented.

Other investigators have considered the differential response to psychologic testing and mental status examinations by depressed and demented patients. Post (1975) found that patients with depression usually have the onset of their symptoms before the appearance of cognitive dysfunction. In patients with dementia the onset of depressive symptoms usually follows the development of cognitive failure. He also observed that "near miss" responses to the mental status examination suggested organic brain dysfunction, whereas "don't know" answers were more typical of depression. Folstein et al (1975) tested a number of patients who were depressed but who also had cognitive dysfunction. They found that individuals with cognitive deficits improved after their depressive symptoms remitted.

Wells wrote a seminal article in 1979 on the problem of diagnosing pseudodementia (Wells, 1979). He described 10 patients with pseudodementia and compared the clinical features of the disorder with those of true dementia. Although the pseudodemented patients had varying psychiatric disorders, they all exhibited certain personality traits. The most striking common feature was a marked dependency on physical care and emotional support. The interaction of cognitive deficits and demands on the care of others was apparent in all of these patients. The major clinical features differentiating pseudodementia from dementia, adapted from Wells, are presented in Table 9-1. A history of the clinical course of the condition and multiple interviews of the patients are critical in distinguishing pseudodementia from dementia.

In contrast to patients with pseudodementia, demented patients appeared unaware of the extent and severity of their cognitive dysfunction and they frequently used stratagems to conceal their dysfunction from other persons. Pseudodementia "is not so closely related to depressive disorders as has been suggested by earlier authors . . . The syndrome of pseudodementia . . . occurs in a variety of psychiatric disorders other than depression, is not confined to the aged, and is not necessarily associated with underlying brain damage" (Wells, 1979). Depressive affect was pervasive in seven of his ten patients.

Hypochondriasis

Hypochondriasis is a frequent disorder among the elderly (Busse and Blazer, 1980). As noted previously, anxiety, a depressed mood, and compulsive personality traits are

TABLE 9-1. Characteristics Distinguishing Depression (pseudodementia) from Dementia

Dementia	Depression
Insidious and indeterminant onset	Rapid onset
Symptoms usually of long duration	Symptoms usually of short duration
Mood and behavior fluctuate	Mood is consistently depressed
"Near miss" answers typical	"Don't know" answers typical
Patient conceals disabilities	Patient highlights disabilities
Cognitive impairment relatively stable	Cognitive impairment fluctuates greatly

Adapted from Wells CE: Dementia, pseudodementia and dementia praecox. In Fann WE, et al (eds): *Phenomenology and Treatment of Schizophrenia*. New York, Spectrum Publications, 1978.

common in this condition. Unlike the mood disorders, the course of hypochondriasis is usually chronic with fluctuation in symptoms over time but not nearly to the degree seen in the remission and exacerbation of the mood disorders.

Since persons with mood disorders in late life may have exaggerated fears and worries about their bodies, it is not easy to make the differential diagnosis between depression and hypochondriasis. A number of investigators report the prevalence of hypochondriac symptoms to be high in the depressed elderly. De'Alarcon (1964) found that, of 152 depressed patients, 66% of men and 62% of women older than 60 had hypochondriac symptoms, the most common being constipation. These symptoms took on special significance in that elders with hypochondriac complaints proved to be at significant risk for attempted suicide (25% of individuals with hypochondriac symptoms attempted suicide, whereas 7% of those free of such symptoms did so).

Clinical features that assist the clinician in distinguishing hypochondriasis from depressive disorders are presented in Table 9-2. A long and extensive medical history with frequent "doctor shopping" is characteristic of the hypochondriac patient, whereas the depressed patient does not follow this chronic course. One of the most effective means of differentiating an exaggeration of hypochondriac complaints from the onset of a significant major depressive episode is the quality and degree of complaints reported by the patient. Only experience with an individual patient will permit the clinician to accurately assess the severity of a symptom complex.

Hypochondriac patients, in contrast to those suffering from major depressive disorders, do not tolerate antidepressant medications well. Side effects are often exaggerated and may become so severe that the patient presents an entirely new spectrum of complaints, which may persist for many months after the discontinuation of the antidepressant medication. Therefore the clinician must take care when deciding to prescribe antidepressant drugs, further necessitating an accurate diagnosis of a major depressive episode.

TABLE 9-2. Differential Diagnosis of Patients with Depressive Disorders and Hypochondriasis

Depressive disorders	Hypochondriasis
Appear to suffer from their symptoms	Despite numerous reported symptoms, do not appear to suffer significantly
Anger directed inward	Anger directed outward
Social withdrawal is prominent and often dysfunctional	Social interaction is often decreased but not dysfunctional
Will discuss feelings and social life with minimal coaxing	Insist on discussing their physical ailments to the exclusion of intrapersonal and interpersonal issues
A history of episodes of somatic difficulties less frequent in middle life	Frequent episodes of somatic difficulties in mid-life
Condition tends to be cyclic over time	Condition tends to be persistent over time
Tolerate the side effects of antidepressant medications as well as other elderly patients	Do not tolerate the side effects of antidepressants
Suicidal thoughts are common	Suicidal thoughts are rare

Adapted from Blazer DG, Seigler I: *Working with the Family of the Older Adult Patient.* Menlo Park, CA, Addison-Wesley, 1981.

Sleep Disturbances

Changes in the requirements for sleep and the quality of sleep continue throughout the life cycle (Roffwarg et al, 1966). Older persons require less sleep on average than individuals at earlier stages of life. Most individuals older than 60 require around 7 hours of sleep per night, yet sleep requirements of the elderly vary to a considerable extent. The sleep of older persons is lighter and associated with frequent awakenings. The problem of nocturia, especially for men, contributes to these frequent nocturnal awakenings.

The normal changes in sleep with aging can be disturbing to the older person. Many elders are concerned that a decreased amount of sleep will lead to serious illness. They complain of difficulty falling asleep, insufficient sleep, restless sleep, and frequent awakenings. Relatives and friends also become disturbed about the sleep problems in elders. True sleep disorders do present in late life (see previous discussion). Idiopathic insomnia (i.e., insomnia that has no known cause but that is documented by a diagnostic workup in a sleep laboratory) is most common, however. Both acute and chronic organic mental disorders can lead to sleep disturbances. An especially troublesome problem is the "sundowning" syndrome. Frequent awakenings in a darkened room associated with agitation and occasional paranoid or delusional thinking occur in individuals who have difficulty orienting themselves both at home and at the hospital during the night. This condition is further complicated by awakening during rapid eye movement (REM) or dream sleep (i.e., they may awaken and not be able to distinguish the dream from reality).

Depression significantly affects the sleep patterns of elderly persons as it does persons at other stages of the life cycle (Mendels et al, 1966). Therefore the clinician must distinguish the patient with a depressive disorder and the patient with a primary sleep disturbance of another source. This distinction is often a complicated one because depressed older persons frequently concentrate on their sleep disturbance to the exclusion of other complaints. Clinical lore that sleep problems secondary to depression present as early morning awakening does not hold true. Older depressed patients often have difficulty falling asleep, awakening during the night, suffering a fitful and disturbed sleep, as well as awakenings early in the morning. Concentration on the sleep disturbance to the ex-

TABLE 9-3. Differential Diagnosis of Patients with Depressive Disorder and Sleep Disorders

Depressive disorder	Sleep disorders
Sleep complaints one of a symptom complex with other symptoms	Sleep problems, lethargy, and concern about sleep predominate in the symptom presentation
Sleep problems, although severe, often are not spontaneously reported as a major complaint	Sleep problems always predominate as the chief complaint
Affect usually worse in the morning and improves throughout the day	Affect does not vary significantly during the day. Patients may report increased lethargy as the day progresses
Long daytime naps are infrequent	Long daytime naps are frequent
Sleep problems usually of recent onset	Sleep problems often reported for many years

clusion of other symptoms will usually prove unfruitful in yielding the correct diagnosis. Rather, the underlying mood of the patient is the key factor for the differential diagnosis. Patients with sleep disorders are disturbed by their sleep problems, but this disturbance does not invade the total life of the patient as does depression. Depressed patients rarely complain of sleep to the exclusion of other symptoms. Weeks or months into the depression, the sleep problem often fades into the background and other problems surface. A comparison of sleep problems and depressive disorders is presented in Table 9-3.

REFERENCES

Akiskal HS: A biobehavioral approach to depression. In Depue RA (ed): *The Psychobiology of the Depressive Disorders: Implications of the Effects of Stress.* New York, Academic Press, 1979, pp. 407-437.

Angst J, Marikangas K, Scheidegger P, Wicki W: Recurrent brief depression: a new subtype of affective disorders, *Journal of Affective Disorders,* 19:87-98, 1990.

Blazer D: Clinical features in depression and old age: a case for minor depression, *Current Opinion in Psychiatry,* 4:596-599, 1991.

Blazer DG, Hughes D, George LK, Swartz M, Boyer R: Generalized anxiety disorder. In Robins LN, Regier DA (eds): *Psychiatric Disorders in America: The Epidemiologic Catchment Area Study.* New York, Free Press, 1991, pp. 180-203.

Broadhead WE, Blazer DG, George LK, Tse CK: Depression, disability, and days lost form work in a prospective epidemiologic survey, *Journal of the American Medical Association* 264:2524-2528, 1990.

Busse EW, Blazer DG: Disorders related to biological functioning. In Busse EW, Blazer DG (eds): *Handbook of Geriatric Psychiatry,* New York, Van Nostrand Reinhold, 1980, pp. 390-414.

DeAlarcon R: Hypochondriasis and depression in the aged, *Gerontological Clinics,* 6:266, 1964.

Diagnostic and Statistical Manual of Mental Disorders (ed 3). Washington, DC, American Psychiatric Association, 1980.

Diagnostic and Statistical Manual of Mental Disorders (ed 3—revised). Washington, DC, American Psychiatric Association, 1987.

Duckworth GS, Ross H: Diagnostic differences in psychogeriatric patients in Toronto, *Canadian Medical Association Journal,* 112:847, 1975.

Folstein MF, Folstein SE, McHugh PR: "Mini-Mental State": a practical method for grading the cognitive state of patients for the clinician, *Journal of Psychiatric Research,* 12:189, 1975.

Grinker RR, Jr, Miller J, Sabshin M, Nunn R, Nunnally JC: *The Phenomena of Depressions.* New York, Paul B. Hoeker, 1961.

*The International Classification of the Diseases-*10th Revision. Draft of Chapter V (Categories F00.F99/Mental, Behavioral and Developmental Disorders, World Health Organization, Division of Mental Health, Geneva, Switzerland, 1986.

Kahn RL: Memory complaints and impairment in the aged, *Archives of General Psychiatry* 32:1569-1572, 1975.

Kiloh LG: Pseudodementia, *ACTA Psychiatrica Scandinavica* 37:336, 1961.

Lowenthal MF, et al: *Aging and Mental Disorder in San Francisco.* San Francisco, Gossey-Bass, 1967.

Mendels J, Hawkins DR, Scott J: *The Psychophysiology of Sleep and Depression.* Paper presented at the Annual Meeting of the Association for Psychophysiological Study of Sleep, Gainesville, FL, March, 1966.

Post F: Dementia, depression and pseudodementia. In Benson DF, Blumer D (eds): *Psychiatric Aspects of Neurologic Disease,* New York, Grune and Stratton, 1975.

Roffwarg HP, Muzio JN, Dement WC: Ontogenetic development of the human sleep-dream cycle, *Science* 152:604, 1966.

Spitzer RL, Endicott J, Robins E: Research diagnostic criteria. Rationale and reliability, *Archives of General Psychiatry,* 35:773-782, 1978.

Wells CE: Pseudodementia, *American Journal of Psychiatry,* 136:896, 1979.

Categories of Depressive Disorders of Late Life

10

Bipolar Disorder

The study of bipolar disorder in late life is relatively recent, possibly because depressive episodes predominate bipolar disorder in late life. Most elders appear to experience their first manic episode after one or more depressive episodes. Shulman and Post (1980) evaluated 67 older bipolar patients. Nearly one third of these persons initially suffered a depressive episode, and more than 50% of those whose bipolar disorder began with a depressive episode had three more episodes of depression before the first manic episode. On average, 10 years lapsed between the first depressive episode and the first manic episode. Most of these persons experienced episodes of depression in mid-life and the onset of mania in later life. Although manic episodes are relatively uncommon in the elderly and 90% of bipolar patients experience their first manic episode before age 50, manic episodes are by no means nonexistent and may appear for the first time in late life, either as the first sign of the onset of a bipolar disorder or the natural evolution of a bipolar disorder through time.

In a clinical sample of 14 elderly bipolar patients, Spar et al (1979) conclude that bipolar mood disorder may be misdiagnosed frequently in older persons. Inaccurate historical data, atypical course of the illness, and atypical clinical presentation all may contribute to diagnostic error. Older persons admitted to the hospital experiencing a manic episode are frequently poor historians. When past history is a key to accurate diagnosis, the older person (and even the spouse) has frequently forgotten or distorted previous episodes of illness, and family members (e.g., children and siblings) are often geographically dispersed and difficult to contact for additional information. Despite these diagnostic problems, bipolar disorder manifests in late life as it does throughout the life cycle in that (1) there is some genetic contribution to the etiology; (2) there is a good response to lithium; (3) the gender distribution is approximately equal; and (4) the first episodes of the illness usually occur early in life (and therefore there is a history of mood disturbance that can be used to improve diagnostic accuracy). Sibisi (1990), using data from the United Kingdom, shows some differences between the genders and the age-specific inception rates for mania. Although women had a higher inception rate than men during their middle years, cumulative admission rates for manic illness were equal between the genders. The inception rate in the 65 and older group was approximately equal to that in the younger age groups.

The prevalence of bipolar disorder in community populations is low (less than 0.5%), regardless of age (Myers et al, 1984). In geriatric psychiatry units the prevalence is higher. Yassa (1988) studied the prevalence of mania with onset after the age of 60 in 217 patients admitted to a geriatric psychiatry unit in Canada. Nearly 5% of all subjects exhibited symptoms of mania overall, and 9% of the persons suffering a mood disorder were admitted because of manic symptoms.

In a retrospective study of 92 elderly patients admitted to a psychiatric unit in a manic episode, Stone (1989) found that 26% had no prior history of affective illness, 30% had only experienced depression previously, and one half of those with previous depression had at least three episodes of depression before the onset of the first manic illness (finding similar to Shulman and Post, 1980). In the study, patients with a family history of mood disorder had a significantly earlier age of onset of illness. There was evidence of cerebral organic impairment in 24% of the patients, and this group had a significantly later onset of illness. The finding of an association between manic illness and cerebral pathology in older patients reinforced early observation by Stotsky (1973) that becoming manic after age 60 implied organicity unless otherwise proven. Despite the cerebral organic changes, prognosis was good. Lithium prophylaxis, however, was not as effective as earlier in life, since lithium did not alter the number of readmissions and many of these patients suffered lithium toxicity. In contrast with other investigations, Snowden (1991) found few of the 75 elderly psychiatric inpatients with bipolar mood disorder that he examined had experienced a manic episode before the age of 40. The mean onset of the mood disorder was 46 years of age and the mean age of onset of the first manic episode was 60 years of age. Cerebral insults before the onset of first manic attacks were documented in a substantial number of cases. Family history of any mental illness was less common in the older bipolar patients than younger bipolar patients. He concluded that, although the prevalence of bipolar mood disorder is minimal in community populations, bipolar affective disorder is relatively common reason for readmission of elderly patients to geriatric psychiatry units.

In this chapter a case of an older person with a typical manic episode is presented, followed by a discussion of the characteristics of bipolar disorder in late life and a review of the differential diagnosis of bipolar disorder as it applies to older persons, as well as a presentation of the diagnostic workup, the treatment, and the prognosis.

■ CASE PRESENTATION

Mrs. N., a 76-year-old woman, was admitted to a local psychiatric unit in a small rural community with confusion, agitation, and psychotic behavior. She was taking no medications at the time of admission. The family noted that she had become progressively worse over the 6 months before admission. A thorough diagnostic workup revealed no medical problems, yet she exhibited significant cerebral atrophy on CT scan. A sister of the patient had suffered early onset Alzheimer's disease. Local physicians diagnosed Alzheimer's disease and discharged the patient to a nursing home. The patient become progressively more difficult to manage in the nursing home because of agitation and confusion, thus prompting family members to seek referral to a university hospital.

On admission to the university hospital, her symptom presentation was similar to that 2 months before at the local hospital. Medical workup was normal. On review of her history with the family, it was discovered that she had suffered "two nervous breakdowns" in the past. No family members could document the nature of the psychiatric disorder that led to hospitalizations at a state hospital facility (the hospitalizations occurred when the children were young). One daughter remembered, however, that a local doctor had placed the patient on lithium approximately 20 years before the index admission. Lithium was continued for a short time and then stopped. Lithium therapy was therefore reinstituted (300 mg bid) along with the antipsychotic thioridazine (10 mg bid and 50 mg po qhs) on admission.

The patient's lithium level quickly exceeded 1.0 μmol/L and the lithium dose was reduced to 150 mg po bid. The patient tolerated both drugs well, but her symptoms did not improve. After consultation, the patient was referred for electroconvulsive therapy (ECT). After seven treatments, the patient's agitation was dramatically reduced. Two days after completion of the course of ECT (nine treatments total), the patient experienced confusion and difficultly with memory but tolerated this cognitive impairment well. Agitation and psychotic behavior had totally disappeared as symptoms. She was placed on lithium 150 mg po bid as a prophylactic medication 1 week after the last ECT treatment. Approximately 6 months after discharge, cognitive function had not returned to normal, yet the patient still scored 25 out of 30 on the Mini-Mental Status Examination. She was living at home with her son, a single male, age 34, who was working locally. She suffered a mild relapse episode of mania 1 year after ECT, but this episode was responsive to a transient increase in medication.

This patient represents older adults with atypical presentation of manic symptoms. Without knowledge of the rapid onset of her symptoms and the vague history of previous psychiatric disorder (as well as the use of lithium in the past), it would have been impossible to distinguish the symptom picture of this patient from a case of late Alzheimer's disease with psychotic features and agitation. The lack of response to lithium and thioridazine is also typical of individuals suffering severe manic episodes in late life (i.e., such episodes are resistant to pharmacologic intervention). ECT is an appropriate treatment for pharmacologic-resistant, severe cases. The likelihood of relapse is high in bipolar patients, but forms of therapy that are effective previously are usually effective in treating subsequent episodes.

■ PRESENTATIONS OF MANIC SYMPTOMS IN LATE LIFE

Many investigators have commented on the atypical presentation of mania in older adults. Yassa et al (1988) suggest many different presentations in the elderly. In addition to the classical manifestations of mania (i.e., hyperactivity, decreased sleep, flight of ideas, grandiose delusions, and hypersexuality), these authors describe a number of atypical presentations. They describe mania in which the predominate symptom presentation was paranoid delusions. The frequent clinical intuition that older persons with mania present more often with paranoia and fragmented flight of ideas, as opposed to an elated affect, has not been confirmed in control studies (Post, 1982). Mania may also present as a syndrome of reversible cognitive impairment, which appears much like an Alzheimer's type of dementia (as illustrated in the case described previously). Symptoms of pseudodementia in mania usually are severe, and these patients are difficult to manage. Confusion, agitation, and incomprehensible loud verbalizations are typical of these individuals.

Another presentation of mania in older adults is that of irritability and anger without evidence of elated affect (Pitt, 1974). Most investigators, however, do not find irritability and anger to be more common in late life bipolar disorder than in manic episodes earlier in life (Glasser and Rabins, 1984).

Another presentation in older adults is dysphoric mania. Epstein (1978) suggests that depressive thoughts associated with symptoms of mania are more common in late life than earlier in the life cycle. Other investigators, however, do not report the so-called mixed manic episodes to be more common in late life (Glasser and Rabins, 1984; Yassa et al, 1988). Post et al (1989) note that many patients at the peak of a manic episode exhibit substantial dysphoria and anxiety. Dysphoric manics typically have a greater number of previous hospitalizations and display less rapid cycling, both in the year before and during the index hospitalization. Although dysphoric manics may have a poor prognosis compared with other manics and respond less well to lithium carbonate, Post et al (1989) suggest that they may respond better to carbamazepine. They did not find age to be associated with dysphoric mania, although they studied mostly younger manics.

■ THE ETIOLOGY OF MANIC DISORDERS IN LATE LIFE

Few question the hereditary predisposition to manic episodes, regardless of age. Yet most investigators do not believe that the genetic predisposition to bipolar disorder is as great in late life as in early stages of the life cycle (especially for first onset bipolar disorder). Hopkinson (1964) found that early onset psychotic episodes are more than twice as likely to be associated with a first-degree family member suffering a bipolar disorder as late onset (after age 50) psychotic episodes. Glasser and Rabins (1984) found that nearly 25% of a group of 42 persons with late onset mania (first episode of mania occurring at an average of 51 years) had a positive family history of a mood disorder in a first-degree relative. Those bipolar episodes that are driven predominately by heredity usually present for the first time early in the life cycle. Other etiologic factors may therefore be more prominent with increased age.

Despite the biologic predisposition to bipolar illness, life events also contribute to the onset of manic episodes. Glasser and Haldipur (1983) studied 46 patients with bipolar disorder to determine the association of age of onset of the disorder and stressful life events. Persons 20 years of age and older were more likely to report a stressful event before the first and before subsequent manic episodes than persons with onset in adolescence. Dunner et al (1979) found that two thirds of patients with a first-onset manic episode reported a stressful event associated with the onset of the episode. Yassa et al (1988) found 7 of the 10 persons with late-onset mania reported life events associated with the onset of the episode that were severe enough to disrupt usual activities of daily living. It is difficult to determine whether stressful life events play a greater role in the onset of late life manic episodes than at earlier stages of life.

Medications also precipitate manic episodes. Yassa et al (1988) reviewed medications that can lead to manic episodes, including corticosteroids, levodopa, decongestants, bronchodialators, phencyclidine, and thyroid replacement. Illnesses may also contribute to the onset of manic episode (Yassa et al, 1988). These illnesses include B12 deficiency, end-stage renal disease, and dramatic interventions for treatment serious illnesses, such as surgical procedures and renal dialysis. Krauthammer and Klerman (1978), in a review of the literature, note that secondary mania (i.e., secondary to medical and pharmacologic precipitants) was more likely to occur later in life than primary or idiopathic mania and was likely to be associated with a positive family history. In other words, exogenous factors are more likely to precipitate a manic episode in a person predisposed by hereditary factors.

Cerebral pathology may contribute to manic episodes in late life. Shukla et al (1987) studied 20 patients who developed mania after head trauma. Association was found between the severity of head trauma (based on the length of the posttraumatic amnesia), posttraumatic seizure disorder, and the type of bipolar disorder. Manic episodes were characterized by irritable mood rather than euphoria. Psychosis occurred in only 15% of the sample, and 70% had no prior depressive episodes. Bipolar disorder was absent among all of the first-degree relatives. Although most of these patients were young (average age of 25), the finding is relevant to manic episodes in the elderly.

Spicer et al (1973), in a national survey of the British Isles, conclude that some cases of mania among the elderly may be attributable to dementia. Shulman and Post (1980) found that an association between cerebral vascular accidents and mania in the elderly. McDonald et al (1992), in a retrospective study of 12 elderly patients with manic symptoms, compared age- and gender-matched controls, found the manic patients demonstrated a significantly greater number of large subcortical hyperintensities on magnetic resonance imaging (MRI), particularly in the middle third of the brain parenchyma. In contrast to MRI changes in late life depression, these subjects exhibited no differences in the size of the ventricles nor the presence of perventricular hyperintensities.

■ DIFFERENTIAL DIAGNOSIS

Numerous nomenclatures have evolved to classify the major mood disorders. A comparison of the usual systems of classifications is presented in Table 10-1. The orientation of diagnoses based on etiology, as reflected by DSM II, dramatically changed with the development of the genetic taxonomy of unipolar and bipolar disorder. DSM III-R deviates only slightly from the genetic taxonomy, yet is compatible. There have been no studies in the literature that apply this system specifically to older patients in terms of frequency or symptoms distribution. Yet the symptoms of bipolar mood disorder are known to change with aging, as noted previously.

Older persons most commonly suffer bipolar I or bipolar II disorder (the relative prevalence of the two disorders is not known). The diagnosis of the older adult with bipolar disorder is based, as noted in the description of the subtypes, on symptom presentation, an accurate past history, and family history.

The differential diagnosis of bipolar disorder in the older adult must first include differentiation of a manic episode from an agitated depression. Since older persons are less likely to exhibit euphoric symptoms in the midst of a manic episode, the agitation and irritability typical of manic episodes may be confused with agitated depression. Course of the illness and the lack of response to antidepressant medications (coupled with a accurate past history) should alert clinicians to the possibility of a manic episode.

A second disorder that must be distinguished from a manic episode is a dementing disorder with significant agitation and paranoid symptoms. As exemplified in the case described previously, manic episodes may accompany mild-to-moderate cognitive im-

TABLE 10-1. Diagnostic Classification Systems of the Major Affective Disorders

DSM-II	GENETIC TAXONOMY	DSM-III-R
Manic-depressive illness, manic type	Unipolar mania At least one hospitalization for mania but no depressive episodes	Bipolar disorder, manic Currently in a manic episode
Manic-depressive illness, circular type	Bipolar I Both manic and depressive episodes that require treatment	Bipolar, depressed Past history of a manic episode
Manic-depresive illness, depressed type	Bipolar II Family history of mania or hypomania and depressive episodes that require treatment; manic symptoms that never lead to hospitalization	Bipolar disorder, mixed NOS Major depressive episode and at least one episode of hypomania
	Bipolar III Family history of mania or hypomania; no personal history of mania or hypomania but at least one hospitalization for a depressive episode	Major depression No history of a manic episode; currently in a major depressive episode

From DePue and Monroe, 1979.

pairment, and in the midst of a severe episode the older person appears to suffer a severe demeaning disorder with marked agitation and paranoia. Language may deteriorate to a word salad.

The diagnosis of a manic episode can be made only when it is established that an organic factor has not initiated and maintained the manic-like behavior. Organic mood disorder with manic symptoms may derive from psychoactive substances, such as amphetamines or steroids, or to other known physical problems, such as multiple sclerosis (APA, 1987). Both of these causes, however, are rare in older adults. When an episode of mania is precipitated by an organic factor, such as a antidepressant medication (or even), the correct diagnosis is a manic episode if the symptoms persist after the organic agent is removed (e.g., discontinuing the antidepressant medication).

Some schizophrenic disorders (especially the paranoid type) are characterized by irritability, anger, and psychotic symptoms that are difficult to distinguish from a manic episode in late life (DSM-III-R). In these situations, however, past history generally permits the clinician to distinguish the disorders. During the acute phase, both can be treated successfully with antipsychotic medications. Lithium is essential in the prevention of recurrent episodes of bipolar disorders, yet is of little benefit in preventing recurrence of paranoid symptoms in schizophrenic disorders.

■ DIAGNOSTIC WORKUP

The diagnostic workup of the patient suspected to be in a manic episode presented in the box on p. 179. The key to an accurate diagnosis is a history of the patient's past and present symptoms and a family history of mood disorders. Therefore family members from at least two generations should be interviewed, if possible, to corroborate reports from

Diagnostic Workup for Suspected Bipolar Mood Disorders

Patient's History

Symptoms and signs
Previous episodes of mania or depression
Previous treatment of mania or depression
   Hospitalization or outpatient
   Response to specific medications or electroconvulsive therapy
Family history of mania, depression, suicide, alcohol abuse, or psychiatric treatment
Assessment of functioning in present living environment
Assessment of suicidal thoughts, gestures, or attempts
Social adaptation, including marital status, socioeconomic status, and the support network
Premorbid personality

Data from Two Family Members

History of mania, depression, suicide, alcohol, or psychiatric treatment in family

Mental Status Examination

Affect, mood
Psychomotor behavior
Evidence of a thought disorder
Evidence of cognitive dysfunction

Physical Examination

Review of endocrine system
Neurologic examination

Laboratory Tests

Chemical screen of blood
Thyroid panel
Computerized axial tomography scan or magnetic resonance imaging (if questionable dementia)

the patient. The patient frequently is incapable of providing an accurate history of his or her past symptoms or of symptoms experienced by other family members. Previous history of a response to a psychotropic medication or electroconvulsive therapy can provide valuable guidelines to therapeutic management when symptoms recur in late life.

■ TREATMENT OF BIPOLAR MOOD DISORDER IN LATE LIFE

A decision tree for the psychobiologic treatment of manic episodes in late life is presented in Figure 10-1. As with the patient suffering from a depressive episode, the first decision to be made by the clinician is whether the patient requires hospitalization or not. If the manic behavior is so disruptive as to severely inhibit the patient's ability to manage daily activities or personal relationships, hospitalization is indicated. Civil commitment proceedings against the manic patient should be avoided, if possible. The older

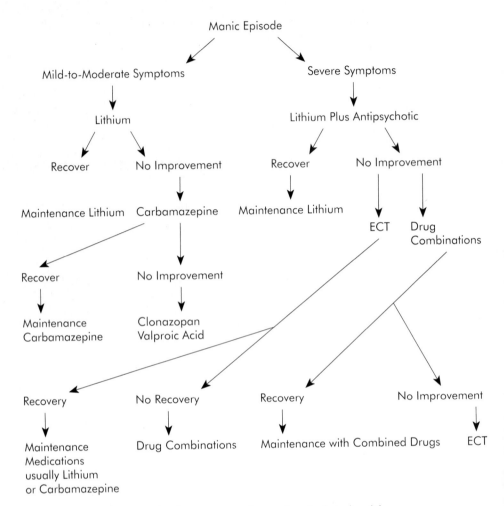

Figure 10-1. Decision tree for the treatment of a manic episode in late life.

manic can be most convincing to judges or magistrates who determine the appropriateness of the commitment (especially during a euphoric and less-agitated manic episode). If the clinician is convinced that hospitalization is necessary, an alliance with patient and family usually facilitates voluntary hospitalization. The clinician can discuss with the patient, in the presence of the family, his or her concerns about the patient's behavior. A plea to the patient to accept hospitalization for the sake of the family, although the patient may not believe hospitalization is necessary, is often a successful tactic.

Antipsychotic medication is the first-line treatment for acute agitated behavior in the manic patient. The drugs of choice are haloperidol or thioridazine (depending on the cardiovascular status of the patient). The potential cardiovascular side effects of thioridazine must be considered when one is choosing a medication for the treatment of manic episodes in elderly persons. Agitated behavior and changing dietary status invariably alter the patient's ability to metabolize the antipsychotic drug, so pharmacotherapy must proceed with caution. The acute symptoms of mania are usually brought under control within 24 to 72 hours with antipsychotic drugs.

Lithium carbonate is the cornerstone of prevention of recurrent symptoms of mania. Lithium therapy should be instituted concurrently with the antipsychotic medication. The renal status of the patient should be determined before lithium therapy is instituted, however. A chemistry screen in patients without a history of cardiac or renal disease is one means of screening renal status. If compromised renal function is suspected, then a 24-hour creatinine clearance can be obtained. However, it may be difficult to obtain estimates of clearance in uncooperative patients. In extreme cases, lithium carbonate may be prescribed in very low doses with close daily monitoring of plasma levels. If the patient is known to experience cardiac or renal diseases that preclude the use of lithium carbonate and symptoms are not controlled by antipsychotic medications, the therapeutic alternative is ECT. Lithium carbonate is an excellent medication for the control of symptoms of acute manic episodes, but the onset of lithium effects may take from 7 to 10 days—much too long to use lithium alone to treat the severely agitated patient.

Elderly patients are subject to the same toxic side effects of lithium carbonate as younger persons (see Chapter 19). The predominant characteristic of lithium toxicity in late life, however, is an acute organic brain syndrome with extreme neuromuscular irritability and impaired consciousness (which on occasion may lead to coma). The symptoms may occur even when lithium is in the high range of the normal therapeutic window (0.8 to 1.2 μmol/L). A lithium level of less than 1.0 μmol/L, however, is generally sufficient not only for the treatment of an acute manic episode but also the prophylaxis of recurrent episodes. Lithium can be maintained in the range of 0.4 to 0.6 μmol/L. Most older adults do not develop toxic symptoms when begun on lithium carbonate 150 mg bid. The daily dose may then be increased by 150 mg qod with close monitoring of blood levels. The maximum daily dose of lithium in older persons rarely exceeds 600 mg qd.

After maintenance lithium is instituted and manic symptoms subside, the patient should be continued on lithium carbonate for 6 to 12 months. If there are no recurrence of symptoms, serious consideration should be given to withdrawal from the medication gradually over 1 to 2 weeks. If recurrence follows withdrawal, the patient's lithium dosage should be reinstituted, and maintenance therapy should be continued indefinitely, with frequent checks. Plasma levels should be checked every 6 weeks to 3 months and a thyroid panel scheduled once a year.

When lithium therapy is ineffective, other medications may be prescribed. Carbamazepine is the most intensively studied of the alternatives to lithium (NIMH, 1989). Carbamazepine may be prescribed with lithium to augment the effects of lithium. Usual dose in the elderly is 200 to 600 mg qd. Carbamazepine may be effective in individuals who cannot tolerate lithium therapy (not an uncommon problem faced by clinicians treating older adults) and in situations where persons are suffering from rapid cycling. Carbamazepine may rarely lead to acute agranulocytosis but is more likely to lead to a transient decrease in the white blood cell count. Therefore periodic blood counts should be obtained. Side effects are less severe with carbamazepine than with lithium, but the nausea associated with the drug can be problematic in older adults. Clorazepam in doses of 0.5 to 2 mg qd is another alternative to lithium therapy but is very sedating when used in late life.

Valproic acid also can be prescribed to augment or replace lithium carbonate in the treatment of manic illness across the life cycle. A number of investigators recommend using either valproic acid alone or in combination with lithium (NIMH, 1989). Organic mood disorder with manic symptoms may be especially responsive to valproic acids. Usual dose does not exceed 500 mg qd in divided doses. Gastrointestinal problems may emerge as with carbamazepine, as can bone marrow toxicity.

If medications are not effective in controlling the manic episode, then ECT is a useful alternative therapy (see case report). ECT is administered by a protocol described in Chapter 20. Since it is most difficult to obtain patient compliance with ECT while the patient is manic, careful work with the family of the patient is important. Usually with the encouragement of the family members, the elderly will agree to ECT without being coerced or threatened. In severe cases, therapy may need be administer without the patient's agreement (e.g., as when the patient is incompetent to make the decision).

The severely manic older adult usually requires hospitalization, at least until medications can be controlled and behavior is acceptable in the outpatient setting. Although civil commitment may be necessary to institute hospitalization, work with the family usually facilitates hospitalization in the uncooperative elder, thus obviating the need for commitment. Periodic visits by family members to the patient while hospitalized and a supportive nursing staff usually render the initial hospitalization experience an accepted one and the elder manic usually, although begrudgingly, cooperates. When civil commitment is necessary, however, it should be vigorously pursued.

Once in the hospital, the manic patient must be monitored carefully. The frail manic elder with extreme agitation is at increased risk for falls and other injuries. When older manics with aggressive and intrusive behavior are hospitalized on general psychiatric wards, younger psychiatric patients, especially adolescents, may react and physically abuse the manic elder. In other cases the manic elder may be dangerous to patients and nursing staff.

Working with the manic elder necessarily involves family therapy. The family should be made aware of the nature of the manic episode, and help should be provided through instruction so they can better tolerate the manic behavior. Time spent with the family, however, should not preclude time spent with the patient. If the patient is hospitalized, the clinician at first should instruct family members to limit the duration of their visits with the patient during the initial days of hospitalization, usually to not more than 15 to 30 minutes per day. Phone calls between the patient and family should be limited by the hospital staff, because family members feel guilty with the pressure or repeated phone calls from manic patients who believe hospitalization is unnecessary.

An issue that the clinician who works with manic elders must face is the accountability of the patient for financial and other business matters. Older manics often desire to cancel an old will and write a new one based on recent events. Although the clinician may believe that the patient's disease has interfered with judgment required to make such a decision, the person legally has a right to change his or her will if the heirs and the extent of property are known. When manic episodes are accompanied by delusional thinking, the patient may actually believe that a son or daughter is no longer family or may underestimate the value of a piece of property, especially real estate holdings. Clinicians should be aware of the laws applicable in the state in which he or she practices. The clinician may express an opinion to the patient about the advisability of making major changes in business or personal affairs but must work within the limits of the law in such matters. The problem should be explained to the family after the patient has granted permission. After the clinician discusses the situation with family members, they may take legal action. The clinician will inevitably be asked to testify in such cases.

The manic patient may summon a lawyer if committed to the hospital. The physician should then obtain the patient's permission to discuss the case with the lawyer and talk with the lawyer only about the patient's illness and what typically can be expected from the illness. Specific discussion of the patient's interaction with family members and views of whether particular actions are justified should be avoided.

■ PROGNOSIS

A number of outcome studies of manic illness in late life have been reported, and these reports do not show marked deviation from studies of the outcome of manic disorders and other stages of the life cycle. Harrow et al (1990) in a follow-up of the psychobiology of depression cohort found a large percentage of manic patients experiencing difficulty in posthospital adjustments. Over 40% experienced manic symptoms during the follow-up. In general, manic patients experienced a poorer outcome than unipolar depressives. Of interest, manic patients taking lithium carbonate did not show a better outcome than those not taking lithium.

Broadhead and Jacoby (1990) followed 35 manic patients who were 60 years of age and older and compared the outcome on clinical and cognitive measures with 35 patients below the age of 40. CT scan comparisons were made between elderly and age-matched normal controls. The elderly were clinically indistinguishable from younger patients except that the younger patients experienced a more severe course of illness. CT and cognitive testing results, in the elderly group, however, showed evidence of changes which support the view that cerebral organic factors play an important role in the genesis of manic episodes in late life.

Young and Falk (1989) studied the relationships between age and clinical signs and symptoms in 40 manic inpatients. Soon after admission, some psychopathologic features were less prominent in older patients. In older patients, after 2 weeks of treatment with lithium and neuroleptics, there was greater residual total pathology, higher ratings of some clinical features and less change in total pathology. Older patients tended to be hospitalized longer and were more likely to be hospitalized during follow-up. In the study, however, the oldest patient was only 66.

Dhingra and Rabins (1991) performed a 5- to 7-year follow-up of elderly individuals hospitalized with manic episodes resulting from a bipolar disorder. A majority of those hospitalized for mania were alive and living independently 5 years after hospitalization. However, 32% had experienced a decline in cognitive function and mortality rates were higher than expected for an aged control population. Of interest, patients with bipolar disorder not only had an earlier age of the onset of the disorder but were less likely to be rehospitalized than patients with unipolar affective disorder.

REFERENCES

American Psychiatric Association: *Diagnostic and Statistical Manual Mental Disorders* (ed 3—revised). Washington, DC, American Psychiatric Association 1987.

Broadhead J, Jacoby R: Mania in old age: a first prospective study, *International Journal of Geriatric Psychiatry* 5:215-222, 1990.

DePue RA, Monroe SM: The unipolar-bipolar distinction in the depressive disorders: implications for stress-onset interactions. In DePue RA (ed): *The Psychobiology of the Depressive Disorders: Implications for the Effects of Stress*. New York, Academic Press, 1979, pp. 23-53.

Dhingra U, Rabins PV: Mania in the elderly: a 5-7 year follow-up, *Journal of American Geriatric Society* 39:581-583, 1991.

Dunner DL, Patrick V, Fieve RR: Life events and the onset of bipolar affective illness, *American Journal of Psychiatry* 136:508-511, 1979.

Epstein LJ: Clinical geropsychiatry. In Raichel W (ed): *Clinical Aspects of Aging*. Baltimore, Williams and Wilkins, 1978, pp. 105-115.

Glasser G, Haldipur CV: Life events in early and late onset of bipolar disorder, *American Journal of Psychiatry* 140:215-217, 1983.

Glasser M, Rabins T: Mania in the elderly, *Aging* 13:210-213, 1984.

Harrow, M, Goldberg JF, Grossman LS, Meltzer HY: Bipolar disorder: a naturalistic follow-up study, *Archives of General Psychiatry* 47:665-671, 1990.

Hopkinson G: A genetic study of affective illness in patients over fifty, *British Journal of Psychiatry* 140:244-254, 1964.

Krauthammer C, Klerman GL: Secondary mania, *Archives of General Psychiatry* 35:1333-1339, 1978.

McDonald WM, Krishnan KRR, Doraswami PM, Blazer DG: The recurrence of subcortical hyperintensities in elderly subjects with mania, *Psychiatry Research* 40:211-220, 1992.

Myers JK, Weissman MM, Tichler GL, Holcer CE, Overshell H, et al: Six month prevalence of psychiatric disorders, *Archives of General Psychiatry* 41:959-967, 1984.

National Institute of Mental Health: *Report from the NIMH Workshop on Treatment of Bipolar Disorder*. Bethesda, MD, NIMH Division of Clinical Research, NIMH Division of Intramural Research, 1989.

Pitt B: *Psychogeriatrics*. Edinburgh, Churchill Livingstone, 1974, pp. 69-75.

Post F: Affective disorders in old age. Paykel, ES (ed): *Handbook of Affective Disorders*. New York, Gilford Press, 1982, p. 393-402.

Post RM, Rubinow DR, Uhde TM, Roy-Byrne PP, Linnoila M, et al: Dysphoric mania: clinical and biological correlates, *Archives of General Psychiatry* 46:353-358, 1989.

Shukla S, Cok BL, Mukherjee S, Godwin C, Miller MG: Mania following head trauma, *American Journal of Psychiatry* 144:93-96, 1987.

Shulman K, Post F: Bipolar affective disorder in old age, *British Journal of Psychiatry* 136:26-32, 1980.

Sibisi CD: Sex differences in the age of onset of bipolar affective illness, *British Journal of Psychiatry* 156:842-845, 1990.

Snowden, J: A retrospective case-note study of bipolar disorder in old age, *British Journal of Psychiatry* 158:45-49, 1991.

Spar JE, Ford CV, Liston HE: Bipolar affective disorders in aging patients, *Journal of Clinical Psychiatry* 40:504-507, 1979.

Spicer CC, Hare EH, Slater E: Neurotic and psychotic forms of depressive illness: evidence from age incidence in a national sample, *British Journal of Psychiatry* 123:535-541, 1973.

Stone K: Mania in the elderly, *British Journal of Psychiatry* 155:220-224, 1989.

Stotsky BA: Psychosis in the elderly. In Einsdorvr C, Fann WE (eds): *Psychopharmacology and Aging*. New York, Plenum Press, 1973, pp. 193-203.

Yassa R, Nair NPV, Iskendar H: Late-onset bipolar disorder, *Psychiatric Clinics of North America* 11 (1):117-131, 1988.

Yassa R, Nair V, Nastase C, Camille Y, Belzile L: Prevalence of bipolar disorder in a psychogeriatric population, *Journal of Affective Disorders* 14:197-201, 1988.

Young RC, Falk JR: Age, manic psychopathology and treatment response, *International Journal of Geriatric Psychiatry* 4:73-78, 1989.

11

Major Depression

The majority of older adults admitted to psychiatric hospitals or to psychogeriatric units for symptoms of a mood disorder are diagnosed with unipolar mood disorder (i.e., major depression). Dysthymic disorders, bereavement, and minor depression are much more common in community settings and primary care facilities, although major depression is a frequent diagnosis in these settings as well. Since major depression is the core depressive syndrome that has been studied across the life cycle (from epidemiology to psychobiology), a review of epidemiology, etiology, and the diagnostic workup of major depression would be redundant, since there are chapters on epidemiology, biologic origins, psychologic origins, social origins, and diagnostic workup elsewhere in this book. Therefore the focus in this chapter is on the diagnosis, differential diagnosis, and treatment of the older adult experiencing major depression.

■ CASE PRESENTATION

Mrs. Washington was admitted to a psychiatric unit after a 3-month history of progressive decline in her physical function, suspiciousness regarding her sister, and frequent crying spells. She was initially evaluated by a primary care physician, at the insistence of her sister (with whom she lived for many years), and he immediately referred her for hospital psychiatric evaluation given the dramatic change he witnessed in her behavior.

On admission to the hospital, Mrs. Washington reported that she had done well until 3 months before admission. At that time, her sister sold some property that she owned, and the patient became quite concerned that the financial transaction was detrimental to her sister, which in turn meant that the patient would become financially responsible for her. The financial transaction appeared reasonable to other members of the family. The patient withdrew from her sister and began to doubt that she could trust her. She also reported difficulty sleeping (primarily early morning awakening and frequent awakenings during the night), decreased appetite (she had lost about 4 pounds), and loss of interest in her usual activities of cooking, house cleaning, and working at a store owned by the patient, her sister, and her brother in a small North Carolina community. She stopped going to church after almost perfect attendance for nearly 50 years and refused to invite others to her home, a behavior unlike Mrs. Washington and disagreeable to her sister (who had always relied on the patient to initiate social contact with others). The patient began to feel "anxious" and spent much of the day pacing throughout the house. Previously accurate "to a fault" in keeping the financial records of the family, the patient, over the 2 months before admission, neglected to pay a number of bills, which led to a temporary discontinuation of her health insurance policy.

During the mental status examination, the patient was an alert, oriented, and pleasant but obviously disturbed and depressed woman. She spontaneously expressed her disappointment and concern regarding her sister's behavior and, although she did not believe that she suffered from a psychiatric illness, nevertheless recognized that "something is the matter." She made no protest against being admitted to a psychiatric unit and interacted well with patients on the unit from the day she was admitted. Early in her admission, however, she would not leave her room except with the encouragement of the nursing staff.

Mrs. Washington, a widow, had never suffered an episode similar to the one that she described on admission. She was grieved at the death of her husband when she was very young (age 24), but she had adapted to this loss well, moving at that time to live with her sister. She began work after 4 years of living as a homemaker. Always outgoing and a "take charge person," the patient's behavior complemented the life-style of the sister, and the two had related extremely well over many years. The patient was well-known in her community for her work at the church and with the local garden club.

On admission, the patient received a medical workup. She was found to be in excellent health with no previous serious physical problems. Her electrocardiogram was normal. A thyroid panel showed a slight increase in thyroxine, but this was repeated 10 days later and was found to have returned to normal. Her dexamethasone-suppression test results were negative (a postdexamethasone cortisol of 0.3 μg/dl). There were no neurologic abnormalities and therefore no imaging studies were obtained.

After admission and the diagnostic workup, the patient was begun on nortriptyline 25 mg po qhs, which was increased over 5 days to 75 mg po qhs. Almost immediately, the patient responded to the medication well, with improved sleep and an improved appetite. Approximately 10 days after the initiation of pharmacotherapy, the patient subjectively recognized that she was "doing better," and the negative feelings toward her sister gradually disappeared. She continued to believe that the sister's business judgment was not good but reflected philosophically that "it is her money and she can do with it what she likes. Actually, she is quite well off financially and should have no problem in the future." The patient never referred to her previous fear that she would be forced to become a caretaker for the sister.

She participated in a cognitive psychotherapy group while hospitalized and not only enjoyed the group but, according to the therapist, participated actively. The patient was discharged from the hospital after 2 weeks. She was followed at 1 month, 3 months, and 6 months after hospitalization. At each visit, she reported that things were going "great" and that she had not felt so well in many years. After 9 months, the patient requested that she be taken off the medication. The nortriptyline was gradually withdrawn over a 1-month period. The patient responded well to the withdrawal (with no return of sleep difficulties or depressive symptoms). She was seen again 1 year after discontinuation of the drug and was doing well. At that point, the patient was discharged from therapy.

The patient returned a call to the psychiatrist 6 years later. She reported, at that time, that she was beginning to feel "those same funny feelings I experienced before." On this occasion, the symptoms were slightly different in that she was experiencing more somatic problems (especially pain in her leg). She had undergone major surgery for lower back pain, and the slow recovery from this surgery, she believed, had led to the recurrence of the "problem with my nerves." She was immediately begun on nortriptyline 75 mg po qhs, to which she responded well. In the interim the patient's sister had died and, 18 months after her sister's death, the patient had married. The marriage had been somewhat stressful, since her husband suffered significant physical problems. Nevertheless, the patient had adapted to both the death of her sister and her husband's illnesses without a recurrence of the depressive symptoms. The patient continued on nortriptyline for 9 months and once again withdrew from the medication without difficulty.

■ DIAGNOSIS AND DIFFERENTIAL DIAGNOSIS

The symptoms of a major depressive episode are outlined in the box below. The symptoms of major depression must not be secondary to a substance, such as medications or elicit drugs, and is not accounted for by uncomplicated bereavement. In addition, although psychotic symptoms may be present, the depressive episode should not be better classified as a schizoaffective disorder, schizophrenia, schizophreniform disor-

---

Diagnostic Criteria for a Major Depressive Episode

The older adult must report five or more of the following symptoms lasting for at least 2 weeks or more. One of the symptoms reported must be either anhedonia (loss of interest or pleasure) or a depressed mood. Anhedonia is a more frequent symptom of major depression in later life than at younger ages.

Criteria Symptoms

Depressed mood (older adults often report feeling empty or hopeless).

Loss of interest or pleasure in usual activities (anhedonia is a common symptom of major depression in late life, especially major depression with melancholia).

Significant weight loss or weight gain (older persons suffering from major depression rarely report weight gain. Weight loss is usually less than at earlier stages of the life cycle, but a 3- to 4-pound weight loss in a person who has maintained weight for many years is clinically significant).

Insomnia or hypersomnia (hypersomnia is rare in late life major depression).

Psychomotor agitation and retardation (symptoms similar to those at earlier stages of the life cycle).

Fatigue (fatigue is a common symptom of major depression and is no more common in the elderly than at other stages of the life cycle).

Feelings of worthlessness or guilt (guilt is less common as a symptom of depression in late life).

Diminished ability to think or concentrate (older adults do not complain more of difficulty concentrating when suffering from major depression but are more likely to exhibit abnormalities on detailed psychologic depression secondary to diminished cognitive abilities than younger persons during a depressive episode).

Recurrent thoughts of death or suicidal thoughts (older persons are less likely to report suicidal thoughts, although they are likely to report during a depressive episode that they have little interest in remaining alive).

Adapted from DSM-III-R.

der, or delusional disorder. A major depressive episode may be part of a unipolar disorder.

The major depressive episode may be diagnosed as with or without melancholia and with or without psychotic features. There is considerable debate among phenomenologists regarding the characteristics of melancholia that should be included in the diagnosis. The more common lists include the following: loss of interest or pleasure in most activities; lack of reactivity to usual stimuli; diurnal variation (depression worse in the morning); early morning awakening; psychomotor retardation or agitation, as observed by others; significant weight loss; previous episodes of depression that remitted completely; and a previous response to somatic therapies (e.g., antidepressants or electroconvulsive therapy [ECT]). Investigators working with DSM-IV are debating whether criteria for the subtype of melancholia should include treatment response. Regardless, symptoms of melancholia are common in late life depression, but the diagnosis of melancholia does not appear to be more common among persons admitted to psychiatric units for major depression in late life than at other stages of the life cycle. Psychotic depression is diagnosed when individuals report mood-congruent psychotic symptoms. Although psychotic mood disorders are usually more severe than nonpsychotic mood disorders and are less likely to respond to antidepressant therapy (thus requiring ECT or combination antidepressant/antipsychotic drugs), there is no evidence that psychotic depression is necessarily a more severe depressive episode. In other words, one can suffer a severe major depression with melancholia without receiving the diagnosis of a psychotic depression. aIn contrast, persons such as Mrs. Washington may suffer a psychotic major depressive episode that is moderately severe and does respond to antidepressant medications.

Other subtypings of major depression have emerged, including rapid cycling (multiple episodes [usually four or more] of major depression that meet criteria within a 12-month period) and major depression with a seasonal pattern. Seasonal pattern is probably less frequent in late life than earlier in life. There is no evidence that rapid cycling is more or less common in late life that at other stages of the life cycle.

Perhaps the most significant suggestions for changing the nomenclature in DSM-IV regarding major depression is the addition of longitudinal core specifiers (American Psychiatric Association, 1991). Many persons across the life cycle, but especially in late life, do not report a return to full functioning and to their previous mood state after an episode of major depression. In addition, other persons who enter an episode of major depression have suffered a less severe disturbance in mood before the episode. Therefore the DSM-IV task force is suggesting a number of possible modifiers for major depression, which include the following: single episode with antecedent dysthymia; single episode without antecedent dysthymia; recurrent episode with antecedent dysthymia with full recovery; recurrent episode with antecedent dysthymia without full interepisode recovery; recurrent episode without antecedent dysthymia with full interepisode recovery; and recurrent episode with antecedent dysthymia and without full interepisode recovery. The task force also recommends longitudinal core specifiers for bipolar disorder to provide the clinician the ability to designate the antecedent mood state and whether the individual recovered fully from the episode.

Regardless of the subtyping of major depression, the treatment plan is usually standard and follows that presented in Figure 11-1. The one exception to the figure is the

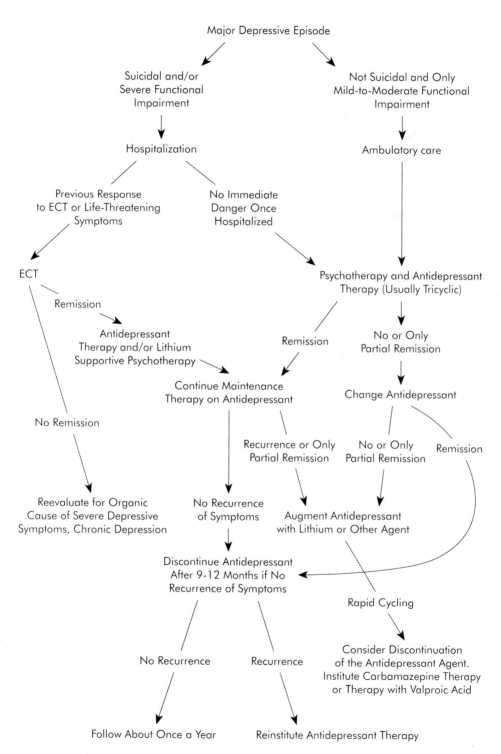

Figure 11-1. Therapeutic tree for treating a major depressive episode.

belief by some that major depression without melancholia of only mild-to-moderate severity should not be treated with antidepressant medications initially. Rather, these investigators suggest that a course of psychotherapy (e.g., cognitive or inner personal therapy) should be initiated before antidepressant therapy. There are no set rules, however, for when to prescribe an antidepressant medication. Even individuals with mild to moderately severe nonmelancholic major depression in late life may respond to antidepressant therapy. In contrast, some persons with more severe major depression (with or without melancholia) do not respond to medications or other somatic therapies. The clinician must, therefore, decide on the appropriate therapy based on previous experience with individual patients, presence or absence of physical health problems that may preclude somatic therapies, presence or absence of extenuating circumstances (e.g., severe stressful life events that may be associated with the onset of the depressive episode), and a trial-and-error approach to therapy.

The first decision to be made by the clinician, once the diagnosis of major depression has been established, is whether the individual can be treated in an outpatient setting. Most often, the older adult can be treated without great difficulty as an outpatient. Support from family members (see Chapter 18) is essential, however, to ensure compliance with therapy and to monitor the outcome of therapy. If the clinician is concerned about suicide, then he or she should admit the patient to the hospital. Even if the older adult protests admission, a frank discussion with the family regarding the risk of suicide is usually sufficient to encourage the patient to be hospitalized. Rarely is civil commitment necessary once the family is convinced that inpatient treatment is necessary.

Other than the risk of suicide, the main factors which must be considered in the decision to hospitalize or not are the functional status of the depressed elder and the difficulty of implementing and monitoring therapies (especially somatic therapies). Most depression rating scales correlate with function but are not analogous to function.aOlder adults may be severely depressed (Hamilton Depression Rating scores of 30 or more) but may be maintained at home because they continue to eat, can toilet themselves, and have around them a supportive family environment. In other cases a less severe depression may manifest with appreciable functional impairment. For example, the older adult (for whatever reason) may not be willing to fix proper meals, maintain hygiene, or take medications that are necessary for maintenance of physical health. In such cases, hospitalization is essential.

Hospitalization is also recommended when somatic therapies are difficult to monitor and/or ECT is to be prescribed. To administer proper antidepressant therapy, the older person may need to be withdrawn from a number of psychotropic medications, a difficult task in the outpatient setting. In addition, the elder may have exhibited many adverse side effects to antidepressants in the past. In other cases the elder may be prescribed adjunct therapies, such as lithium, in the presence of physical health problems, such as renal disease. In each case, daily (or hourly) observance may be necessary to institute therapy effectively. If the older person has experienced problems with postural hypotension, sitting and standing blood pressures can be checked frequently in the hospital.

Once the setting for therapy has been established, therapy for major depression usually consists of a combination of psychotherapy and antidepressant therapy. If the elder suffers from a major depression with melancholia, the clinician may elect to begin with pharmacotherapy alone. If significant psychosocial factors are believed to be contributors to the depressive syndrome, a combination of therapies is usually indicated. (As noted previously, psychotherapy alone may be recommended for less severe and non-melancholic late life depression). The tricyclic antidepressants, especially desipramine and nortriptyline, are the drugs of choice initially. Despite the advent of new generation antidepressants (see Chapter 19), tricyclics remain the drugs of choice. Dosage usually begins at 25 to 50 mg and all of the medication can be given at night. The dose is gradually increased and, in each case, the clinician can monitor therapeutic blood levels. A test dose of medication is usually not necessary and the first blood level usually should be drawn approximately 5 days after what appears to be an optimal dose of the drug has been taken.

Initial response to the medication usually includes improved sleep, decreased agitation, and possibly an increased appetite. At the same time, the clinician should monitor for adverse side effects (especially postural hypotension and significant anticholinergic effects).

Only after 3 to 4 weeks will the older adult report a significant change in mood secondary to the medication. By that time, the hospitalized depressed elder may have been discharged and therefore the clinician must explain to the elder that improvement from the drug does not occur totally within the first weeks of therapy. After 6 to 8 weeks, the clinician can evaluate effectively the response of the elder to the antidepressant. A successful response at that time includes not only improvement in melancholic symptoms (e.g., diurnal variation in sleep patterns, sleep difficulties, and decreased appetite). By 6 to 8 weeks, the elder should report that his or her mood has improved and he or she has reestablished former interests and former relations. If the depressive disorder has persisted for many months before treatment, however, the elder may require a number of months after the initiation of therapy to reintegrate into his or her previous life-style. Frequently, clinicians are impatient that the depressed elder has not returned to his or her previous life-style quickly.

If the older person is severely depressed and requires hospitalization and especially if the elder is suffering from a psychotic depression, ECT may be selected as the initial treatment. The indications (and contraindications) for ECT are presented in Chapter 19. If ECT is effective, the older person suffering major depression is then placed on maintenance antidepressant therapy and/or lithium carbonate. Supportive psychotherapy, once again, is essential to treatment. The severely depressed elder often has difficulty in reintegrating into life, even once his or her mood has improved. In addition, the potential for relapse after ECT is high, and the use of maintenance medication and possibly of psychotherapy significantly reduces the risk.

If the older person responds to the combination of antidepressants and psychotherapy, maintenance therapy should be continued for at least 9 to 12 months, if the episode is a first episode. On the other hand, if the elder has suffered repeated depressive episodes, then indefinite maintenance therapy on an antidepressant and/or lithium should be considered. Maintenance doses of medications do not need be as high as treatment doses and can be decreased after 3 to 4 months of initial therapy. For example, if the older person responds to nortriptyline 75 mg po qhs, maintenance therapy of 25 to 50 mg po qhs is usually sufficient. The drug should be withdrawn gradually, however, and the elder carefully instructed regarding the emergence of a recurrent depression. Distinguishing a recurrent depression from the side effects of rapid withdrawal (e.g., difficulty sleeping) can be difficult, which necessitates a slow withdrawal of the medication. If the elder responds well to antidepressant therapy during an initial episode of major depression then gradual withdrawal from the medication is indicated 9 to 12 months after the episode. The older person should be seen a few weeks after withdrawal from the medication and approximately 1 year later. If there is no evidence of a return of depressive symptoms, then the older person can be discharged from therapy. If the depression recurs, then antidepressant medication should be reinstated (psychotherapy is usually not necessary at this time) and continued indefinitely.

If the ambulatory elder does not respond well to initial psychotherapy and antidepressant medications, the physician faces a quandary. First, the physician should consider a second antidepressant, usually with a different mode of action. For example, if the initial drug prescribed was desipramine (a selective norepinephrine uptake inhibitor), then the second drug might be fluoxetine or sertraline (i.e., selective serotonin uptake inhibitors [SSR1]). The clinician may also elect to prescribe monoamine-oxidase inhibitor at this time (although these drugs are less likely to be prescribed as second-choice agents given the advent of the selected serotonin uptake inhibitors). If the elder exhibits obsessive symptoms in the midst of the depressive episode, prescription of cloimipramine, fluoxetine, or sertraline is indicated. If side effects have been problematic with the tricyclic antidepressant, especially anticholinergic effects, then trazodone, buproprion, fluoxetine, or sertraline are good alternative drugs. On the other hand, if the elder has experienced considerable sedation and postural hypotension, then fluoxetine would probably be the alternative drug of choice. Although data are not available, one clinical impression is that fluoxetine often is beneficial for mild-to-moderate ambulatory cases of major depression that have not been responsive to tricyclic antidepressant therapy. In the more severe tricyclic-resistant depressions, fluoxetine generally is not helpful.

Another choice is to treat the tricyclic antidepressant resistant major depression by augmenting the tricyclic drug. For example, lithium carbonate, methylphenidate, T3, and even propranolol have been suggested as agents that may augment these drugs. Approximately 40% of individuals who are treatment resistant to a single tricyclic antidepressant and/or monoamine-oxidase inhibitor may respond to augmentation with lithium carbonate. The augmenting dose of lithium can be low, usually 300 mg qd in the older adult (see Chapter 19).

At times, the clinician faces an equally difficult dilemma, rapid-cycling depression. In the midst of rapid cycling, it is often difficult to determine whether the antidepressant therapy is effective or not (because the person is cycling in and out of depressive episodes quickly). In late life the clinician is as likely to find individuals who cycle between relatively normal mood state and severe depressions as to find cycling between manic and depressive states. If the clinician cannot establish that the antidepressant medication is effective in treating depressive episodes in the midst of rapid cycling, then antidepressants should be discontinued. Rather, the clinician can prescribe lithium carbonate, carbamazepine, clonazepam, or valproic acid. In the midst or rapid cycling a trial-and-error approach to medications (or a particular combination of medications) is indicated as there are no clear guidelines as to which medications may be effective in controlling rapid cycling in which individuals. Carbamazepine has been demonstrated to be effective in controlling rapid cycling among persons who have previously been treated with a combination of lithium carbonate and a tricyclic antidepressant.

A person with treatment-resistant but only moderately severe depressive episode is not a candidate for ECT. Many clinicians (and patients) are tempted to institute ECT for mild-to-moderate but refractory cases of major depression. Not only does ECT rarely effect a reversal of the depressive episode in such cases, it may lead to further complications (e.g., difficulties with memory).

If the clinician cannot, through following the decision tree described, adequately treat the depressive episode, then he or she should search for organic causes that may have gone unnoticed before the initiation of therapy. For example, thyroid abnormalities may contribute to treatment-resistant depression. In addition, the older person may suffer brain changes, such as an organic mood disorder (a disorder that is much more difficult to treat than usual major depression).

The nursing staff faces a particular problem when treating the severely depressed older adult within the hospital. When the patient refuses to eat or becomes mute or negativistic in response to nursing personnel, behavioral techniques must be instituted. If the patient refuses to eat, the nursing staff, in conjunction with the psychiatrist, psychologist, and dietician, should establish a daily requirement of caloric intake. For example, the dietician discusses dietary intake with the patient, who then is given control of food selection, but this selection must total a certain number of calories per day. If the patient refuses to select an appropriate diet, the dietician plans a diet of a minimum caloric level, which is then available to the patient. If the patient refuses this food, a protein-caloric supplement in liquid form is offered to the patient. If the supplement is refused, a nasogastric tube may need be instituted for feeding. Initially, the tube is removed after each meal and the patient is given a choice between oral or tube feedings. If the patient continues to refuse to eat, the nasogastric tube is left in place until the patient's symptoms improve.

The patient should be required to remain out of the hospital room in the public area during waking hours, except for brief visits to the room if physical health permits. Occasionally, the desire of the patient to sleep or sit alone makes it necessary to keep the patient locked out of the room during certain hours of the day.

The patient with a combination of depression and dementia with severe depressive symptoms is frequently at risk for suicide within the hospital setting. The patient with a unipolar disorder with agitation is more likely to commit suicide than is an individual with a retarded depression (Jamison, 1979). After the patient is admitted to the hospital, one-to-one nursing coverage may be necessary. If the older patient has made a suicide attempt, is not communicative about feelings and thoughts and is unwilling to discuss control of suicidal impulses, one-to-one nursing coverage is essential. To further reduce the risk of suicide on the psychiatric ward, a room search for potentially dangerous weapons, such as a razor blade, rope, and stowed away medications, is often necessary. The purpose of the room search must be explained to the patient (i.e., the clinician is ordering the search because of concern for the well-being of the depressed patient). Although the patient may insist on maintaining responsibility for his or her own life, the clinician should claim a medical and legal responsibility that cannot be compromised. Patients remain in the room during the search and any objects that are dangerous are removed to the nursing station and are carefully labeled, to be returned to the patient at the end of the crisis.

Once the clinician and the patient can reliably enter into brief contracts concerning suicidal impulses and behavior, the stringent nursing restrictions can be lifted, and privileges can be gradually increased. A patient who does not have cognitive impairment rarely enters honestly into a contract and then violates that contract. Yet contracts do carry risks, since there is no means by which suicide can be absolutely prevented, except one-to-one coverage. Such coverage cannot be maintained indefinitely. The patient with both a severe depressive episode and dementia is particularly at risk as noted previously. If depressive symptoms continue to the point that the prime motivation is a will to self-destruction, suicide may occur when the medical nursing staff least expects it. The family should be warned of the potential for suicide attempts, but this warning should not be phrased in a sensationalistic term.

When suicide occurs, the clinician should schedule an interview with the family. This interview allows the family to work through their feelings about this tragic occurrence. The treatment team should also meet to work through their own feelings and review the case. In almost every circumstance the team can be assured that poor patient care was not the cause of the suicide. Most clinicians feel hurt, guilt, and anger after a patient's suicide and these feelings should be expressed. Yet the clinician must work closely with risk-management experts whenever an elderly patient becomes a serious risk for suicide, attempts suicide, or completes a suicide. Refraining from making critical clinical decisions in isolation not only ensures that optimal clinical care is provided, it also ensures that no one person assumes too much responsibility for care.

REFERENCES

American Psychiatric Association: *DSM-IV Options Book: Work in progress.* (Task Force on DSM-IV). American Psychiatric Association, 1991.

Diagnostic and Statistical Manual of Mental Disorders (ed 3— revised). Washington, DC, American Psychiatric Association, 1987.

Jamison KR: Manic depressive illness in the elderly. In Kaplan O (ed): *Psychopathology of Aging.* New York, Academic Press, 1979, pp. 79-95.

CHAPTER

12

Dysthymia and Minor Depression

After two decades of clinical and community-based investigation into the mood disorders, which focused on bipolar disorder and major depression, an interest in less severe depressive syndromes has emerged. Dysthymic disorder (chronic but less severe depression) is a common syndrome in older adults and is as prevalent in late life as mid-life in contrast to the lower prevalence of depression in late life (see Chapter 1). Converging evidence from a number of studies and clinical experience suggests that minor depressions, including dysthymic disorder, may be useful diagnostic categories for resolving many of the epidemiologic and diagnostic dilemmas that confront nosologists and epidemiologists who study late life depression.

The DSM-IV task force (1991) is considering the possibility of including minor depressive disorder and recurrent brief depressive disorder within the mood disorders section. Since the threshold for severity and duration of the DSM-III-R depressivedisorders are arbitrary and not based on firm empirical evidence, studies document that persons who do not meet criteria for DSM-III-R major depression or dysthymic disorder nevertheless exhibit significant clinical impairment, use health services more frequently, and experience greater disability in the work place (Broadhead et al, 1990).

Snowden (1990) criticizes the Epidemiologic Catchment Area (ECA) studies of late life depression, which estimated a much lower prevalence of mood disorders in the elderly compared with younger adults (see Chapter 1). He compared the ECA findings with other studies in which clinical depression was found to occur at higher prevalence among older adults than found in the ECA studies and also noted the frequent association of depression and physical health problems in elders, a factor that is not easily disaggregated in the ECA studies. Snowden concludes that the awareness of "masked" depression in elders with physical symptoms should increase the sensitivity of clinicians to diagnose depressive disorders. Blazer et al (1987) found a significant portion of elders in the ECA study from North Carolina reported depressive symptoms yet did not receive a diagnosis of a depressive disorder. About 4% of the community-based elders experienced significant depressive symptoms that were not classified as either dysthymia or major depression. Koenig (1988) found that, in addition to the 10% of hospitalized elders in a Veterans Administration Hospital diagnosed with major depression, nearly 20% experienced significant depressive symptoms that did not meet criteria for a major depression or dysthymia (i.e., they could be classified as suffering minor depression).

Parmalee et al (1989) identified a similar burden of depressive symptoms in a long-term care facility. Over 12% of the sample met criteria for major depression and another 31% reported less severe but nonetheless significant depressive symptoms. Oxman (1990) found the prevalence of major depression in elderly outpatients to be relatively low (less than 5%) yet minor depression, as diagnosed by the Research Diagnostic Criteria, was diagnosed in approximately 10% of the sample.

Therefore the combination of dysthymic disorders and minor depression probably accounts for a much higher percentage of depressed elders in both institutional and community settings than do episodes of major depression. Yet minor depression and dysthymic disorder have been studied infrequently.

■ CASE REPORT

Mrs. Danforth, a 72-year-old woman, was referred to a psychiatrist by her primary care physician. She had experienced a 2-year history of periodic episodes of "panic" and loss of interest in her activities. She also reported difficulty sleeping compared with her earlier life. A review of her symptoms revealed that she did not suffer from panic disorder but rather experienced infrequent episodes of moderately severe anxiety associated with a fear that she was losing her memory. The most prominent presenting symptoms were anhedonia accompanied by sleep difficulties.

The patient stated that she had spent a productive life as a mother, wife, and bank teller and looked forward to retirement, since she had many interests that she had planned to pursue, including art work, music, and enrolling in continuing education courses. Over the 6 months before evaluation, however, she found little interest in these pursuits, although she had plenty of time to pursue them. Nevertheless, she had enrolled in a continuing education course and periodically would work on her painting. She also maintained an active social schedule with her husband.

The patient's mother had died with memory difficulties in her 80s (probably because of Alzheimer's disease). The patient was fearful that her lack of concentration and memory difficulties represented the beginning of Alzheimer's disease. She was tested psychologically and no abnormalities were identified.

Given her symptoms, the psychiatrist placed her on nortriptyline 50 mg po qhs. She exhibited a partial response within 4 weeks, noting that her sleep was definitely improved and the anxiety episodes disappeared (in part because of the realization that she was not suffering from Alzheimer's disease). Her activities increased somewhat after initiation of nortriptyline therapy. Nevertheless, she continued to complain of anhedonia.

In retrospect the psychiatrist believed that his initial diagnosis of major depression was not "accurate" in that she did not meet symptom criteria for the diagnosis. Because she had responded partially, he suggested that she begin psychotherapy. She was referred to a cognitive therapist and completed 20 sessions of cognitive therapy. After these sessions, she returned to the psychiatrist for a regular medication check. At that time, she reported that she found the therapy experience educational but did not believe that her mood had improved.

The psychiatrist continued to follow her for medication checks over an ensuing 3 years. Her condition did not improve but she functioned normally and expressed no additional complaints during this period of follow-up. When fluoxetine was introduced to the US market, the patient was placed on fluoxetine for a therapeutic trial after discontinuation of the nortriptyline. Initially, she experienced a "marked" improvement in her mood and disappearance of the anhedonia. Unfortunately, she experienced considerable agitation within 5 weeks of the initiation of fluoxetine therapy and a return of the anhedonia. Given the agitation, the patient elected to return to taking nortriptyline. She later was tapered off the nortriptyline and experienced a return of the anxiety and sleep difficulty, as well as a worsening of the anhedonia. Nortriptyline therapy was reinstated.

The patient remained on nortritpyline for an additional 2 years and, during regular medication check visits, reported no change in her mood and little change in her activities. A typical visit revealed the patient to be sleeping well, to have a good appetite with no weight change, to complain of mild difficulties in concentration (but never enough to interfere with her usual activities or reading), persistent yet moderate anhedonia, but no other symptoms of depression. At each visit, she expressed that she was functioning well and had much to be thankful for. Nevertheless, she insisted that her mood was not like her usual state (since the anhedonia persisted over 7 years of follow-up). If she were not depressed, she believed that she would become more active outside the home. The patient was retested for cognitive impairment every 2 years and no evidence of impairment emerged.

■ THE PHENOMENOLOGY OF MINOR DEPRESSION

There are no adequate studies in the literature to establish the diagnostic criteria for minor depression. Blazer et al (1989) performed one of the few objective studies of community and clinical samples. Grade of membership analysis (a statistical procedure similar to factor and cluster analysis) was applied to symptom data to determine the degree to which individuals met criteria for a series of "pure types" of statistically defined depressive syndromes. One cluster of symptoms or pure type was virtually identical to the DSM-III-R criteria for major depression with melancholia. Five additional pure types emerged, including the following:

1. A relatively asymptomatic symptom cluster;
2. A symptom cluster with symptoms of both major depression and generalized anxiety;
3. A cluster (found predominantly in older persons) that was symptomatically defined by depressed mood, psychomotor retardation, difficulty concentrating, and problems performing on the mental status examination, as well as difficulty concentrating;
4. A symptom cluster characterized by depressed mood, sleep problems, and symptoms of generalized anxiety; and
5. A cluster characterized by depressed mood, weight gain, and sleep disturbance found almost exclusively in females (and possibly analogous late luteal phase dysphoric disorder).

The symptom cluster found almost exclusively in the elderly was characterized by depressed mood, psychomotor retardation and difficulty concentration, constipation, and poor perceived health yet few of the individuals who manifested this cluster met the criteria for a diagnosis of major depression similar to the patient described previously.

Therefore these older persons in community and clinical settings suffered a minor depression syndrome of late life often associated with physical illness and cognitive difficulties. This syndrome did not replace other moods because older persons also manifested classic symptoms of major depression, bipolar disorder, and dysthymic disorder. The distribution along this symptom cluster, however, was continuous, suggesting that most of the persons experienced some but not all of the criteria and no clear demarcation (i.e., no bimodal distribution) of symptoms emerged that would inform the nosologist regarding the specific symptoms nor general severity of minor depression.

Oxman et al (1990), using the Research Diagnostic Crieria for the diagnosis of minor depression, found that among the elderly, those meeting criteria for minor depression were almost equally distributed between episodic minor depression and chronic minor depression. The most common symptoms of minor depression in this sample were worry (84%), blaming self (79%), decreased energy (79%), everything an effort (68%), irritability (63%), disturbed sleep (53%), crying (53%), and feelings of hopelessness (53%). Both psychologic and somatic symptoms therefore characterized the elders diagnosed with minor depression in this outpatient clinical sample.

Angst et al (1990) suggest criteria for a variant of minor depression (i.e., recurrent brief depression). Angst's criteria, however, probably do not fit the construct of minor depression discussed in this chapter, since the episodes of depression that he described, although brief, reached the severity of major depression. The requirement for length of a brief, recurrent depressive episode was reduced to less than 2 weeks. He found that individuals who were categorized as experiencing brief, recurrent depression related an age of onset, family history, longitudinal course, and level of impairment similar to those with major depression.

Wood et al (1990) surveyed 48 patients referred to an inpatient geriatric service. Nearly half (44%) exhibited a significant flattening of affect. Characteristics of this affective flattening included unchanging facial expressions, decreased spontaneous movements, paucity of expressive gestures, poor eye contact, affective nonresponsivity, and lack of vocal inflection. This low grade "anhedonia" is suggestive of a chronic minor depression with predominantly somatic symptoms, as exhibited by the patient described in the case study.

In summary the extant studies shed little light on the specific symptoms that may characterize minor depression. Current studies of minor depression, therefore, would best focus on subsyndromal depression (as opposed to applying specific diagnostic criteria) to determine if other factors, such as outcome, response to therapy, and level of impairment over time, might enable clinicians to disaggregate the syndromes of minor depression. Yet various investigators have established criteria for minor depression and these criteria are presented next.

Snaith (1987) suggests that minor depression is primarily biogenic and, although not meeting criteria for major depression, is likely to respond to antidepressant therapy. A central feature of mild biogenic depression for Snaith is anhedonia. In contrast the criteria proposed for mild depression in the International Classification of Diseases (ed 10 or ICD-10) emphasizes lowered self-esteem, feelings of guilt and worthlessness, and absence of biologic symptoms. Criteria proposed by both the Research Diagnostic Criteria and DSM-III-R take an intermittent position. The Research Diagnostic Criteria require two or more criteria symptoms (i.e., poor appetite, sleep difficulties, loss of energy, self-pity, and dependency) and a duration of a week for probable and 2 weeks for definite minor depression. DSM-III-R, in the category "Not Otherwise Specified" suggests the following two criteria for the diagnosis of minor depression:

1. A recurrent, mild, depressive disturbance that does not meet the criteria for dysthymia;
2. Non–stress-related depressive episodes that do not meet criteria for a major depression.

Unfortunately, none of these diagnostic categories are based on empiric data and do not provide guidelines for clinical investigators to explore more thoroughly minor depression. The Research Diagnostic Criteria for minor depression are as reasonable as any for performing epidemiologic and clinical studies of minor depression.

Dysthymia or depressive neurosis, in contrast to minor depression, is a long-lasting chronic disturbance of mood that lasts for 2 years or longer by definition (DSM-III-R, 1987). Dysthymia rarely begins in late life but may persist from mid-life into late life. If the initial onset of dysthymia directly follows an episode of major depression, the correct diagnosis would be major depression in partial remission rather than dysthymia. Typical symptoms of dysthymia include the symptoms of major depression plus less activity and social withdrawal, inability to respond positively to praise or rewards, low self-esteem, self-depreciation, a perceived difficulty in coping with usual activities of daily living, and a pessimistic attitude about the future along with regret regarding the past. Dysthymia differs in concept from minor depression in terms of its chronicity and its psychogenic etiology, since minor depression may be of either biogenic or psychogenic etiology.

Minor depression and dysthymia are not easily distinguished, yet most investigators are convinced that more than one subtype of these syndromes that are less severe than major depression exist and that through better phenomenologic studies and outcome studies, they can be identified. The differential diagnosis of dysthymia and minor depression includes cyclothymia, adjustment disorder with depressed mood, and organic mood disorder. The diagnosis of cyclothymic disorder should not be made unless both major depression and bipolar disorder have been eliminated and have never occurred in the history of the patient. To meet criteria, an individual must have both numerous episodes of hypomania and numerous periods of depressed mood. Although no data are available, most clinicians believe that cyclothymic disorder is less common in late life than at earlier stages of the life cycle. The disorder is usually thought to begin in adolescence or early adult life and to exhibit an attenuation of the hypomanic episodes with aging. Most syndromes of minor depression and dysthymia are not accompanied by hypomanic episodes.

Minor depressive episodes in late life may be secondary to organic mood disorder, but it is uncommon for clinicians to directly relate minor fluctuations in mood to clear organic etiology. When such a relation is observed, treatment of the underlying organic illness is the correct course of action. An adjustment disorder with depressed mood may manifest with symptoms of minor depression or the symptoms may reach severity of a major depressive episode. In either case the reaction is clearly related to an identifiable psychosocial stressor (including a physical illness). By definition, adjustment disorder should not last longer than 6 months. In the development of DSM-IV, however, the criteria may be changed, specifically the criteria will state that the symptoms should not persist for more than 6 months after the termination of the stressor (or its consequences). Therefore, as is often the case in late life, a depressive reaction to a chronic physical illness may be classified as an adjustment disorder with depressed mood. Most cases of minor depression and dysthmia are not associated with stressors that account for the disturbance in mood.

■ TREATMENT

The nature of minor depression and dysthymic disorders suggests that psychosocial interventions would be appropriate. Nevertheless, empiric literature provides very little evidence for the success of psychosocial therapies. The lack of data regarding the effectiveness of psychosocial therapy is undoubtedly due to the absence of clear diagnostic categories in the case of minor depression and chronicity in the case of dysthymia. Clinicians who have worked with depressed older adults with intermittent and less severe episodes of depression tend not correlate therapeutic intervention with improvement in mood, for fluctuation in mood occurs so frequently. Dysthymia on the other hand, is a chronic condition that usually does not respond to psychosocial or pharmacologic intervention, except after many months or perhaps years of therapy.

Therefore the empiric literature on the treatment of minor depression has focused on treatment with antidepressant medications. Paykel et al (1988) reviewed the benefits of amitriptyline as a therapy for minor depression in a general practice population (all ages). In this study, persons with major depression were compared with persons with mild or minor depression, as defined by the Research Diagnostic Criteria. A minimum duration of 1 week for symptoms was required to be entered into the study. Amitriptyline was found to be superior to placebo for persons experiencing probable or definite major depression but not for minor depression. Amitriptyline was also superior to placebo in subjects with initial scores on the Hamilton Depression Rating Scale that were above 12 but not for individuals who initially scored between 6 and 12. The problem inherent in this study is obvious. Specifically, the severity of symptoms, and therefore the possibility for documenting improvement, were lower in minor depression and therefore change in symptoms among minor depressive did not reach statistical significance.

The study does not rule out the possibility that antidepressant medications, especially low doses of tricyclic antidepressants, may not be effective for treating minor forms of depression. Most psychiatrists do not encounter these milder depressive syndromes, since these individuals seek help from primary care physicians. Primary care physicians often prescribe low doses of antidepressant medications and intuitively conclude that the medications are successful. The intermittent nature of minor depression, with the natural decrease in depressive symptoms over time, render these conclusions suspect, however. It is questionable whether the improvement in symptoms can be attributed to the medication or to the natural history of the disorder. Many clinicians also report a decrease in episodes of depression over time in persons with minor depression prescribed antidepressant medications.

Quitken et al (1990) investigated the use of imipramine and phenalzine in a control study of over 400 adult patients. A significant number of these individuals scored 10 or less on the Hamilton Depression Scale yet showed significant improvement in their symptoms with phenalizine (compared with imipramine). These investigators therefore concluded that persons who are chronically and persistently depressed, even if they do not meet criteria for major depression, should be treated with antidepressants. Perhaps patients using medications, such as MAO inhibitors (e.g., phenalzine), and new generation antidepressants (e.g., fluoxetine) are more likely to respond with a decrease in depressive symptoms than with the traditional tricyclic antidepressants.

■ PROGNOSIS

Broadhead et al (1990) review the outcome of persons with subsyndromal depressive symptoms (minor depression) and a diagnosis of major depression in the North Carolina ECA study. Compared with asymptomatic persons, those with major depression were at nearly five times greater risk for disability at 1-year follow-up and persons with minor depression had nearly two times greater risk. Minor depression was defined as having at least two symptoms of depression but not meeting criteria for a major depression or dysthymic disorder. Because of the higher prevalence of minor depression compared with major depression in this community sample, individuals with minor depression accounted for 51% more disability days in general in the community than persons with major depression. Broadhead et al divide minor depression into those with and without "mood disturbance" (i.e., individuals who suffered symptoms of depression but were disaggregated according to self-report of depressed mood). Minor depression without mood disturbance was more frequent in the elderly group than any of the remaining age groups.

Any study of the outcome of minor depression, however, must take into account the longitudinal course of major depression. In the suggestions for changes in the DSM-III-R criteria for major depression with DSM-IV, longitudinal course specifiers are included (American Psychiatric Association, 1991). These include a single episode of major depression with antecedent dysthymia, a recurrent episode of major depression with antecedent dysthymia, a recurrent episode of depression with antecedent dysthymia without full interepisode recovery, and a recurrent episode of major depression without antecedent dysthymia and without full interepisode recovery. In other words, many cases of minor depression identified in a cross-sectional study may represent antecedent major depression or partial recovery from an episode of major depression.

Comprehensive study of depression in late life must consider subsyndromal or minor depression (i.e., depressive symptoms that do not meet criteria for major depression or dysthymic disorder). Although these syndromes are more common in primary care than in mental health specialists' offices, epidemiologic data document the significant prevalence and the public health burden of the disorders. Minor depression, however, is probably not a single entity. Current data suggest that many syndromes, such as the persistent anhedonia described by Snaith (1987), the recurrent brief depressive disorders described by Angst (1990), and the chronic minor depressive disorders associated with cognitive impairment described by our group (Blazer et al, 1990) are captured by the construct of minor depression. Virtually no data are available regarding the psychosocial treatment of these minor depressive disorders. Data regarding the pharmacologic treatment of minor depression are conflicted. Well-described control studies are needed to document whether tricyclic antidepressants are effective in these less severe depressive disorders. Possibly new generation antidepressants, such as fluoxetine and other selective serotonin uptake inhibitors, may significantly improve depressive symptoms in this group.

REFERENCES

Angst J, Merikangas K, Scheidegger P, Wicki W: Recurrent brief depression: a new subtype of affective disorders, *Journal of Affective Disorders* 19:87-98, 1990.

Blazer D: Clinical features and depression in old age: a case for minor depression, *Current Opinion in Psychiatry* 4:596-599, 1991.

Blazer DG, Hughes DK, George LK: The epidemiology of depression in an elderly community population, *The Gerontologist* 27:281-287, 1987.

Blazer D, Woodbury M, Hughes DC, George LK, Manton KG, et al: A statistical analysis of the classification of depression in a mixed community and clinical sample, *Journal of Affective Disorders* 16:11-20, 1989.

Broadhead WE, Blazer DG, George LK, Tse CK: Depression, disability days and days lost from work in a prospective epidemiologic survey, *Journal of the American Medical Association* 264:2524-2528, 1990.

DSM-IV Options Book: Work in Progress. Washington, DC, American Psychiatric Association, 1991.

Diagnostic and Statistical Manual of Mental Disorders (ed 3—revised). Washington, DC, American Psychiatric Association, 1987.

Koenig HG, Meador KG, Cohen HJ, Blazer DG: Depression in elderly hospitalized patients with medical illness, *Archives of Internal Medicine* 148:1929-1935, 1988.

Oxman TE, Barrett JE, Barrett J, Gerber T: Symptomatology of late-life minor depression among primary care patients, *Psychosomatics* 31:174-180, 1990.

Parmelee P, Katz IR, Lawton MP: Depression among institutionalized aged: Assessment and prevalence estimation, *Journal of Gerontology* (MS)44:22-29, 1989.

Paykel ES, Hollyman JA, Freling P, Sedwick P: Predictors of therapeutic benefit for amitriptyline in mild depression: a general practice placebo-control trial, *Journal of Affective Disorders* 14:83-95, 1988.

Quitken FM:Can mildly depressed outpatients with atypical depression benefit from antidepressants? *American Journal of Psychiatry* 149:615-619, 1992.

Snaith RP: The concepts of minor depression, *The British Journal of Psychiatry* 150:287-293, 1987.

Snowden J: The prevalence of depression in old age, *Psychiatry* 5:141-144, 1990.

Wood KA, Nissenbaum H, Livingstone M: Affective flattening in elderly patients, *Age and Aging* 19:253-256, 1990.

CHAPTER

13

Bereavement

Every clinician who has worked with older patients has witnessed the depressive symptoms occurring after a significant loss, especially after the loss of a loved one or the loss of physical function. Reactive depressions may become more frequent with aging, whereas neurotic disorders appear to be less frequent when compared with persons in mid-life (Verwoerdt, 1976). Depressive reactions do not usually extend beyond the severity of uncomplicated bereavement. Patients experiencing these reactions to loss are usually resistant to psychopharmacologic agents and electroconvulsive therapy but do respond to psychotherapeutic intervention.

Normal bereavement is ubiquitous with living (Clayton, 1968). Most older persons who experience a loss grieve that loss appropriately and grow from the experience. The grief experience, however, at times can lead to serious adverse outcomes. Poor outcome from bereavement (i.e., abnormal bereavement) is a major concern of the clinician working with the bereaved elderly. Many risk factors for abnormal bereavement have been documented (Jacobs and Kim, 1990). Predisposing factors for abnormal bereavement after a loss include poverty (during young age), low self-esteem (especially a belief that one has poor internal controls), difficulties in prior relationships with parents, and multiple previous losses. The relationship of the bereaved elder to the deceased may also contribute to poor outcome from bereavement (Parkes and Weiss, 1983). Situations that can contribute to poor outcome include the following: the lost loved one was a spouse (especially when a husband loses his wife), the bereaved was dependent on the deceased, the deceased was overly dependent on the bereaved, or the bereaved had ambivalent feelings toward the deceased.

The type of death leading to bereavement may also contribute to bereavement with poor outcome (Jacobs and Kim, 1990; Duke, 1980). An unexpected or untimely death, a long terminal illness, the bereaved being unaware of the diagnosis or prognosis of the deceased, the bereaved being remote from the dying patient at the time of death, grieving a loved one who committed suicide, or grieving a loved one who was a victim of murder or manslaughter can contribute to difficult bereavement. Poor social supports also may contribute to abnormal bereavement (Jacobs and Kim, 1990; Parkes and Weiss, 1983). When there is no child or family near, or when the family is seen as unhelpful, the elder may experience a difficult bereavement.

Older persons also experience considerable depressive symptoms in response to the loss of nonspousal family members. In a study of 825 elderly men and women, Siegel and Kuykendall (1990) found loss of social network members other than family to be related to a high level of depressive symptomatology in men but not women. Both the presence of a spouse and membership in a church or temple moderated the impact of loss on depression in men. This study illustrates how social support (both spousal and through membership in social groups) can buffer loss by the elderly. Retirement has also been postulated to contribute to bereavement in older adults (Portnoy, 1983). Retirees who undergo other significant stressful life events (e.g., physical illness or loss of a loved one) appear to be at greater risk for developing a depressive disorder. Retirement uncomplicated by other stressors, however, does not usually contribute to depressive symptoms in older adults.

The symptoms of bereavement do not vary across the life cycle (Clayton et al, 1968; Fasey, 1990). Breckenridge et al (1986), however, in a study of bereaved subjects, 20 to 80 years of age, found depressive symptoms less frequent in the over 55 age group.

The symptoms of normal and abnormal bereavement are presented next. A case history of an elderly man who experienced bereavement is then presented as an illustration. The diagnostic workup and management of bereavement are reviewed next with particular emphasis on the need to facilitate normal bereavement to avoid lapse into abnormal bereavement. Finally, the outcome of bereavement is reviewed.

■ NORMAL BEREAVEMENT

Although the more severely and abnormally bereaved patients are referred to psychiatrists, primary care physicians are likely to encounter those individuals who experience the normal symptoms of grief. Lindemann (1944), whose work is described in more detail in a later section, symptomatically distinguished the normally and the abnormally bereaved (see box on p. 205). The clarity of his description of symptoms in 101 subjects, each of whom had lost a close relative in the Coconut Grove fire in Boston, renders his report of the emotional sequeleae of the disaster a classic.

Clayton et al (1968) interviewed relatives of deceased hospital patients and found that only three symptoms—depressed mood, sleep disturbances, and crying—occurred in more than one half of the bereaved subjects. Three other symptoms—difficulty concentrating, loss of interest in television or news, and anorexia and weight loss—occurred less frequently. No differences in symptoms were found in relation to gender, age, length of the deceased's illness, and relation of the bereaved to the deceased. Approximately 2 to 4 months after the initial interview, 81% were improved, and only 4% were worse. Approximately 98% of the subjects did not seek psychiatric assistance during the period of grief. Bereavement, regardless of age, usually manifests itself as mild and predictable symptoms that improve spontaneously.

Parkes (1972) studied the longitudinal aspects of bereavement in London widows. Most of the persons had not anticipated the loss of the spouse. After the death of the spouse, the widows entered a phase of numbness, followed by a period of yearning during which the "pangs" of grief occurred. "Yearning" was associated with "protest," a rest-

---

Symptoms of normal and abnormal bereavement

Symptoms of Normal Bereavement

Sensations of somatic distress (e.g., tightness in the throat, shortness of breath, sighing respirations, lassitude, loss of appetite)

Preoccupation with the image of the deceased

Guilt

Irritability and hostile reactions

Loss of patterns of usual conduct (e.g., push of speech, restlessness, inability to sit still, lack of capacity to initiate and maintain organized patterns of activity, clinging to routine prescribed activities)

Appearance of traits of the deceased in the bereaved's behavior

Symptoms of Abnormal Bereavement

Delayed grief reaction

Distorted reactions (e.g., overactivity without a sense of loss, acquisition of symptoms belonging to the last illness of the deceased, psychosomatic illness, alteration of relationship to friends and relatives, hostility toward specific persons, persistent loss of patterns of social interaction, self-defectory activities, agitated depression)

Adapted from Lindemann E: *American Journal of Psychiatry,* 101:141-148, 1945.

less irritability or bitterness toward the self and others. Tearfulness and acute anxiety were the first features to decline during the first year. Preoccupation with memories of the lost spouse, as well as general restlessness and tension, declined gradually throughout the year.

The reaction of grief appears deeply imbedded in both humans and primates. McKinney (1986) reviewed the relevance of primate separation studies (in monkeys) to bereavement in humans. When monkeys were separated from their parents, heart rate and body temperature decreased almost immediately. If a young monkey was returned to the parents soon after separation, heart rate and body temperature returned to normal. If time until the return is prolonged, the body changes may become permanent. Harlow (1971) found that young animals separated from their mothers progress through predictable stages, often labeled as *protest* and *despair*. In the protest stage the young animal is agitated and often sounds distressed. Oral behavior, such as feeding and touching the lips, increases. During the stage of despair the young animal decreases its activity, huddling in the corner of a cage, thereby withdrawing from its social surroundings.

In the third edition (revised) of the *Diagnostic and Statistical Manual* (APA, 1987), uncomplicated bereavement is described as a normal reaction to the death of a loved one. Although the full depressive syndrome may be seen, with symptoms such as poor appetite, weight loss, and insomnia, other symptoms of depression, such as morbid preoccupation with worthlessness, prolonged and marked functional impairment, and marked psychomotor retardation, are uncommon. Guilt, according to DSM-III-R, is chiefly focused on things done or not done by the bereaved at the time of the death. Thoughts of the bereaved's own death are usually limited to the persons thinking that they would be better off dead, or wishing he or she had died with or instead of the deceased person (as opposed to suicidal ideation). Normal bereavement generally occurs within the first 2 months, although it may not begin immediately after the loss.

Gallagher and Thompson (1989) summarized the literature on the stages of grief by abstracting three distinct stages (Blazer, 1990). The first is shock and disbelief, which is usually associated with feelings of numbness, confusion, and emptiness. The immediate details surrounding the death of the loved one usually dominate the thoughts of the bereaved. Anxiety, as opposed to depression, is the most common symptom during this first stage and may lead to marked fluctuations in mood during the first few days after the loss. Physical symptoms are also common during this stage. This initial phase of shock or disbelief is often more pronounced if the death is sudden, unexpected, and/or unnatural.

The second phase is depression. Depression usually emerges as the predominate stage 4 to 6 weeks after the loss, although no schedule can be imposed on the grieving older adult. Friends and families become less available and less helpful a few weeks after the loss, as they return to their own activities, possibly forgetting that the bereaved elder must gradually undertake the difficult adjustment to a life without the loved one. Decreased attention for loved ones coupled with the recognition of the finality of the loss leads to crying, sleep problems, fatigue, decreased energy, and social withdrawal.

Brief visual and auditory hallucinations of the lost loved one are not uncommon and may be normal during this phase of bereavement. The bereaved may have a strong sense of the presence of the deceased and become preoccupied with this presence. Older persons hear their names being called or believe they have received a message from the lost loved one that, possibly, all is well. Clinicians must not interpret such experiences as abnormal, since they are apt to be brief and may actually assist the older adult in progressing with the grief work, which includes confronting the denial of death and the reality of being alone. During this stage, unresolved anger toward the lost loved one and guilt regarding neglect of the loved one often emerge.

The second or depressive stage of bereavement often persists for at least a year. Although no schedule can be imposed on the grieving process, usual milestones are useful in marking the progress of bereavement (Blazer, 1990). The most severe period of depression usually occurs 1 to 2 months after the loss. A second but less severe period occurrs about 4 months later. Improvement in symptoms and outlook and the reduction of dysfunction often occur during the second 6 months, until the first anniversary of the loss. The first-year anniversary often precipitates a recurrence of symptoms, referred to as the "anniversary reaction." The anniversary of the death is not the only anniversary that can precipitate increased symptoms, however. Birthdays, wedding anniversaries, special holidays, or dates of special planned events that were never realized may also contribute to an exacerbation of grieving, especially during the first year of bereavement.

After the anniversary of a loss, the third phase of bereavement generally predominates (Gallagher and Thompson, 1989; Blazer, 1990; Fasey, 1990). During the third phase, the grief process gradually resolves. Different authors have labeled this period of resolution as acceptance, identity reconstruction, and reintegration. Social contacts are increased and life is reorganized around events that did not involve the lost loved one. Brief periods of depression, often manifested by crying and feelings of emptiness, are not uncommon and they generally resolve after a few hours or a day at the most. The physical symptoms of grief, such as loss of energy, loss of appetite, and loss of sleep, usually resolve completely during the first year of bereavement. The acceptance phase, however, may require as much as a year before a relatively normal life-style and mood state have been reestablished.

Older adults do not march step through these stages. Rather, they may fluctuate from one to the other. Denial, in one form or another, may persist for many months after the death of a loved one. Depression, especially when the death has been preconceived, may be the first symptoms to appear. For some older adults, the process of adaptation and reintegration into a new life may occur early and may be appropriate. Although relatives often become concerned when a bereaved older adult remarries quickly (perhaps a few months after the loss of a spouse), these marriages may be appropriate and adaptive.

Zisook and Shuchter (1986) followed a group of grieving men and women for 4 years. The most severe symptomatic distress occurred during the first month after the death of the loved one. Anger and guilt, rather than depression, were the most frequent symptoms. Anger among persons who perceived themselves responsible for their loved ones' deaths was a more lasting symptom than guilt. Depression, although not as severe in the initial months, persisted throughout the 4 years of follow-up. All symptoms become much less severe in the latter years of this follow-up study. In the view of the bereaved, function returned to normal after the first year of bereavement, and social involvement increased dramatically after the first anniversary of the death.

■ ABNORMAL BEREAVEMENT

Persons who experience abnormal bereavement are of much greater concern to the clinician than the normally bereaving older adult. Yet a thorough understanding of the normal process of bereavement is essential if the clinician is to accurately identify the older adult experiencing abnormal bereavement.

■ CASE PRESENTATION

A 72-year-old woman was referred because of her propensity to fall on standing. Her inability to stand had precipitated an admission to a long-term care facility for 1 year before the referral. Family members suspected that she would require indefinite institutionalization, but they wished to obtain a further evaluation to rule out possible psychologic influences.

The patient had lived at home and functioned well, maintaining self-care until 2 years before her hospital admission. Her youngest son died at that time, and the patient began to "fall apart" according to the family. She ceased many of her activities and progressively relinquished self-care until neighbors noticed the neglect and reported her to the family. She was evaluated in the geriatric unit of a local hospital and was then placed in the long-term care facility. During the intake interview, the patient complained that she no longer could care for herself and was losing her mind. She directed frequent questions to the interviewer about where she was, his profession and background, and her sons. The patient answered most questions with "I don't know" or "you tell me." She revealed that she had a problem with constipation, markedly decreased appetite, and weight loss of 33 pounds. She also noted that she had no interest in some of her previous activities (mainly reading), was restless most of the day, and had falling episodes (the symptom for which she was referred). She complained of problems with her sleep, yet her family stated that she slept well. When asked if she felt depressed or sad, she stated that she was losing her mind and that memory problems were her major concern. She did admit, however, to sadness after the death of her son.

During the mental status examination, the patient was observed to be a sad, agitated woman who would smile occasionally; she was clearly experiencing a depressed mood. She did not cry or tear during the interview, however. Her thought content was dominated by denial, grief, and depressive symptoms. She focused on her body with frequent expressions of helplessness and uselessness. She refused to cooperate with tests of cognitive functioning, stating that she "couldn't remember."

On physical examination, the patient appeared older than her stated age and demonstrated marked weight loss. She was found to suffer from a marked impaction of feces. All admission laboratory tests were normal.

Past history revealed that the patient was a native of North Carolina and not moved from her hometown since birth. She married soon after graduation from high school. After working for 2 years, she gave birth to five sons and devoted herself to her children. One of these sons died at a young age. At age 46, her husband divorced her after finding a "younger woman." The patient then returned to work and continued to work until she retired at age 67. Her younger son moved away from home when she was 50 years old and she lived alone until the onset of the present illness.

The family dated the onset of the patient's difficulties to the death of one of her sons 2 years before the evaluation. This son had been a favorite of the patient's, since he had been physically ill most of his life and had developed chronic renal disease secondary to diabetes. His condition deteriorated during the 6 months before his death, such that the physicians had advised the family against further treatment, specifically hemodialysis. A family conference was held, excluding the mother but including the son's wife and his brothers. They decided against continuing hemodialysis. (At that time, the ill son was not competent to make decisions regarding his health care.) The patient later learned of the conference and was very angry with the family. She attempted to have her son's hemodialysis restarted but was unsuccessful. The son died soon afterwards. The patient did not attend the funeral and expressed little overt grief at his death. She would neither talk about her deceased son nor visit his grave. Her behavior deteriorated remarkably soon after his death, however, leading to a psychiatric admission.

After evaluation during the index hospitalization, it was determined that the patient should be readmitted to the hospital for further tests and therapy. During the first few days of hospitalization, the patient became opposed to attempts to encourage her to eat. She refused to eat solid foods and was started on a liquid dietary supplement. During interviews she continually deflected the conversation away from herself, usually by commenting about other patients on the ward. When she noticed others observing her, she would begin to stumble and fall into chairs. On one occasion she missed the chair and was slightly bruised, but otherwise her falling behavior did not lead to injury.

With time, the patient began to discuss her family and her past. She praised her living children, stating that they were "fine sons" but did express disappointment that they could not take her into one of their homes, electing instead to place her in a long-term care facility when she was unable to remain in her own home. When the sons visited her on the ward, she increased her falling behavior and was less responsive to them than to the nursing staff. In particular, she complained of their attempts to bring her presents, clothes, and other items. She belittled their choice of clothes, stating that they knew nothing about shopping and could not obtain the assistance of their wives to help them in shopping.

Later during the hospitalization, she discussed her deceased son, noting that he had been a "fine boy" who suffered greatly during his life. He had experienced weakness, decreased appetite, dizziness, and his wife had not appeared to show concern about his condition. His wife did not notice when her son almost fell on standing. The patient herself had experienced many hardships during her adult years, which she gradually began to reveal. Her anger toward her divorced husband persisted, since she felt he left her at a time when she had overwhelming parental responsibilities with few economic resources available to her. She enjoyed her work as a clerk, but when she retired, she had no life outside her home.

The symptoms and signs presented by this patient are consistent with the diagnosis of a major depressive episode. Yet the patient's clinical picture is characteristic of the prolonged and complicated bereavement at times experienced by the depressed elderly. Goldfarb (1974) outlined a number of complaints and behavior patterns seen in frightened or angry persons whose feelings of helplessness have led to a maladaptation, namely a search for aid, dependency striving, or attempts to establish personal relationships that will bring protection, care, and security. These behavior patterns may overlap with the symptoms of a major depressive episode in a bereaved elder. This patient exhibits these symptoms dramatically. First, such patients are often apathetic, listless, and without initiative. They withdraw, are slow in speech and movement, and enter into conversations reluctantly. Basic problems are denied and during instances when the patient interacts with social network, a token compliance, frequently followed by protest and even angry resistance, characterizes the interaction. This symptom pattern is reminiscent of pseudoanhedonia.

Pseudoanhedonia, according to Goldfarb (1974), is a mechanism by which a patient speaks as if to say, "I'm without feelings, nothing matters, you can do whatever you want with me." Clinicians frequently note the irony in these statements, since such patients are rarely compliant with therapeutic techniques, often insisting on being left alone and not being pushed into activities. Pseudoanhedonia is self-punitive and punitive to others. The behavior in some ways justifies one's existence and, at least, for a short while, elicits sympathy from the social network. A third symptom described by Goldfarb is the display of helplessness. Patients advertise their weaknesses, their ineptitude, or their memory problems. If real illness exists the patients exacerbate their conditions by self-destructive behaviors and self-neglect. Other patients complain of an inability to carry out routine activities of daily living and, if left alone, may refuse to cook, clean the house, or maintain personal hygiene. Still others complain vehemently that they have lost their minds. Such patients are most frustrating to work with through any type of therapy, since they do not maintain attention, and when important issues are discussed, they often deny remembering the nature of the conversation.

Closely associated with pseudoanhedonia is somatic preoccupation. Complaints of pain, constipation, weakness, and various malfunctions of organ systems may be the only subjects that the patient will discuss in conversation. Depressive symptoms usually include anhedonia, loss of interest, loss of purpose and motivation, and preoccupation with their sad state. Anorexia, constipation, sleep disturbances, and loss of libido are common symptoms of prolonged, complicated grief reactions.

Manipulative and coercive behaviors are also exhibited by older adults with maladaptive bereavement. Implicit and explicit requests include the following examples: statements such as "If you don't take me into your house, I'll just die" or "There's no use living since the children have lives of their own" or attempts to modify the environment to meet their dependency, such as a request to add a guestroom to a child's house, which the elder intends to move into once completed. These requests are coupled with anger toward family members, which is displaced from the lost loved object. Most family members recognize these attempts to control their behavior, yet these attempts provoke anger in the family.

Passive-aggressive behavior (aggression toward an external object expressed indirectly and effectively through passivity, masochism, and turning against the self) is another common symptom in abnormal bereavement. Passive-aggressive behavior is usually determined by premorbid personality style and therefore will not be a component of every abnormal grief re-action. The patient described demonstrates passive-aggressive behavior toward family and those who are working with her. Resistance to eating and to self-care in the hospital evokes considerable frustration among the nursing staff.

The patient's depression is primarily the result of a reaction to the events surrounding the death of her son. She was left out of a life-and-death decision, which led to anger that could not be expressed openly. The symptoms and dynamics in this patient also fit Verwoerdt's (1980) description of "vindictive depression." There are many regressive and hysteric mech-anisms present, such as hysteric exaggeration of her physical symptoms through falling, which border on a conversion disorder.

This patient also demonstrates many of the symptoms of abnormal grief described by Lin-demann (1944). Her grief was delayed and she acquired many of the symptoms of her de-ceased son during the terminal phase of his chronic renal failure, especially decreased food intake, complaint of a lack of appetite, and weight loss. The falling behavior is reminiscent of the deceased son's episodes of dizziness. Much of her anger at the loss of her child was displaced onto her living children, with considerable attention focused on their decision to exclude her from the final discussion of whether to continue the hemodialysis, exaggerating her feelings of uselessness. Her obstinate behavior caused relationships with friends to de-cline dramatically, and her passive-aggressive behavior precipitated the admission to a long-term care facility (where the patient least wished to live).

What leads to these maladaptive symptom patterns after a significant loss? Goldfarb (1974) emphasizes the role of regression in producing the symptom complex described. Although no significant physical or cognitive deficit was noted in the patient, the gradual decrease in functional capacities led her to recognize her need for care in the future. Distress over the loss of her son, a disruption of her support network, and the realization of increased depen-dency may have produced a constellation of symptoms as a means of signaling distress, de-spair, and helplessness, which were undoubtedly associated with an expression of protest. Symptoms of physical and mental impairment were easily incorporated into the personality as a mode of communication and served the psychologic purpose of resolving the interper-sonal conflicts over dependency, anger, and guilt.

Weinberg (1959) suggests that withdrawal and apathy are defensive maneuvers to avoid being overwhelmed. This patient faced many difficult decisions and issues, including con-frontation with her family, her daughter-in-law, and others. She effectively avoided direct confrontation after her symptoms had been manifested.

Verwoerdt (1976) traces the experience of many reactive depressions in late life to mid-life crises. He notes that the "involutional grief reaction" secondary to failure to obtain ide-als, realization of one's transience, relinquishing illusions of parental success, and other dis-illusionments, as well as biologic and social stresses, merge during this period. Therefore the mid-life grief reaction may become the first in a series of episodes of grief secondary to the repeated losses of later life.

Under certain circumstances, grieving can then "unravel" into a neurotic or major de-pression. The persistence of depressive symptoms is not to be interpreted as chronicity but reflects a succession of superimposed losses and episodes of grief without appropriate reso-lution. Although the loss of the son precipitated the patient's depressive symptoms, the real-ization that her sons would not care for her in their homes and the decline of her own phys-ical and emotional health were superimposed. Verwoerdt (1976) notes three dynamic factors that contribute to these persistent and aggravated periods of depression. First, if the individ-ual possesses ambivalent feelings about the lost object, a grief reaction comes to an impasse. The patient undoubtedly was relieved to some extent when the son died after a long and painful illness. Energy, time, and worry directed toward this child during much of his adult life and the abandonment by the husband (partially caused by his inability to cope with the child), undoubtedly led to unconscious resentment of the son. Yet the son had been kind and considerate to the mother and was a "favorite" of hers. Therefore she experienced a major loss with his death. Affectionate feelings toward the son led to introjection or identification, as evidenced by the patient taking on the symptoms of the dead son. Negative feelings of hostility and resultant guilt influenced the "selection" of those symptoms of the son with which the patient identified. Therefore the patient identified with the painful and difficult features of the son's illness and helplessness.

Older persons who experience significant losses may overreact to these losses. After one loss is experience the older adult may feel more easily threatened and develop an attitude of anticipating frequent losses. These anticipated losses are not realistic but have an intrapsychic reality. There may also be a process of generalization of a specific loss to general losses. For example, the loss of the son and exclusion from the life-and-death decision about her son led this patient to conclude that all of her children had deserted her and would not repay the many years of effort she had contributed to their upbringing. The minor declines in her physical health resulted in the generalization that she was physically ill and was "losing her mind."

Verwoerdt (1976) further notes that the depressed older adult may withdraw, and this withdrawal represents a protection against the potential for being hurt again. The partial resolution of grief leaves "an emotional, sensitive scar." Avoidance of further object relations may lead to somatization or even a narcissistic self-absorption. Neglect of interpersonal contacts and self-centeredness further places the patient at risk for alienating the social contacts of value. Zetzel (1965) describes a depressive anxiety related to loss. This anxiety is associated to the primitive meanings of anxiety that occur in the helpless and dependent young child who fears the loss of parental support and love. Fear of object loss in a vulnerable person is more likely to be seen during the aging process so that feelings of helplessness and weakness return. Fears of being left alone throughout life may predispose an individual to develop this "depressive anxiety."

Fasey (1990) suggests that abnormal grief can be classified as chronic, inhibited, or delayed. Chronic grief is a reaction to loss, persisting beyond the expected duration and of greater severity than the loss would warrant. Inhibited grief is a reduced expression of distress, with many symptoms of grief being minimal or absent. Symptoms may be substituted, especially somatic symptoms or emergent symptoms late in the course of grief that are not associated with the loss. Delayed grief occurs when a response of denial and numbness do not emerge and a period of overt normality begins almost immediately and persists for weeks or even months after the loss. Persons who must cope with complex social and economic changes after a loss may temporarily focus exclusively on these changes, thus delaying the expression of their feelings.

Abnormal bereavement can also lead to an increased use of medications and alcohol (Bornstein, 1973). However, medications may be appropriately used by the clinician treating a recently bereaved older adult (e.g., brief use of a sedative hypnotic agent), yet prolonged isolation, depressed affect, and anxiety associated with bereavement may lead to the onset of the use of alcohol or anxolytic agents that persists and even increases over months and years after the loss.

■ DIAGNOSTIC WORKUP OF THE BEREAVED ELDER

The diagnostic workup of the bereaved older adult derives from an understanding of the broad spectrum of bereavement and the context in which bereavement occurs

(Blazer, 1990). A number of questions should be included in the history obtained from both the bereaved elder and the family. These questions include the following:

1. What is the physical health and psychiatric history of the bereaved elder?
2. Is the bereaved elder currently taking any medications. Are there any recent changes in medications?
3. Was the death of the loved one natural or unnatural?
4. Was the death expected or unexpected?
5. Are there unique stressors or complications accompanying the loss?
6. Given the loss experienced by the bereaved elder, are the symptoms appropriate, excessive, or muted?
7. Has the course of bereavement followed the usual expected course?
8. Have family and friends responded to the bereaved older adult? Has the response been appropriate and supportive?
9. Do family and friends view the response of the elder to the loss as normal or abnormal?
10. What particular changes in behavior or function have been noted in the bereaved individual?

The clinician should attend to an assessment of physical health in some detail. Adequate dietary intake, physical exercise, and maintenance of personal hygiene are often neglected during bereavement. As the older person experiences symptoms suggesting the emergence of health problems (e.g., chest pain, excessive weakness) particular attention should be directed to medical status. If the elder experiences prolonged symptoms of anxiety of depression, such as difficulty sleeping, decreased appetite, weight loss, excessive diarrhea, or constipation, the possible emergence of a psychiatric disorder should be explored. Medication used by the older person should be screened carefully to determine which medications were used by the elder before the bereavement and what changes in medication use have occurred during the process of bereavement. Health habits of the bereaved elder should be examined for changes. For example, if the bereaved elder has increased smoking or alcohol use, these changes should be carefully documented.

Since males usually adjust less well to bereavement than females, professionals working with bereaved elders must especially take care in evaluating the older male who now lives alone. Given the mortality rates of older men and women in the latter twentieth century, males are less likely to lose a spouse and therefore less likely to expect the loss of a spouse. Women married to older men, although they may not discuss it, have usually rehearsed in their minds how they will adapt to the loss of their spouse. Men, on the other hand, are much less likely to consider the necessary adaptations if they lose their wives. Men (at least in the latter twentieth century) are also less capable of caring for themselves in the home. They may have never learned to cook or manage the household. Tasks such as managing a household budget and shopping may be especially difficult for a man after the loss of his spouse. Men are also at greater risk for social isolation, given that they usually do not express their feelings openly and do not have close friends with whom they can share their deepest thoughts.

In the evaluation of the bereaved elder the clinician should carefully evaluate social network and social interaction, since the network is the greatest ally with the clinician in recognizing the onset of abnormal bereavement and alerting the clinician to abnormal symptoms. The social network includes family, friends, other professionals (e.g., lawyers, clergy), and persons with whom the elder is engaged in business. The clinician should inquire about social interactions (e.g., number of phone calls per week and number of visits with others during the week). Does the older adult leave his or her house daily to perform regular chores, such as shopping, banking, and personal care? Does the bereaved elder belong to social groups or clubs, such as religious groups, and does the elder continue to attend the activities of these groups during the period of bereavement? During the first year of bereavement, a vacation may be especially beneficial to revitalize the bereaved elder. Does the older person who has lost a loved one have family or friends who can accompany the elder on a vacation?

There are no routine laboratory tests in the diagnostic evaluation of the elders suffering from uncomplicated bereavement. As noted, older persons who are bereaved exhibit symptoms similar to those of major depression. Kosten et al (1984), in a study of 13 older adults who had lost a loved one within 6 months before the study, found that cortisol levels after administration of dexamethasone were higher than expected but not as high as found in persons suffering from major depression not associated with bereavement. Cortisol levels were correlated with the severity of the depressive symptoms.

■ TREATMENT OF ABNORMAL BEREAVEMENT IN LATE LIFE

Treatment of the bereaved older adult who suffers from abnormal bereavement must be multidimensional. Ancillary procedures for care are usually instituted before considering psychotherapy as a treatment. Guidelines for ancillary therapy are presented in the box below. A decision to hospitalize the patient is usually based on the patient's ability to maintain himself or herself in the present living arrangements or the patient's willingness to participate in therapy. The use of antidepressant medications is usually not necessary. Although symptomatic guidelines for the use of somatic therapies with the bereaved are not always clear (since bereaved elders may experience a major depressive episode), prolonged administration of antidepressant medications should be avoided when possible. Psychotropic medications may be useful for certain patients but the greater the reactive component, the less the impact of the tricyclic antidepressant.

Medications may be useful in augmenting sleep and in improving appetite. Low-dose tricyclic antidepressants with sedative effects, such as 25 mg of amtriptyline or nortrip-

---

Guidelines for ancillary therapy for the bereaved older adult

Prescribe medications judiciously and monitor their use carefully.
  Attempt to maintain the patient in the most independent living arrangement reasonable.
  Movement to extended-care facilities or into the home of a friend, sibling, or child should be temporary.
Assist the patient in engaging in new activities and establishing new relationships.
Suggest resources to the patient for dealing with the administrative and legal problems surrounding the death.
Include the family in the therapeutic process.
Institute behavioral approaches to therapy when necessary.
Encourage appropriate physical activity.

tyline, can be used rather than benzodiazepine compounds. If medications are prescribed, they should be monitored carefully and should be only continued for a short period of time (a few days). The clinician should especially monitor the emergence of side effects, such as confusion or excess sedation.

In contrast to bereavement at earlier stages of life a significant interruption in self-care of the elderly bereaved places them at high risk for hospital admission and placement in long-term care facilities. Attempts should be made from the outset of therapy to plan for and encourage the most reasonable living arrangements for the bereaved older adult. These attempts may fail, but they should be made nevertheless. Coordination of efforts between the family and medical staff is essential for ensuring the success of movement from the hospital or long-term care facility back into the home.

Behavior modification techniques are often used within the hospital and in the outpatient setting to encourage the bereaved older adult to become more independent and self-sufficient. Whenever positive reinforcement can be used as an incentive for more independent behavior, it should be implemented. If behavior modification can be considered within a broader framework, many activities applicable to both hospital and home are included. Materials of interest to the patient can be made available to the bereaved elderly, such as books and materials for arts, crafts, and hobbies. Recommendations of clubs, religious or social groups, and support groups, can be implemented. When attention-getting behaviors emerge, such as the falling behavior described in the case study, this behavior should be ignored by the family and staff after it has been established that the patient is at little danger for injury. Direct confrontation of these patients by family is not generally useful and may increase the patient's need to get attention. Under these circumstances, verbal reward of positive behavior often eliminates the attention-getting symptoms.

Guidelines for psychotherapy of the bereaved older adult are presented in the box below. Resistance may prevent the older adult from expressing deep feelings of loss and

---

Guidelines for psychotherapy for the bereaved older adult

Permit and help the patient to put into words and nonverbal expression the pain, sorrow, and finality of bereavement.

Review the relationship of the patient with the deceased (i.e., a life history approach).

Encourage the patient to discuss feelings of love, guilt, and hostility toward the deceased.

Help the patient recognize the alterations in cognition, affect, and behavior secondary to bereavement.

Work with the patient to find an acceptable balance for the future intrapsychic representative of the deceased.

Avoid interpretations of long-dormant, highly charged intrapsychic conflicts.

Support existing coping mechanisms.

Reassure the patient that the suffering and pain are transient.

Allow a positive, even parental transference to evolve.

Facilitate the transfer of dependency from the deceased to other sources of gratification when necessary.

Decrease sessions with the patient on improvement but avoid abrupt termination.

anger about the deceased loved one. Encouraging review of past history (i.e., the "life review") often provides a window into the relationship of the patient with the deceased. The task of the life review is to integrate life as it has been lived and how it might have been lived, a task so similar to the task of psychotherapy with the bereaved that one usually overlaps with the other. Family photo albums, videotapes, and audiotapes can be useful in accomplishing this task.

Of special importance in the therapy of the bereaved older adult is the relationship with the therapist. A transference may develop rapidly, and most often this transference is initially positive. Equation of the therapist with the deceased is not uncommon, especially if the deceased was approximately the same age as the therapist (often occurring when the older adult loses a child). If the patient develops a positive, dependent transference, the therapist should not discourage this relationship and should be cautious of pushing independence too quickly. The usual therapeutic goal with the young and middle-aged adult is independence from the therapeutic relationship. This assumes that the adult is capable of independent living, both physically and psychologically. Older adults may, for various reasons, not be able to maintain an independent life-style. The dependent transference should not be overinterpreted in therapeutic work with such patients, and the patient should be reassured that the relationship will continue with the therapist. Treatment sessions may decrease over time, but permanent termination usually is not necessary.

Kavangh (1990) proposes a cognitive-behavioral intervention for adult grief reactions that is appropriate for older adults. First, he suggests that the intervention recognize the benefits obtained from understanding personal and social rules about mourning. A healthy respect for usual strategies of mourning should be established before new strategies are implemented. Next, the bereaved are encouraged to gradually confront environmental and cognitive stimuli that are associated with the bereavement. This type of intervention is especially important when the bereaved has avoided bereavement. For example, the bereaved elder should not avoid situations or places that remind him or her of the lost loved one. For example, returning to a religious service after a death and sitting in the same place where the bereaved elder for years sat with the lost loved one is a means of gradually exposing oneself to bereavement. The therapist also encourages the bereaved elder to engage in activities that temporarily distract him/her from the loss and substitutes moments of pleasure. More traditional approaches to traditional cognitive therapeutic approaches are also used. The therapist should inquire about the evidence for negative cognitions (see Chapter 5) regarding the lost loved one and events surrounding the death. A frequent focus in such an intervention is the blame the bereaved elder places on himself or herself.

Bruhn (1984) emphasizes the therapeutic value of hope in the patient-therapist relationship. Hope is most important after an acute loss. Hope enables the bereaved elder to look to the future, review the pain of the past, and go forward and search for increased growth and development. Components of hope often include a close attachment with surviving kin (a desire to live their lives such that their friends and relatives are benefitted), an intense drive to survive, and a sense of religious experience. The therapist should encourage hope in the bereaved older adult. Bereaved elders expect that their therapist will express a caring and hopeful attitude. A shared expectation that the older adult will adapt to the loss is essential for successful therapy, although hope should not interfere with the natural pain of grief.

■ THE OUTCOME OF BEREAVEMENT IN LATE LIFE

Madison and Viola (1968) studied the health of widows in the first year after bereavement. These widows (all under the age of 60) reported many more complaints about their physical health during the year after bereavement than in matched nonbereaved population during a similar period of follow-up. Parkes (1964) reports that younger widowers consulted the general practitioner because of psychiatric symptoms more than three times as often during the 6 months after bereavement than they had the 6 months before bereavement. He suggests that a heightened dependency on the doctor may play a role in the increased frequency of office visits. Yet these bereaved women were often physically ill, although psychiatric symptoms were the most common for them to report during these visits. Symptoms, such as insomnia, nervousness, and a reduced capacity for work, were the most common.

Fasey (1990) reviewed the current literature on mortality in grief. A number of studies have demonstrated the increased risk of death among the widowed, especially among the widowed males. According to Fasey, the following possible explanations of these results emerge: (1) health is not independent from marital status, since unhealthy widow and widowers are less likely to remarry; (2) unhealthy people may tend to marry one another; (3) spouses share adjoining environment so that the adverse effects of diet, smoking, and other factors impact both partners; (4) both partners may die of a common illness, such as infection or accident; (5) widowers are often underrepresented in sampled surveys and overrepresented in mortality statistics. Nevertheless, most well-designed studies show an increased risk of mortality among the bereaved, especially in the 6 months immediately after death (Rees and Lutkins, 1967; Helsing et al, 1982).

REFERENCES

Blazer DG: Bereavement. In Blazer DG (ed): *Emotional Problems in Later Life: Intervention Strategies for Professional Caregivers.* New York, Springer, 1990, pp. 201-219.

Bornstein P, Clayton PJ, Halikes JA, Maurice WL, Robins E: Depression of widowhood after thirteen months, British Journal of Psychiatry 122:561-566, 1973.

Breckenridge JN, Gallagher D, Thompson LW, Peterson JA: Characteristics of depressive of bereaved elders, Journal of Gerontology 41:163, 168, 1986.

Bruhn JG: Therapy of hope, *Southern Medical Journal* 77:215-219, 1984.

Clayton PJ, Desmarias L, Winokur G: A study of normal bereavement, American Journal of Psychiatry 125:168-178, 1968.

Diagnostic and Statistical Manual of Mental Disorders (ed 3—revised). Washington, DC, American Psychiatric Association, 1987, pp. 361-362.

Duke D: A *Study of the Effects of Bereavement.* Newcastle, England, Newcastle Polytechnic, 1980 (thesis).

Fasey CL: Grief in old age: a review of the literature, *International Journal of Geriatric Psychiatry* 5:67-75, 1990.

Gallagher D, Thompson LW: Bereavement and adjustment disorders. In Busse EW, Blazer DG (eds): *Geriatric Psychiatry.* Washington, DC, American Psychiatric Press, 1989, pp. 459-473.

Goldfarb AI: Mild maladjustments of the aged. In Ariti S (ed): *American Handbook of Psychiatry.* (vol. 1) New York, Basic Books, 1974, pp. 820-860.

Harlow HF, Suomi SJ: Production of depressive disorders in young monkeys, *Journal of Autism and Childhood Schizophrenia* 1:246-263, 1971.

Helsing KJ, Comstock GW, Szklo M: Causes of death in a widowed population, *American Journal of Epidemiology* 116:524-532, 1982

Jacobs S, Kim K: Psychiatric complications of bereavement, *Psychiatric Annals* 20:314-317, 1990.

Jacobs S, Ostfeld A: The clinical management of grief, *Journal of the American Geriatric Psychiatry* 28:331-335, 1980.

Kavangh DJ: Towards a cogntive-behavioral intervention for adult grief reactions, *British Journal of Psychiatry* 157:373-383, 1990.

Kosten TR, Jacobs S, Mason JW: The dexamethasone suppression test during bereavement, *Journal of Nervous and Mental Disease* 172:359-360, 1984.

Lindemann E: Symptomatology and management of acute grief. *American Journal of Psychiatry* 101:141-149, 1944.

Madison D, Viola A: The health of widows in the year following bereavement, *Journal of Psychosomatic Research* 12:297-306, 1968.

McKinney WT: Primate separation studies: referenced to bereavement, *Psychiatric Annals* 16:281-287, 1986.

Parkes CM: *Bereavement, Studies of Grief in Adult Life*. London, Pelican, 1972.

Parkes CM: The effects of bereavement on physical and mental health; A study of the case records of widows, *British Medical Journal* 2:274-279, 1964.

Parkes CM, Weiss RS: *Recovery from Bereavement*. New York, Basic Books, 1983.

Portnoy VA: Post-retirement depression: myth or reality, *Comprehensive Therapy* 9:31-37, 1983.

Rees DW, Lutkins SG: Mortality of bereavement, *British Medical Journal* 4:13-16, 1967.

Siegel JM, Kuykendall DH: Loss, widowhood, and psychological distress among the elderly, *Journal of Consulting and Clinical Psychology* 38:319-324, 1990.

Verwoerdt A: *Clinical Geropsychiatry*. Baltimore, Williams and Wilkins, 1976.

Verwoerdt A: Personal Communication. 1980.

Weinberg J: *Research in Aging*. Veterans Administration, 1959.

Zetzel ER: Dynamics of the method of psychology of the aging process. In Berzin MA, Kath SH (eds): *Geriatric Psychiatry: Grief, Loss and Emotional Disturbances in the Aging Process*. New York, International Universities Press, 1965.

Zisook S, Shuchter SR: The first four years of widowhood, *Psychiatric Annals* 16:288-294, 1990.

14

Depressive Disorders Associated with the Physically Ill Elderly

Depression is the most frequent psychiatric syndrome among the physically ill elderly. Studies of older male inpatients reveal a prevalence of significant depressive symptoms of 40%, with 10% or more meeting criteria for diagnosis of major depression (Koenig et al, 1988). Depressive symptoms also increase the morbidity of physically ill elders, jeopardize their survival after hospitalization, and increase the use of health services (especially increased length of hospital stay). Yet depression is often unrecognized by clinicians in inpatient settings. Rapp et al (1988) found the detection by house staff officers of depression among elderly medical inpatients to be extremely low (less than 10%), although these depressed elders were readily identified by using self-rating instruments, such as the Beck Depression Inventory and the Geriatric Depression Scale.

Depressive symptoms are also frequently associated with physical illness in older persons living in the community. Palinkas et al (1990) found the prevalence of significant depressive symptoms in over 1600 community dwellings to be 5.2%. Depressive symptoms were associated with several risk factors in both genders, especially self-perception of poor current health status, chronic diseases, medication use, and decreased physical activity.

The association between physical illness and depression is complex. Depression has been documented to be associated with a variety of physical disorders, including thyroid disorders, cancer, vitamin B12 deficiency, chronic pain, cardiovascular disorders, malnutrition, general functional disability, and the use of medications to treat physical illnesses. Depression has also been associated with general physical debility. For example, Katz et al (1989) found depression associated with decreased serum albumin in a residential sample of elders. In addition, older persons may react to physical illnesses with certain symptoms of depression, such as loss of a sense of control and increased dependency. Major depression may be precipitated by the onset of a physical illness in a previously healthy older adult who has a past history of a mood disorder. The personality styles of individuals, as they mold adaptive strategies to chronic illness, may lead to depressive symptoms. Exaggeration of physical problems, such as observed in somatization and hypochondriasis, may mask a depressive disorder. Therefore the diagnostic workup of the medically ill depressed older adult deserves special attention in any discussion of depression among the elderly.

The treatment of depression in the medically ill elderly is not as effective as in uncomplicated late life depression. As with other depressive disorders, however, a combined approach using psychotherapy and pharmacotherapy along with social and family support is essential. Management of the medical illness associated with the depressive disorder may be the key to the treatment of late life depression. If intervention is to be successful, it is essential that such intervention occur early in the course of a depression associated with medical illness. Not only has late life depression been associated with increased mortality among medically ill elders, it may also lead to other health problems, such as hip fracture and increased susceptibility to infection. Depression also extends recovery time and prolongs hospitalization (Mossey, et al, 1990).

■ CASE PRESENTATION

Mr. LJ, a 72-year-old retired businessman was referred to a psychiatrist for chronic depressive symptoms after having been forced to retire from work 3 years before the evaluation. The patient, a tall and thin Caucasian male, had been a smoker during most of his life and did not suffer significant health problems until later in life. Almost simultaneously, he began to have difficulty with his breathing and with lower back pain. These symptoms forced him to retire from work at age 67 (he had planned to work until he was at least 75). His work was relatively nondemanding and was most enjoyable to him (work was his major interest in life). On initial evaluation, it was found that the patient suffered from significant emphysema. He immediately ceased smoking. Nevertheless, chronic progressive pulmonary changes complicated by osteoarthritis led to a decreased lung capacity over 3 years. The lower back pain was diagnosed as osteoporosis, and he subsequently experienced three extremely painful compression fractures of his vertebrae.

The patient was treated aggressively with analgesics and nonsteroidal antiinflammatory agents for the arthritic pains and was also treated aggressively for the osteoporosis. He gradually improved symptomatically but never to the point that he could return to his previous work. About 1 year before the psychiatric evaluation, when he was functioning better, he returned to his place of employment and learned that the company had no plans for him to return to work.

Sleep problems, loss of appetite, loss of weight, and general discouragement were symptoms that prompted his primary care physician to prescribe imipramine 25 mg qhs (which improved his sleep). The depressive symptoms continued, however, and he was subsequently referred to the psychiatrist.

On evaluation the patient did not appear acutely ill, but evidence of the chronic medical illness was apparent in his gait and in the pain he experienced on standing or sitting. In addition, he was short of breath even at rest. During the initial evaluation the patient focused his discussion on a business venture that had failed when he was in his late thirties. He had sold his interest in a shoe manufacturing company and had moved to another city where he had bought into another shoe company. The company that he sold continued to do reasonably well (although did not dramatically succeed as a business and later was merged into a larger firm). The company that he bought into struggled financially throughout its brief history and the patient later sold his interest. After this, and with the strong encouragement of his wife, the patient sought employment with a local business firm in which he had no ownership. He was salaried and worked on commission. During the remaining 25 years of his working career the patient had been financially successful, although he never made the money that he had hoped to make in business. He was well accepted and appreciated in the local business community, belonging to many civic clubs.

When forced into retirement the patient initially spent almost 1 year in bed with the combined problems of emphysema and osteoporosis. When he finally regained some function, he found that most of his former associates were no longer available to him socially, since virtually all of them were business associates. Although his wife continued to work and he did not suffer significant financial impairment, nevertheless, he acutely experienced social isolation and loss of status in his community.

During therapy, it became apparent that this patient's depression derived from his unwillingness to accept that the disability associated with his physical illness had caused him to lose his job. He could psychologically better adapt to failing at something over which he perceived he had control than to admit that he was impaired by problems over which he had no control. Although he could speak realistically about the impairments associated with the physical illness, he had great difficulty in accepting that his life had been a successful one until the physical problems became so acute.

During the course of therapy the patient was withdrawn from imipramine. Depressive symptoms persisted and he was prescribed fluoxetine 20 mg po every other day. Although he experienced some late-night agitation while on fluoxetine, he became more active and experienced a lifting of the depressed mood. As therapy progressed, he rarely referred to his former business *failures* and appropriately grieved the loss of his physical function secondary to his illnesses.

Mr. LJ is typical of many older persons who suffer chronic and moderately severe physical illnesses for which they can expect only partial improvement, even with the best of medical therapies. For physically ill elders who have previously been healthy, the need to confront and adapt to a chronic physical illness is one of the most challenging prob-lems of late life. Depression is a frequent accompaniment of the adjustment process. Most elders recognize that the depressive mood is associated with the process of grieving for former health and therefore do not require intervention. Others, however, tend to deny that the physical problems are a concern and focus on other issues, often perceived failures from the past; therefore the depressive symptoms become exaggerated. On reviewing perceived past failures with family members, rarely do these perceived failures appear to have greatly influenced the course of the person's life despite the reinterpretation in late life.

Medically ill older persons, such as Mr. LJ, often respond to low doses of antidepressant medications, if the medical illness is not severe and antidepressant therapy is not contraindicated for medical reasons. Antidepressant medication is usually much more effective in the medically ill outpatient than in the medically ill inpatient. Regardless, the selection of a medication must depend on the need to avoid troublesome side effects. Anticholinergic effects are especially troublesome in the medically ill elderly and therefore selecting a drug relatively free of these effects, such as fluoxetine or trazodone, is preferred. Bupropion may be used safely and effectively in medically ill elderly patients, especially those who experience sexual dysfunction while taking fluoxetine.

■ PHYSICAL ILLNESSES THAT CAN CAUSE DEPRESSIVE SYMPTOMS IN LATE LIFE

Thyroid Failure

Hypothyroidism is a common disorder among older adults. (Rosenthal et al, 1987) In one study, thyroid-stimulating hormone (TSH) levels were elevated in 13% of healthy elderly subjects. Over a 4-year follow-up, one third of these subjects developed biochemical thyroid failure. Clinical manifestations of the hypothyroidism frequently include depressed mood and anergia (Whybrow et al, 1969). Psychiatric symptoms may be the only manifestations of thyroid dysfunction in older adults. Therefore the appearance of subclinical hypothyroidism (evidenced by an elevated TSH level) suggests the need for a comprehensive thyroid evaluation.

A majority of patients with hypothyroidism suffer from autoimmune thyroiditis as evidenced by increased plasma titers of antimicrosomal antibodies. The prevalence of circulating autoantibodies in general and thyroid antibodies in particular increases significantly with age. Most elders with high-titer thyroid antimicrosomal antibodies eventually become overtly hypothyroid. The supplementation of naturally produced thyroid hormone with levothyroxine (Synthroid) often will correct the problem of hypothyroidism and improve depressive symptoms.

Hyperthyroidism may present clinically as withdrawal or depression in older persons, often called *apathetic thyrotoxicosis* (Thomas et al, 1970). Treatment of the thyroid disorder appropriately usually reverses the depressive symptoms.

Cobalamin Deficiency

Deficiency of cobalamine (vitamin B12) has been long associated with depressive symptoms. In a recent study (Lindenbaum et al, 1988), among 141 patients with neuropsychiatric abnormalities because of cobalamine deficiency, 28% had no anemia or microcytosis on the initial evaluation. Characteristic features of cobalamine deficiency in these patients included a variety of neurologic symptoms (neurosensory loss, ataxia, and memory loss), as well as weakness, fatigue, depressive symptoms. Most of these patients were over the age of 65 and equally distributed between males and females. All but one of the patients in this study responded to cobalamine therapy with improvement in their neuropsychiatric symptoms, including depressed mood.

Bell et al (1991) compared B-complex vitamin status at time of admission in 20 geriatric and 16 young adult nonalcoholic inpatients with major depression. About 28% of the subjects were deficient in B2 (riboflavin), B6 (pyridoxine), and/or B12 (cobalamine). None were deficient in B1 (thiamine or folate). In fact the geriatric sample had significantly higher serum-folate levels. Psychotic depressives had lower B12 than nonpsychotic depressives.

Cardiac Symptoms and Depressive Disorders

Cassem and Hackett (1977) found a depressed mood in 50% of patients immediately after a myocardial infarction. More than 70% of these patients continued to be depressed 1 year after initial evaluation. Depression in these cardiac patients was commonly associated with inability to return to work or to previous activities, to sexual difficulties, and to readmission to the hospital. In another study, patients who had suffered a depressive episode in the past were the most likely to become depressed after a myocardial infarction (Lloyd and Cawley, 1983; Schleifer et al, 1989).

Dovenmuehle and Verwoerdt (1962) found that 64% of 62 cardiac patients, 41 of whom were older than 60 years of age, experienced moderate-to-severe depressive symptoms. These symptoms were frequently associated with a lowered self-esteem and anxiety but not irritability or death wishes. Prominent biologic symptoms of depression were absent in the group. Neither age nor gender contributed to a differentiation between the depressed and nondepressed. The authors conclude that the symptom complex of depression in cardiac patients can best be understood as a depressive reaction to physical illness similar to a grief reaction or an acute situational depression. A patient with cardiac disease must work through the anticipatory threat of possible death and the loss of potential for certain role functions in life. Cardiac disease often calls for a mandatory acceptance of the sick role in the elderly, and grief results from this role transition.

Cancer in Depression

The association of depression and cancer is well established (Massie and Holland, 1990). At least 25% of hospitalized cancer patients will meet criteria for major depression disorder with depressed mood. Individuals who are at the greatest risk for developing depression when suffering cancer are those with a history of mood disorder or alcoholism, a more advanced stage of cancer, poorly controlled pain, treatment with medications, or concurrent illnesses that produce depressive symptoms.

Diagnosing major depression may be more difficult in the cancer patient. Kathol et al (1990) found that the diagnosis of major depression in 152 cancer patients differs as much as 13%, depending on the diagnostic system used. Screening instruments were useful for identifying potential cases but frequently misclassified those who had no major depression according to one or more of the criteria-based diagnostic systems. Evans et al (1986) attempted to determine whether the dexamethasone-suppression test and the thyrotrophin-releasing hormone (TRH) stimulation test for diagnosing major depression would be useful in identifying depression among 83 women hospitalized for gynecologic cancer. The mean age of these patients was 53, with the oldest being 86. The sensitivity and specificity of the DST were 40% and 88%, respectively. There was no relationship between DST findings and TRH test results. The authors conclude that the routine use of the DST and TRH test was not indicated at this time for the diagnosis of major depression in cancer patients.

Much attention has been directed over the years to depression as a predisposing factor to the development of cancer and/or depression as the first symptom of cancer. Whitlock and Siskind (1979) followed a group of subjects 40 years of age and older with a primary diagnosis of depression for 2 to 4 years. During this period, nine male and nine female patients (most of whom were over 65 years of age) died. Six of these patients died from cancer not diagnosed at the time of psychiatric admission, with male cancer deaths being significantly higher than expected. Linkins and Comstock (1990) performed a 12-year follow-up of a community sample originally evaluated for depressive symptoms. Although there was only a slight association of depressed mood and subsequent cancer among the total population, the association was stronger among cigarette smokers. Older patients, although more likely to develop cancer, were less likely to exhibit a relationship between depressed mood initially and development of cancer on follow-up. One possible linkage between depression and cancer is that persons who have experienced frequent episodes of depression throughout their lives may have subsequently been more prone to smoke cigarettes.

Fras et al (1968) found that symptoms of a depression, anxiety and feelings of a premonition of serious illness, were valuable as an aid to the early diagnosis of carcinoma of the pancreas. These findings resulted from a systematic study to verify earlier reports that psychiatric symptoms, especially depression, were the first manifestations of carcinoma of the pancreas. Parmoa and Gershon (1984) reported a case of a recurrent and treatment-resistant depression with a positive dexamethasone-suppression test in an individual in whom carcinoma of the pancreas was eventually diagnosed. After excision of the tumor, there was an increased therapeutic response to antidepressants and normalization of the DST. The authors suggest that the active adenocarcinoma could have played a role in not only the depressive symptoms but also the lack of responsiveness to traditional therapies for depression.

Postmenopausal Depression

Menopause is associated with a decline in circulating estrogen because of decreased ovarian and adrenal function. Decreased circulating estrogen has been associated with depressive symptoms, but the results in the literature are conflicting. Ballinger et al (1979) suggest that the intervening factor of life events during the menopause may play a major role in the development of depression in those women who enter the postmenopausal era and suffer significant depressive symptoms. They found that estrogen levels in a group of women, postmenopausal with depression presumably associated with high psychologic stress, was significantly lower than those with lower reported stress. They also found that estrogen levels increased in women as they recovered from depressive illness. These investigators therefore conclude that women may experience a low estrogen level secondary to depression (not the other way around) and that successful treatment of depression in turn leads to an increase in estrogen levels during the postmenopausal years.

Chronic Pain

Chronic pain and depression are frequently associated (Romano and Turner, 1985). Chronic pain is more frequent in mid-life than late life, with a mean age of onset of 39 years (Blumer and Heilbronn, 1982). Romano and Turner (1985) concluded, after reviewing the literature, that there is support for an association between the syndromes of chronic pain and depression, with a suggestion that coexisting pain and depression is the final common presentation reached by a number of pathways. The majority of persons with comorbid pain and depression probably experience a secondary depression after the development of a chronic pain syndrome. In other cases, pain may occur as a symptom of depression or may mask a primary mood disturbance.

Colenda and Dougherty (1990) studied three groups of older patients—those with chronic pain, those with major depression, and those who were healthy. Even though the defense mechanisms and self-esteem reports for the three groups were not that different, depressed patients used greater levels of projection and demonstrated lower levels of self-esteem. The investigators conclude that personality and coping patterns are similar for individuals with chronic pain and depression in late life and confirm previous results that somatic or illness behavior (specifically chronic pain behavior) is not an expected result of the aging process but rather is related to physical illnesses. These results also confirmed the impression that chronic pain problems in late life associated with major depression are less frequent than in mid-life.

Functional Disability

Regardless of the specific illnesses studied, functional disability has been clearly associated with depression in the elderly. The proportion of persons who can maintain their usual daily routines of caring for themselves and remaining mobile decreases significantly with increasing age, especially after the age of 85 (Gurland et al, 1988). Although older persons are, in general, less likely to suffer major depression than younger persons (see Chapter 1), there is a clear association between functional disability and depression in the elderly. In the most functionally impaired elderly (persons in the hospital and in long-term care facilities), depressive symptoms and the diagnosis of depressive disorders are significantly higher than found in the general population.

In their review of the literature, Gurland et al (1988) acknowledge the relationship between depression and functional disability, but they do not believe it is possible to describe what types or characteristics of depression and disability are related. They do find, however, that disability is the most important determinant of the frequency and outcomes of depression and that the relationship between depression and disability is a reciprocal one, since the cause of pathways may go in either direction. Treatment of disability can be keyed to the effective treatment of depression and that, conversely, treatment of depression may improve functional status in older persons. They also found that the association between disability and depression appears to become less clear as age advances. Advancing age may bring with it an enhanced ability to cope with adversity.

Closely related to functional status and depression is the association of physical activity and depression. In a longitudinal study, Camacho et al (1991) found that among persons who were not depressed at baseline, those who reported a low activity level were at greater risk for depression at follow-up. This study controlled for physical health status and other health habits. Exercise programs, as described in a later section, may not only be of benefit in treating the medically ill depressed; they also may be of benefit in preventing depression in late life.

Nutritional Deficits

Nutritional deficits are a common result of depressive disorders in late life, as well as a cause of depressive symptoms. Depression frequently causes anorexia and weight loss, whereas undernutrition or a purposeful deprivation of food can lead to depressive symptoms (Garetz, 1976). Once the process begins, a vicious cycle ensues with, in severe cases, a failure to eat that can lead to death. In a 1973 Minnesota study, 38 people over 65 years of age died of starvation that was unrelated to conditions such as cancer, alcoholism, or a lack of availability of food (Minnesota State Board of Health: Minnesota Health Statistics, 1973). Depression may lead to overeating as well and, in turn, obesity can contribute to depressive symptoms. Among elderly persons, however, the association between depression and overeating is much less frequent that at other stages of the life cycle.

Depressive symptoms may arise from a number of deficiency states, including cachexia, weakness and mental slowing secondary to starvation, vitamin deficiencies, and deficiencies of important minerals (e.g., iron deficiency and anemia). The signs of undernutrition, listed in the box below should be evaluated carefully by the clinician during the diagnostic workup of the depressed older adult.

There are a number of potential causes of undernutrition in older persons. These are presented in the box on p. 226. Loss of interest in the social environment, decreased appetite, and decreased mobility are the major depressive symptoms leading to undernutrition. Many older persons, however, simply lose their taste sensation, which leads to the poor food intake. Depressed older persons, especially the severely depressed, occasionally develop peculiar food preferences. Some desire only milk or milk products. The desire for milk products may result in a return to a more regressive and dependent stage of life (i.e., early childhood) (Natow and Heslin, 1980). Other elders avoid certain foods, most commonly meats or eggs, because of fear or guilt about eating these foods. There is no evidence that lowering cholesterol in persons 65 years of age and older significantly lowers cardiac mortality risk. Suggestions for improving food intake in the elderly are listed in the box on p. 226.

Medications

Many medications may cause depressive symptoms and the full-blown major depressive episodes. These symptoms may derive either from side effects of the drug or withdrawal from the medications. Drugs that commonly lead to mood disorders are listed in the box on p. 227.

The Signs of Undernutrition

Loss of natural shine and dryness of hair
Loss of skin color with malar and supraorbital pigmentation
Tenting of skin on pinching
Petechiae
Dryness of skin with dyspigmentation
Cornea soft, dull, and scarred
Circumcorneal injection
Nails spoon-shaped and brittle
Lips red and swollen, with fissures at corners of mouth
Tongue swollen, smooth, and raw, with purplish color
Cavities of teeth and bleeding gums
Muscles wasted, weak, and tender
Bones brittle
Tachycardia
Elevated blood pressure
Liver enlargement
Irritability and confusion
Burning and tingling of hand
Loss of position and vibratory sense

Adapted from Natow AB, Heslin J: *Geriatric Nutrition,* Boston, CBI, 1980.

Potential Causes of Undernutrition and Overnutrition in Depressed Older Adults

Undernutrition

Lack of knowledge about nutrition
Social isolation
Alcholism
Economic impairment
Medical illnesses that interfere with intake, absorption, storage, and use of food
Decreased mobility
Neglect of dental problems
Poor gustatory sensations
Peculiar food preferences

Overnutrition

Agitation
Social isolation
Feelings of emptiness
Reduced activity

Suggestions for Improving the Food Intake of the Depressed Elderly

Season foods well
Emphasize the favorite meal of the older person
Create a social atmosphere at mealtime
Select foods preferred by the patient
Assist the older person in eating, but do not force dependence
Attempt to accommodate cultural, class, and religious beliefs
Monitor the interactions of drugs and diet

■ DIFFERENTIAL DIAGNOSIS OF DEPRESSION ASSOCIATED WITH PHYSICAL ILLNESS IN THE ELDERLY

Adjustment Disorder

Adjustment disorders, according to DSM-III-R, are maladaptive reactions to identifiable psychosocial stresses occurring within 3 months after the onset of the stressor. Physical illness is the most common precipitant of an adjustment disorder with depressed mood in later life (Rodin and Voshart, 1986). Because somatic complaints are frequent accompaniments of depressive symptoms in adjustment disorders, these persons are sometimes difficult to distinguish from persons suffering from a major depressive episode secondary to medical illness. Adjustment disorder usually does not require the use of antidepressant medication.

Cassell (1979) suggests a number of reasons why persons suffering physical illness respond with a maladjusted mood disorder. Sick persons suffer a disconnection from their

---

Commonly Used Medications that Can Lead to Depressive Symptoms in Late Life

Amphetamines and anorectic agents—when the drugs are withdrawn

Benzodiazepines—depressive symptoms are common, especially with chronic use

Cimetidine—usually with higher doses and more often in older persons and individuals suffering from renal dysfunction

Clonidine—early depression may resolve with continued use

Disulfiram—the depressive symptoms may or may not be related to concurrent alcohol abuse

Ibuprofen—depression is rare with this drug, which is very commonly used in late life

Indomethacin—depression, confusion, and anxiety are especially common in the elderly

L-Dopa—depression or manic symptoms may occur and are more frequent in late life than during other stages of the life cycle

Methyldopa—severe depression can occur in older adult patients

Propranolol—severe depression can occur with usual doses

Reserpine—depression is common when given a dose of 0.5 mg or more daily, depression may persist after the drug is stopped

Barbiturates—depression is common with usual doses in older persons, with hyperactivity and excitement occurring on withdrawal

Vinblastine—depression is an occasional side effect

---

usual world, a loss of their sense of indestructibility (omnipotence), a loss of the competence and completeness of their reasoning, and a loss of control over themselves and their world. The environment in which sick older persons are cared for adds to the physical losses of the illness. Unnecessary restrictions on the medically ill, such as forced dependence in a hospital through riding in a wheelchair or restriction to the bed, emphasize the patient's helplessness and inability to be effective. Not including the patient in decisions regarding health care exacerbates the sense of helplessness and loss of control.

Dysthymic Disorder

Dysthymic disorder in DSM-III is a chronic mood disturbance that lasts at least 2 years without interruption for more than a few days or weeks. Chronic physical illness is a common precipitant of a dysthymic disorder. If the physical illness does not increase in severity, yet the older adult does not adapt to the disorder, an initial adjustment disorder may lapse into a dysthymic disorder. The traditional psychiatric nomenclature, however, does not assist in such discrimination, since a chronic illness requires continued adjustment, and an adjustment may be adaptive for an older person.

Major Depressive Episode

Medical illness may mimic a major depressive episode (Rodin and Voshart, 1986). The distinction is best made when the dysphoria and anhedonia that commonly accompany major depression in a medical illness do not remit when the physical disturbance is treated effectively. A predominance of physical symptoms, such as lethargy, weight loss, significant sleep disturbances, and poor appetite in the absence of psychologic symptoms, may be useful to distinguish a medical illness from a major depressive episode. The clinician should also explore carefully for a history of previous mood disorders in the depressed and medically ill elderly. A positive history suggests that a significant change in mood in the older person may be secondary to major depressive episode as opposed to a physical illness. The clinician must recognize that major depression may accompany a medical illness, either precipitated by that illness or occurring independent of the illness. In such cases the traditional treatment of the major depressive episode, when permitted by the symptoms of the physical illness, should lead to a remission of the depressive episode.

Organic Mood Disorder

Organic mood disorders are disturbances in mood secondary to an organic brain syndrome. Conditions such as hypothyroidism or possibly pancreatic carcinoma may lead directly to organic mood disorder rather than a depressive reaction secondary to the physical illness.

Personality Types in Response to Physical Illness

Kahana and Bibring (1964) describe the complications that arise when persons with given personality types are confronted with a physical illness. The *dependent and overdemanding* older adult, who has great fear of being abandoned or being helpless, wishes to be nurtured during a physical illness. Therefore he or she will demand more from family and health care providers and become overly dependent during the illness. When demands are not met, the elder may become critical of the lack of attention and depression may ensue. The *long-suffering and self-sufficient* elder strives for love, care, and acceptance through self-sacrifice and self-acceptance. This person experiences excessive guilt and may actually gain pleasure from the pain and suffering secondary to a physical illness. Long suffering elders, may even refuse treatment and rehabilitation and may be thought to suffer from a severe depressive disorder because of their refusal of help. A review of the life-long personality style generally reveals the problem to be of one of personality type rather than a mood disorder.

The *guarded and querulous* elder fears being placed in a vulnerable position in which he or she could be hurt. Fears may be exaggerated by decreased functional capacity and memory impairment. In turn, the elder projects negative impulses onto others. During the course of a chronic illness, these elders are watchful and inclined to be suspicious. They are oversensitive to demands and criticism and may respond with a depressed mood. In contrast to the long-suffering and self-sufficient personality, these elders usually blame others rather than themselves during the illness.

Depression resulting from medical illness not only impacts personality styles, it impacts compliance with medical treatment. Von Dras and Lichty (1990) found, in a sample of Type I and Type II diabetics, that both psychologic and somatic symptoms of depression were both found to be positively correlated with diabetes glucose control. In his sample, however, age was not found to be associated with either depression or glucose control. Compliance may also be compromised by late life delusional disorder or schizophrenia that must be distinguished from depressive disorders.

Depressive Symptoms Associated with Hypochondriasis

Depressive symptoms may frequently be masked as hypochondriac symptoms. Although hypochondriasis is usually associated with an absence of physical illness, in late life, hypochondriac symptoms are often an exaggeration of physical illness and a psychologic response to those illnesses (Costa and McCrae, 1985). Kramer-Ginsberg et al (1989) found that 60% of patients admitted for depression expressed hypochondriac symptoms. About 12% of these individuals were overtly delusional regarding their physical health. Hypochondriac complaints were associated with anxiety and somatic concerns but not with complaints of depressed mood, suicidality, or short-term outcome. Improvement in hypochondriac complaints with treatment occurred, yet symptoms persisted with less intensity after treatment of the depression. No one in this study continued to suffer delusional symptoms at discharge. In contrast, DeAlarcon (1964) found that hypochondriac symptoms were significantly associated with suicidality in depressed older adults. Yet hypochondriasis is not associated with age alone but is found, to some degree, among all ages of general medical outpatients (Barsky et al, 1991).

In a study of 200 patients on a combined medical-psychiatric unit, Stoudemire et al (1985) found that 17% carried a diagnosis of depression on admission after an intensive psychiatric evaluation and nearly 10% received a depression-related diagnosis. The majority of these patients initially presented to their internist with somatic complaints. These investigators suggest that the results reiterate previous observations that significant numbers of patients (many of whom were elderly) had depression that may be underrecognized because of the presence of somatic symptoms and the prominent use of denial, repression, and obsessive-compulsive defenses. Rather than supporting the hypothesis that these physically ill persons suffered from alexithymia, an inability to psychologize their feelings (Sifneos, 1973), the difficulties of expressing affect in these depressed patients with physical illness were thought to be a function of rigid defense mechanisms derived from severe limitations in cultural, psychologic, and educational development. Such physically ill elders need their complaints legitimized by an internist in a medical-oriented treatment setting. Through psychoeducation, much of the resistance diminished during hospitalization.

■ DIAGNOSING DEPRESSION IN THE MEDICALLY ILL

Diagnosing depression in elderly medical inpatients

Differential diagnosis of depressive symptoms in older adults who are suffering medical illness has already been presented. Detection of symptoms secondary to depression in the midst of a medical illness is difficult because many of the same symptoms are associated with the illness and therefore are not associated with the depression (Rapp et al, 1988). A number of investigators have suggested that screening for depressive symptoms with typical inventories, such as the Geriatric Depression Scale, are useful means of identifying persons who may suffer mood disorders in the midst of a physical illness. These screening instruments are time-efficient (they can be administered by a nurse in the waiting room of an outpatient clinic or by a nurse admitting the older adult to a medical unit of a hospital). Such screening highlights for the medical staff the presence of depressive symptoms.

Considerable debate has arisen regarding the criteria for depression in the medically ill. For example, can the criteria of DSM-III-R and the Research Diagnostic Criteria (RDC) be applied in the medically ill (Kathol et al, 1990)? Endicott (1984) suggests altering the RDC for the diagnosis of depression in cancer. She suggests that substituting psychologic symptoms for somatic ones that might be secondary to the physical illness should improve the ability to identify patients with true depression. In a study evaluating the usefulness of the Endicott criteria, Kathol et al (1990) found that the criteria identified a population similar to that identified by DSM-III criteria. However, major depression was diagnosed much less frequently than when DSM-III-R and RDC criteria were used. Schwab et al (1967) used a group of measures in 153 general medical inpatients suffering depression to identify which persons suffering medical illness were more likely to experience a comorbid depressive illness. Depression varied inversely with the severity of the medical illness, appeared most frequently in concurrence with gastrointestinal diseases, and was often related to object loss. Many symptoms used to diagnose depression were not valuable in discriminating depression from symptoms of medical illness. Symptom profiles did emerge, however, in socioeconomic class and gender groupings. For example, clinicians tend to diagnosis depression much more frequently in upper class persons than in lower class persons, although objective measures suggest that depression is equally common regardless of class. Depressive symptoms in lower class patients, in contrast to those in upper class patients, were seen as a futility syndrome which, according to these authors, must be distinguished from the appearance of poverty and little education or apathy. During depressive illness, women tend to somatization, whereas men tend to express their depression with despair. Guilt, crying, loneliness, and anorexia were particularly common symptoms in the medically ill.

■ THE DIAGNOSTIC WORKUP OF THE MEDICALLY ILL DEPRESSED OLDER ADULT

Rodin and Voshart (1986) suggest four steps in the diagnostic workup of the medically ill depressed patient. First, they suggest a complete psychiatric assessment to establish the diagnosis of depressive disorder, evaluate the potential risk of suicide, and identify other psychiatric conditions that may be contributing to the symptom picture. Past history of psychiatric problems in the elderly patient with a medical illness is often important in determining intervention.

Second, they recommend a close scrutiny of psychosocial factors that may have contributed to the depression identified, including the loss of social supports, problems in adjusting to new family roles, decline in sexual functioning, changes in the body image, and symbolic significance of the illness to the older adult. In the midst of a medical illness, older adults often will not report significant life stresses or changes in their social environment. If impaired social support is not systematically assessed, then potential causes of the depressed affect may go unrecognized.

Third, underlying medical conditions that may contribute to the depressive episode should be identified. In the evaluation of 100 patients admitted to a geriatric psychiatry unit, Sweer et al (1988) found 77 new medical diagnoses during the admission. The most common included electrolyte abnormality (6%), bacteriuria (13%), medication reactions (7%), exacerbation of previous thyroid disease (6%), new thyroid function abnormalities (3%), and renal failure, Parkinson's disease, and chronic obstructive lung disease (2% each). They found that a workup of the medically ill depressed elder should include a complete blood count, blood chemistries, urine analysis, and thyroid-function tests (because each of these yielded abnormal results in some of the 100 patients that they reviewed). CT and MRI scanning, electroencephalography, and chest radiography did not yield results that altered management. The history and physical examination proved to be the most important factors in the diagnostic workup.

Finally, the clinician should identify underlying medical conditions that may impact the choice of treatment. Before beginning a tricyclic antidepressant, an electrocardiogram should be obtained. A history of adverse drug reactions should be obtained so that selection of a drug does not repeat previous treatment failures and adverse side effects.

■ THE TREATMENT OF DEPRESSION IN THE MEDICALLY ILL OLDER ADULT

Guidelines for the effective management of the chronically ill elderly patient suffering depression are presented in the box below. The active interpersonal relationship between the clinician and the older depressed patient is essential to effective care. To ensure adequate attention to the depressive component of the illness complex, early psy-

---

Guidelines for the Effective Management of the Chronically Ill Elderly Patient

Schedule regular appointments with the patient to follow the progress of his or her condition.

Perform periodic physical examinations to screen for the appearance of new illness processes.

Engage the patient in a contract that both of you will work together to combat the problems associated with the illness (i.e., give the patient more control in the treatment process).

Avoid analgesics, sedatives, and tranquilizers that are potentially addictive.

Inform the patient at frequent intervals of the changes occurring in his or her body and their cause and prognosis, yet always give the patient some hope.

Concentrate on the patient's immediate comfort and quality of life instead of the long-range prognosis.

Admit the patient to the hospital for a periodic "tune-up" when home management shows signs of significant deterioration.

Explain the limitations of modern medical science.

Assure the patient that you will provide continuing care, regardless of the circumstances.

Maintain contact with the patient during the referral process to a medical specialist.

Set limits when the patient becomes overly demanding.

Encourage the patient to discuss his or her fears repeatedly.

chiatric intervention is indicated. Strain et al (1991) found that admission psychiatric liaison screening of elderly patients with hip fractures results in earlier detection of psychiatric morbidity, better psychosocial care, and earlier discharge from the hospital.

In general, supportive psychotherapy is the treatment of choice, especially in the presence of depressive symptoms and acute medical illness (Koenig, 1991). Empathy and bolstering of defenses that enable the older person to adapt to the medical illness often relieve the acute depressive symptoms. The use of cognitive and behavioral strategies (see Chapter 17) can be helpful and include the following: monitoring thoughts and challenging false assumptions (this illness is going to kill me in the next few weeks); cognitive reframing (although you may need to change your activities, you do not have to eliminate them altogether); and developing scheduled activities (encouraging the depressed elder to leave the home and contact other persons, especially if the older person was socially active).

Time spent by the clinician, especially the primary care physician, is quite valuable and the physician should therefore be willing to listen and show interest in the older person's perception of his/her illness, not just symptoms of the illness. Physician time can be augmented by many other professionals, such as the nurse, social worker, or chaplain.

Viederman and Perry (1980) suggest the use of a psychodynamic life narrative in the treatment of depression in the physically ill. They base the use of this approach on the premise that depression in the medically ill (which is produced by the crisis of illness) is not only more threatening to the medically ill but that such persons are more responsive to interventions. They suggest that the depressed patient be presented with a statement that places the physical illness in a context of his or her life trajectory. For example, the therapist, after listing carefully to the patient, presents the patient with a perspective of his or her life course and the impact and response of the depression within the context of the life course. They find that the presentation of a life narrative helps to support the self-esteem of the older person, creates a sense of order, and contradicts the belief that depression is an inevitable consequence of illness. In addition, the presentation of the narrative assures the patient that he or she is well understood by the therapist.

Most older persons who suffer medical illness tend to decrease their physical activity. Lack of physical exercise has been associated with depression in older adults (Kivela and Pahkala, 1991). Therefore encouraging the elder to become more physically active (even the bedridden elder) is essential in the effective treatment of the medically ill (see box on p. 233). Contact with a physical therapist, the distraction from psychic pain, and a sense of mastering and completing an exercise program all contribute to an enhanced sense of well-being and relief of depressive symptoms in the older person.

The task of treating the depressed older person who has decreased food intake below daily food requirements is a difficult one. Most clinicians prefer to avoid the rather severe means of ensuring accurate caloric intake, such as the insistence on the consumption of high-protein mixtures or the use of a nasal gastric tube. Suggestions for food intake are listed in the box on p. 226, and have been described previously. Special preparations are available that enhance the seasoning of food to partially overcome the decreased gustatory sensations of late life. Attention should also be directed to the peculiar likes and dislikes of the older depressed adult. Some institutions have implemented

---

General Principles of Exercise for the Elderly

Complete a history and physical examination before initiating an exercise program.
Begin with exercises that do not stress the stamina of the older adult.
Prescribe a balanced exercise program with sufficient stretching and flexibility.
Demonstrate the proper technique. Have the older person repeat the exercise for your critique.
Increase the level of exercise slowly.
Emphasize the need to exercise regularly—at least three times per week.
Instruct the older person in checking the resting heart rate and Immediate postexercise heart rate. (The target immediate postexercise heart rate for older adults is approximately 125 beats per minute at age 65, decreasing 1 beat per minute for each additional year of age.)

---

a "happy hour" at around 4:00 PM. Cocktails are served, after which patients go to dinner. This social atmosphere can be of value, but many patients may be offended or may chose not to participate in activities that involve alcohol. Alcohol can precipitate or worsen a depressive episode, as well as interact with medications, especially the anti-anxiety and antidepressant drugs.

Food preferences originate from cultural, socioeconomic, or religious factors. Some older patients who have grown up in poverty may request that they be given foods that represent a higher social class, such as meat and green vegetables as opposed to potatoes and beans. Other patients may, because of religious background, avoid foods on certain days or certain foods altogether. Depressive symptoms on admission to long-term care facilities do not abolish the preference of many Jewish patients for a Kosher diet. These preferences may be overlooked in some cities where the Jewish population is relatively small. The depressed older patient may not request these special diets but may passively oppose their absence by cessation of food intake.

The standard treatment for major depression in the elderly medically ill is the use of antidepressant medications. There are many doubts about the efficacy and safety of antidepressants, especially in the older frail and depressed medical patient (Koenig and Breitner, 1990). A review of prescribed medications and practices of physicians on adult medical and surgical inpatient services reveals that less than 2% of these persons receive tricyclic antidepressant during inpatient admission (Callies and Popkin, 1987), despite the prevalence of major depression among the medically ill of approximately 10%.

Much of the concern regarding the use of antidepressants in the elderly results from contraindications to the use of these drugs in medically ill patients. Koenig et al (1992) found that minor contraindications include the presence of an enlarged prostate (33%), the concurrent prescription of another anticholinergic drug (33%), the use of other drugs with potential for interactions with antidepressants (50%), and the presence of abnormalities on the electrocardiogram, such as minor conduction disturbances and arrhythmias (25%). Other complications include clinically significant bladder outlet obstruction (46%), orthostatic hypotension (21% in untreated and 58% in treated patients), and significant cardiac conduction disturbances, such as left bundle branch block (13%).

In summary, medical complications prevent the continued use of an antidepressant medication in persons with symptoms of major depression in 80% of elderly depressed inpatients.

Although the literature is not definitive, some well-designed studies of tricyclic antidepressant use in the medically ill elderly do indicate that the medications are of value. Lipsey et al (1984) estimate the efficacy of nortriptyline in treating inpatients and outpatients (average age 60) after they suffered a stroke. The average initial dose of nortriptyline was 20 mg per day and the maximum dose was 100 mg daily. Plasma levels of nortriptyline were monitored and when levels were in the window of 50 ng/ml to 140 ng/ml, significant decrease in depressive symptoms were observed. In contrast, Light et al (1986) did not find that doxepin (at an average dose of 105 mg per day) was effective in treating outpatients with chronic obstructive pulmonary disease who were suffering significant depression (although they were not diagnosed as suffering major depression).

Katz et al (1990) found, in a double-blind, placebo-controlled clinical trial for treating of major depression among frail elderly persons that nortriptyline was significantly better in improving symptoms than the placebo. DSM-III-R diagnosis of major depression in the elderly, therefore, remains a valid diagnosis for pharmacotherapeutic intervention. The prevalence of adverse side effects, however, was high, with 34% of the patients being taken off medications before the treatment trial was completed. High levels of self-care disability and low level of serum albumin were both associated with a decreased therapeutic response.

Koenig and Breitner (1990) recommend that antidepressant medications be used in the depressed medically ill elder if certain guidelines are observed. These are outlined in the box on p. 235. Consider alternative therapies, such as psychostimulants (e.g., methylphenidate 5 to 10 mg daily), when patients cannot tolerate any antidepressant drug.

Traditional antidepressant therapies are not contraindicated but should be used with caution. Any clinician treating depressed older persons should be aware of the range of side effects produced by these medications. Psychostimulants provide a useful alternative to treating depression in the medically ill (Kaufmann et al, 1984). These medications may be especially valuable in older persons who have cardiovascular complications or cognitive impairments that rule out the use of traditional antidepressants. Psychostimulants are rarely addictive in depressed elderly persons, especially when used in lower doses. Benefits of the medication, however, may be short-lived.

Pain frequently accompanies medical illness associated with depression in the elderly. Therefore any therapeutic strategy to alleviate depressive symptoms in the medically ill should include a plan for pain management (Ferrell, 1991). As noted in the box on p. 235, the use of analgesics along with antidepressant medications is indicated when pain is severe. There is little if any interaction between nonsteroidal antiinflammatory drugs (NSAIDs), yet NSAIDs frequently lead to abdominal discomfort. In more severe pain syndromes the use of opiate analgesics is indicated but must be used with great caution. Not only are these drugs potentially addictive but they may cause cognitive disturbances, respiratory depression, and constipation. These symptoms often accompany depression and/or the use of antidepressant medications.

Ferrell (1991) suggests that pain should be assessed and treated as a unique syndrome (regardless of its etiology) in the elderly. Principles of pain management for older persons include the following:

Recommendations for the Use of Antidepressants Medications in the Depressed Medically Ill

Begin with much lower doses of the drugs (e.g., 10 mg per day for nortriptyline and 20 mg per day for desipramine)

Gradually increase the dose

Establish lower maintenance doses of the medications (e.g., 50 mg daily of nortriptyline or 75 mg daily of doxepin)

Obtain an electrocardiogram before and after (1 week after) beginning the antidepressant medication

Check sitting and standing blood pressures before and after beginning of medications to screen for orthostatic hypotension

Use caution in prescribing to patients suffering from dyspnea and respiratory disorders to be certain that respiration is not depressed

Antidepressant therapy should be an adjunct, not a replacement, for specific analgesic therapy in older persons suffering chronic pain (e.g., from osteoarthritis or neoplastic disease)

Use antidepressant medications carefully in patients taking drugs that interact with antidepressants, especially antihypertensive (clonidine, guanethidine, and methyldopa), anticonvulsants, and sedative hypnotic drugs

Prescribe antidepressants with caution to persons suffering hepatic disease (monitor liver enzymes)

Use medications with low anticholinergic side effects (e.g., trazodone and fluoxetine) in patients with cognitive impairment

Adapted from Koenig HG, Breitner J: *Psychosomatics* 31:22-32, 1990.

- Always inquire about pain.
- Accept the older patient's word about pain and its intensity.
- Be thorough in the diagnostic assessment of pain.
- Treat pain as a syndrome initially, even while awaiting the definitive diagnosis of the pain.
- Use a combined approach of pharmacotherapy and nondrug strategies.
- Mobilize patients physically as much as possible.
- Use adjuncts for pain therapies, such as biofeedback, relaxation, and even hypnosis, when indicated.

Pain management has become highly specialized and the referral of an older person to a pain management center may be indicated.

Finally, the older medically ill patient suffering from depression is also likely to suffer impaired social supports. Even when supports remain available to the frail older adult, strains between the patient and the family are often significant. The physician should not only encourage the family to maintain frequent contact with the older person, he or she should also work with the family member (with the permission of the patient), explaining the nature of the depressive illness and how it interacts with the physical illness. Families should be warned about the potential for suicide in the depressed older adult (especially those suffering from physical problems). Family members should be cautioned about and monitored for the burden over time of caring for a frail elder as well.

To provide optimal care for the chronically ill older person, attending to the needs of family members may be the most important factor in the therapeutic process.

■ OUTCOME

To determine the impact of comorbid depression in medical illness, both the impact of the medical illness on the prognosis of depression and the impact of depression on the prognosis of the illness must be considered. Schleifer et al (1989) report that 77% of a group of patients with an average age of 61 were diagnosed with major depression within the first 2 weeks of a myocardial infarction had persistent depressive symptoms 3 months later. Poor recovery from depression in this patient group is in contrast to the improvement after appropriate treatment of the depressed elders who were not medically ill (see Chapter 3). In another longitudinal study of hospitalized elders with major depression, only 18% had completely recovered 3 months after hospital discharge (Koenig et al, 1992). Mortality rates were higher in the depressed as well.

Depression may also affect specific outcomes of medical illness. For example, Irwin et al (1988) found that depressive disorders, or even prolonged bereavement, may lead to a reduction of natural killer cells. The mechanism for this relationship may be through stimulation of corticotrophin-releasing factors (CRF), which triggers the release of norepinephrine from sympathetic nerves and in turn reduces the ability of natural killer cells to destroy tumor cells. Therefore the depressed older adult may be at an increased risk of developing cancer. Nemeroff et al (1984) found that depressed patients, when compared with controls and other diagnostic groups, exhibit increased cerebral spinal fluid concentrations of CRF-like immunoreactivity.

Van Vort et al (1990) reported three cases of pathologic osteoporotic hip fractures in elderly females with major depression. Decreased activity and poor food intake (especially dietary calcium deficiency) were among the risk factors for osteoporosis. Mossey et al (1990) found that, in 196 older white females followed for 12 months after hip fractures, persons who reported persistently elevated symptoms of depression were less likely to achieve independence in walking and performed more poorly on a number of routine physical function measures. Massey and Massey (1980) found that 21 of 181 depressed psychiatric inpatients (most of whom were elderly) were found on neurologic examination to have clinical indications of perineal palsy. Weight loss was universal in these individuals. In all cases a positive factor was leg crossing, related to excessive sitting during depressive illness.

In summary, depression that remains untreated in the medically ill elderly can not only lead to a poorer prognosis than is generally seen in depression at other stages of the life cycle, it can also create adverse consequences for the course of the medical illness.

REFERENCES

Ballinger S, Cobbin D, Krivanek J, Saunders D: Life stressors and depression in the menopause, *Maturitas* 1:191-199, 1979.

Barsky AJ, Frank CB, Cleary, PD, Wyshak G, Klerman GH: The relationship between hypochondriasis and age, *American Journal of Psychiatry* 148:923-928, 1991.

Bell IR, Edman JS, Marrow FD, Marby DW, Marages S, et al: B complex vitamin patterns in geriatric and young adult inpatients with major depression, *Journal of the American Geriatric Society* 39:252-257, 1991.

Blumer D, Heilbronn M: Chronic pain as a variant of depressive disease. The pain-prone disorder, *The Journal of Nervous and Mental Disease* 170:381-406, 1982.

Callies AL, Popkin MK: Antidepressant treatment of medical-surgical inpatients by nonpsychiatric physicians, *Archives of General Psychiatry* 44:157-160, 1987.

Camacho FC, Roberts RE, Lazarus HB, Kaplan GA, Cohen RD: Physical activity and depression: evidence from the Almeda County Study, *American Journal of Epidemiology* 134:220-231, 1991.

Cassell EJ: Reactions to physical illnesses and hospitalization. In Usdin G, Lewis JM (eds): *Psychiatry in Medical General Practice*. New York, Macluen Hill, 1979, pp. 103-131.

Cassem NH, Hackett PP: Psychological aspects of myocardial infarction, *Medical Clinics of North America* 61:711-721, 1977.

Colenda CC, Dougherty LM: Positive ego in coping functions and chronic pain in depressed patients, *Journal of Geriatric Psychiatry Neurology* 3:48-52, 1990.

Costa PT, Jr, McCrae RR: Hypochondriasis, neuroticism, and aging. When are somatic complaints unfounded? *American Psychologists* 40:19-28, 1985.

DeAlarcon R: Hypochondriasis and depression in the aging, *Gerontological Clinics* 6:266-267, 1964.

Diagnostic and Statistical Manual of Mental Disorders. Third Edition. Revised. Washington, DC, American Psychiatric Association, 1987.

Dovenmuehle RH, Verwoerdt A: Physical illness and depressive symptomatology. I. Incidence of depressive symptoms in hospitalized cardiac patients, *Journal of the American Geriatric Society* 10:932-947, 1962.

Endicott J: Measurement of depression in patients with cancer, *Cancer* 53:2243-2248, 1984.

Evans DL, McCartney CF, Nemeroff CB, Raft D, Quade D, et al: Depression in women treated for gynecological cancer: clinical and neuroendocrine assessment, *American Journal of Psychiatry* 143:447-452, 1986.

Ferrell BA: Pain management in elderly people, *Journal of American Geriatric Society* 39:64-73, 1991.

Fras I, Lintin EW, Bartholomew LG: Mental symptoms as an aid in the early diagnosis of carcinoma of the pancreas, *Gastroenterology* 55:191-198, 1968.

Garetz FK: Breaking the dangerous cycle of depression in thought and nutrition, *Geriatrics* 31:73-76, 1976.

Gurland BJ, Wilder BE, Berkman C: Depression and disability in the elderly: reciprocal relations and changes with age, *The International Journal of Geriatric Psychiatry* 3:163-179, 1988.

Irwin M, Hauger RL, Brown M, Britton KT: CRF activates autonomic nervous system and reduces natural killer cells cytotoxicity, *American Journal of Physiology* 2:744-747, 1988.

Kahana RJ, Bibring GL: Personality types and medical management. In Zinberg EN (ed): *Psychiatry in Medical Practice in a General Hospital.* New York, International Universities Press, 1964, pp. 103-123.

Kathol RG, Mutgi A, Williams J, Clamon G, Noyes R: Diagnosis of major depression in cancer patients according to four sets of criteria, *American Journal of Psychiatry* 147:1021-1024, 1990.

Katz IK, Lesher E, Kleban M, Jethanandani V, Parmelee P: Clinical features of depression in the nursing home, *International Psychogeriatrics* 1:5-15, 1989.

Katz IR, Simpson GM, Curlik SM, Parmelee PA, Mohly C: Pharmacologic treatment of major depression for elderly patients in residential care settings, *Journal of Clinical Psychiatry* 51 (7, suppl):41-47, 1990.

Kaufmann N, Cassem NH, Murray GB, Genike M: Use of psychostimulants in medically ill patients with neurological disease in major depression, *Canadian Journal of Psychiatry* 29:46-49, 1984.

Kivela SH, Pahkala K: Relationship between health behavior and depressed in the aged, *Aging* 3:153-159, 1991.

Koenig HG: Treatment considerations for the depressed geriatric medical patient, *Drugs and Aging* 1:1-15, 1991.

Koenig HG, Breitner JCS: Use of antidepressants in medically ill older patients, *Psychosomatics* 31:22-32, 1990.

Koenig HG, Meador K, Cohen HJ, Blazer DG: Depression in elderly men hospitalized with medical illness, *Archives of Internal Medicine* 148:1929-1936, 1988.

Koenig HG, Shelp F, Goli V, Meador K, Cohen H, et al: Major depression in hospitalized medically ill older patients: documentation, management and prognosis, *International Journal of Geriatric Psychiatry* 7:25-34, 1992.

Koenig HG, Shelp F, Goli V, Meador K, Cohen HJ: Survival and health care utilization in elderly medical inpatients with major depression, *Journal of the American Geriatric Society* 37:599-606, 1989.

Kramer-Ginsberg E, Greenwald BS, Aicen PC, Brodmiller C: Hypochondriasis in the elderly depressed, *Journal of the American Geriatric Society* 37:507-510, 1989.

Light RW, Merrill EJ, Despars J, Gordan GH, Mutalipassi LR: Doxepin treatment of depressed patients with chronic obstructive pulmonary disease, *Archives of Internal Medicine* 146:1377-1380, 1986.

Lindenbaum J, Healton EB, Savage DG, Brust JCM, Garrett TJ, et al: Neuropsychiatric disorders caused by cobalamin deficiency in the absence of anemia or microcytosis, *New England Journal of Medicine* 318:1720-1728, 1988.

Linkins RW, Comstock GW: Depressed mood in the development of cancer, *American Journal of Epidemiology* 132:962-972, 1990.

Lipsey JR, Robinson RG, Perlson GD: Nortriptyline treatment of post-stroke depression: a double-blind study, *Lancet* 1:297-300, 1984.

Lloyd GG, Cawley RH: Distress or illness: a study of psychological symptoms after myocardial infarction, *British Journal of Psychiatry* 142:120-125, 1983.

Massey EW, Massey JM: Perineal palsy in depressed patients, *Psychosomatics* 24:93-94, 1982.

Massie MJ, Holland JC: Depression in the cancer patient, *Journal of Clinical Psychiatry* 51 (7, suppl):12-17, 1990.

Minnesota State Board of Health: *Minnesota Health Statistics*. Minneapolis. Section of Health Statistics, 1973.

Mossey JM, Knott K, Criak R: The effects of persistent depressive symptoms on hip fractory recovery, *Journal of Gerontology* 45:M163-168, 1990.

Natow AB, Heslin J: *Geriatric Nutrition*. Boston, CBI, 1980.

Nemeroff CB, Widerlov E, Bissette G, Walleush H, Karlsson I, et al: Elevated concentrations of CSF corticotrophin-releasing factor-like immunoreactivity in depressed patients, *Science* 226:1342-1344, 1984.

Palinkas LA, Wingared DL, Barrett-Conner E: Chronic illness and depressive symptoms in the elderly: a population-based study. *Journal of Clinical Epidemiology* 43:1131-1141, 1990.

Parmoa N, Gershon S: Treatment-resistent depression in an elderly patient with pancreatic carcinoma: case report, *Journal of Clinical Psychology* 45:439-440, 1984.

Rapp SR, Walsh DA, Parisi SA, Wallace CE: Detecting depression in elderly medical inpatients, *Journal of Consulting and Clinical Psychology* 56:509-513, 1988.

Rodin G, Voshart K: Depression in the medically ill: an overview, *American Journal of Psychiatry* 143:696-705, 1986.

Romano JM, Turner JA: Chronic pain in depression: Does the evidence support a relationship? *Psychological Bulletin* 97:18-34, 1985.

Rosenthal MJ, Hunt WC, Garry PJ, Goodwin JS: Thyroid failure in the elderly: microsomal antibodies as an discriminate for therapy, *Journal of the American Medical Association* 258:209-213, 1987.

Schleifer SJ, Macari-Hinson M, Coyle DA, Slater WR, Kahn M, et al: The nature and course of depression following myocardial infarction, *Archives of Internal Medicine* 149:1785-1789, 1989.

Schwab JJ, Bialow M, Brown JM, Holzer CE: Diagnosing depression in medical in patients, *Annals of Internal Medicine* 67:695-707, 1967.

Sifneos PE: The prevalence of alexithymia characteristics in psychosomatic patients, *Psychotherapy and Psychosomatics* 22:255-262, 1973.

Stoudemire A, Kahn M, Brown T, Linfor SE, Houpt JL: Mask depression in a combined medical-psychiatric unit, *Psychosomatics* 26:221-228, 1985.

Strain JJ, Lyons JS, Hammer JS, Fahs M, Lebowtiz A, et al: Cost offset from a psychiatric consultation liaison intervention with elderly hip fracture patients, *American Journal of Psychiatry* 148:1044-1049, 1991.

Sweer L, Martin DC, Ladd RA, Miller JK, Karph M: The medical evaluation of elderly patients with major depression, *Journal of Gerontology* 43:M53-58, 1988.

Thomas FB, Mazzaferri EL, Skillman TG: Alphaphetic thyrotoxicosis: a distinctive clinical and laboratory entity, *Archives of Internal Medicine* 72:679-684, 1970.

Van Vort WB, Rubinstein M, Rose RP: Osteopetrosis with pathologic hip fractures in major depression, *Journal of Geriatric Psychiatry and Neurology* 3:10-12, 1990.

Viederman M, Perry SW: Use of psychodynamic life narrative in the treatment of depression in the physically ill, *General Hospital Psychiatry* 3:177-185, 1980.

von Dras DD, Lichty W: Correlates of depression in diabetic adults, *Behavior Health and Aging* 1:79-84, 1990.

Whitlock FA, Siskind M: Depression in cancer: a follow-up study. *Psychological Medicine* 9:747-752, 1979.

Whybrow PC, Prang AJ, Treadway CR: Mental changes accompanying thyroid gland dysfunction: a reappraisal using objective psychological measurement, *Archives of General Psychiatry* 20:48-62, 1969.

15

Depression Caused by Alcohol and Drug Problems

Alcohol is the drug most commonly used by the elderly for its central nervous system effects. Older persons do not use alcohol as frequently and in as large an amount as persons in middle age. The decreased frequency of alcohol use among elders is probably due to three factors: (1) a cohort affect (i.e., members of the current cohort of elders are less likely to have ever drunk alcohol regularly than members of younger cohorts); (2) the increased mortality rate among younger alcoholics (they do not survive until late life); and (3) a spontaneous cessation of drinking among some persons with aging. The relative decrease in the amount of alcohol consumed by elders who do drink is due to the gradual decrease in the elder's ability to metabolize alcohol.

Older people often use alcohol as an antianxiety agent and as a sedative, since one immediate effect of alcohol is the induction of sleep. Unfortunately, the ensuing sleep is often fragmented with awakenings 4 to 6 hours after alcohol intake. Sedation through the night is more easily accomplished by using therapeutic agents from the benzodiazepine class, such as flurazepam and temazepam. Both benzodiazepines and alcohol, however, are subject to addiction and abuse.

Alcohol can easily lead to problems with mood, as well as sleep difficulties. Finlayson et al (1988) reviewed the medical records of 216 elderly persons admitted to the hospital for treatment of alcohol-related problems. Concern of family and friends was the most common factor motivating patients for admission. Patients with late-onset alcoholism were more likely to report an association between a life event (e.g., loss of a loved one) and alcohol problems than persons with early-onset alcoholism. The most common associated psychiatric disorders were tobacco dependence (67%), organic brain syndrome (26%), atypical or mixed organic brain syndrome (19%), and mood disorders (12%). About 14% of the patients also reported a drug abuse or dependence problem, all of whom abused legally prescribed drugs. Of this group, 56% had early onset of their alcohol problems and 43% had either late onset or the onset could not be determined. Seven investigators have suggested that alcohol intake decreases with age (Callahan and Cisin, 1976), whereas others have reported that rates of alcoholism for the elderly are similar to those with the remainder of the population (Schuckit and Pastor, 1979). In the recent Epidemiologic Catchment Area studies the prevalence of both alcohol and drug abuse was much less frequent in late life than at earlier stages of the life cycle (Myers et al, 1984).

Although older persons infrequently abuse "street drugs," such as opiates and psychostimulants, they are at significant risk for abuse of prescription drugs. Older persons are the largest consumers of legal drugs and the largest users of sedative hypnotic agents and benzodiazepines (Schuckit, 1977). By obtaining their medications from a variety of sources, abuse and dependence often go unnoticed by primary care physicians and specialists treating the older adult.

Alcohol problems and depression often coexist in the alcoholic older adult, a so-called dual diagnosis. By taking a careful patient history, it is often (although not always) possible to determine whether the primary diagnosis is a problem with alcohol or depression. The determination of the primary cause of the problem usually shapes the treatment of the disorder. For example, if alcohol is the primary problem, then successful efforts placed on withdrawal and abstinence usually are successful in treating the depression.

■ CASE PRESENTATION

A 60-year-old married woman was referred after evaluation by a neurologist for an acute and severe organic brain syndrome. She stated that she had developed a problem with alcohol 6 months before the evaluation, although she had been a social drinker with periodic episodes of alcohol intoxication during most of her adult life. She had used alcohol more frequently in the recent past to overcome depressive symptoms. Although she had experienced periodic episodes of depression throughout most of her adult life, she had experienced a constant state of depression during the 6-month period before evaluation, during which her alcohol intake had increased. To escape her feelings of depression and loneliness, she began to drink throughout the day and had increased her alcohol intake to approximately one fifth of bourbon per day.

Memory problems and confusion had progressed until the husband could no longer leave her alone, so he scheduled the neurologic consultation. On admission to the hospital and acute withdrawal from alcohol, the patient returned to her usual mood state. On discharge, she abstained from alcohol, her life-style returned to normal, and she reported a dramatically improved ability to remember. However, during follow-up evaluations, the mental status examination of the patient revealed continued difficulties with abstractions and calculations. Returning to her previous social activities, the patient again became discouraged and feared being left alone. Her sleep was disrupted, and she became agitated in the late afternoon. This precipitated a return to alcohol use at which point she was referred to a psychiatrist.

According to the initial evaluation by the psychiatrist, the patient had moderately severe memory problems, including disorientation to time, difficulty abstracting, difficulty calculating, and poor recent memory. However, the patient's depressed mood and expressions of hopelessness dominated the clinical picture. She recognized her problem with alcohol and resolved that she would never drink again. Her husband recognized that she had to cease her alcohol intake and agreed to any steps necessary, including cessation of his own alcohol intake and removal of alcohol from their home, if his actions would be of benefit to the patient. Treatment was begun with withdrawal from alcohol using chlordiazepoxide, 100 mg daily in five daily doses tapering over a 5-day period.

The patient maintained her resolve not to drink at the end of withdrawal, but her mood continued to be depressed, with sleep difficulties, decreased appetite, and a fear of being left alone. Doxepin (25 mg twice daily and 50 mg a night) was prescribed, and the patient was seen biweekly for medication checks initially, decreasing to weekly checks along with supportive psychotherapy. During the 6 weeks after initial prescription of doxepin, the patient's mood improved gradually to the point where she reported that she felt "like my old self." She continued to experience problems with her memory on objective examination. While taking doxepin, her sleep pattern was unbroken, her appetite improved with a concomitant weight gain of 5 pounds, and her energy level improved.

The patient was willing for her husband to return to his usual activities (he had, during the most severe period of alcohol use, accompanied her almost constantly). Approximately 6 weeks after withdrawal, the patient hinted to her husband that she no longer had a problem with alcohol and wished to have alcohol in the house to "serve friends" even though she did not plan to return to drinking herself. Becoming concerned, the husband spoke to the psychiatrist about these comments. The patient was confronted and disulfiram (250 mg daily) was prescribed for the patient, to be given in the morning by her husband. It was agreed that there should be no alcohol in the house. Six months after prescription of disulfiram, the patient and her husband reported that she had abstained from alcohol and continued to show no evidence of depressive symptoms. Still, she noted that alcohol was "not a problem" and thought she should be able to keep it in the house and discontinue the disulfiram. After confrontation by her husband and the psychiatrist, however, she did not press the issue.

■ DIAGNOSTIC WORKUP

The diagnostic workup of the elder in whom alcohol problems are suspected depends on a comprehensive history (Blazer, 1989). The older person should first be interviewed to determine specific effects regarding drinking and drug use. This information should be supplemented by information derived from an interview of family members, preferably from two generations. Frequently, inadequate information is available regarding alcohol use. When information is forthcoming, the clinician should first inquire about the individual drinks and/or what psychotropic drugs the individual ingests. Since drug and alcohol abuse are frequently comorbid in older persons, inquiring about use of alcohol and drugs at the same time is preferable. Then the clinician should determine how often the individual drinks or takes the medication. Does the elder drink constantly? Is there a pattern of binge drinking? Most elders with alcohol and drug problems suffer from dependence as opposed to abuse. Tolerance for binges decreases with age.

The CAGE questions for screening alcohol problems are not as applicable in late life but may be of use:

(C) " . . . felt the need to Cut down on your drinking?"
(A) " . . . ever feel Annoyed by criticism of your drinking?"
(G) " . . . had Guilty feelings about drinking?"
(E) " . . . ever take a morning Eye opener?"

Additional data that may inform the clinician regarding an alcohol problem include in-formation about personal health, family health, interpersonal difficulties (especially emergent difficulties), and difficulties in employment or volunteer work. The clinician should inquire about gastrointestinal symptoms, such as nausea, vomiting, diarrhea, ab-dominal pain, and unexplained gastrointestinal hemorrhaging. Neurologic difficulties are frequent in alcohol abuse during late life and include episodes of amnesia, headaches, and especially peripheral neuropathy. Falls, bruises, cuts, sprains, cigarette burns on the skin, or skin disease often result from neglect of the body secondary to chronic alcohol use.

The details of the psychiatric interview for the depressed older adult, described in Chapter 7, apply to the adult with alcohol problems and should be completed, given the frequent comorbidity of depression and alcohol. When the conditions are suspected to be comorbid, the clinician should especially inquire regarding the cognitive status, history of major depression, bipolar disorder or other psychiatric disorders, anxiety asso-ciated with depressive illness, and psychotic symptoms (delusions and hallucinations). Paranoid thoughts, especially about friends and relatives, are common in older alcohol-ics with severe drinking problems. Suicidal ideation is critical to document, since the older alcoholic who is depressed (or the elder suffering major depression who drinks) is at greater risk for suicide than with either condition alone.

The physical examination of the older alcoholic is often informative as well. As noted previously, signs of personal neglect of hygiene are valuable clues of alcohol problems. The neurologic examination should be performed in detail, with a special attention to peripheral neuropathy. Other signs of chronic alcohol use are often apparent in older adults, such as flushing of the face, injected conjunctiva, tremors, malnutrition, and, in severe cases, spider angiomas.

Cognitive function, especially during acute intoxication, is usually impaired. Even during abstinent periods, however, cognitive functioning may be abnormal. The clini-cian should therefore attempt to keep the older alcoholic abstinent for at least 2 weeks and then perform a detailed psychologic evaluation. Psychologic testing of the older al-coholic is often threatening because deficits may appear on testing that have been pre-viously unnoticed or denied by the elder. These tests are essential, however, to monitor cognitive functioning over time.

The laboratory evaluation of the older alcoholic should include thorough liver-function evaluation (lactate dehydrogenase, serum glutamic-oxaloacetic transaminase, and alkaline phosphate) (Blazer, 1989). A chemical screen is also essential with a special attention to glucose. Low serum magnesium suggests a magnesium deficiency that can occur with alcoholism. Elevated serum and urine amylase suggest chronic pancreatitis. A thyroid panel is useful, and routine evaluation of pulmonary and cardiovascular functioning is essential. Given the infrequent yet serious side effect of cardiac myopathy with chronic alcohol use, an EKG may reveal arrhythmias and atrial fibrillation.

The diagnosis and differential diagnosis of alcohol abuse/dependence in late life does not vary significantly from other stages of the life cycle. The diagnosis is usually not one of differentiating alcohol or drug abuse from other conditions but rather determining what other psychiatric abnormalities may be comorbid with alcohol abuse/dependence. DSM-III-R describes three main patterns of chronic alcohol abuse or dependence (APA 1987). The first is a dependent pattern of daily intake of large amounts. Older persons may decrease their daily intake yet still suffer the consequences of such a dependent pattern. For example, they may have two or three drinks in the evening, but these two or three drinks lead the elder to experience the symptoms of dependence, such as inability to cut down or control the use of alcohol and cross-tolerant drugs, activity in seeking the substance, social and occupational impairment, and symptoms of withdrawal if intake ceases. The second pattern described by DSM-III-R is the regular heavy drinking of alcohol limited to weekends. During the retirement years, this pattern of abuse no longer applies. Nevertheless, some elders may use alcohol heavily on a regular intermittent basis, such as when they visit a weekend vacation home. The third pattern is long periods of sobriety interspersed by binges of daily heavy drinking lasting for weeks or months. This pattern is less common in older persons. Although good data are not available, dependence probably increases in relative frequency with aging and abuse decreases. Nevertheless, older adults may experience the symptoms of abuse with only a moderate increase over usual daily alcohol intake. The decreased tolerance of elders to alcohol leads to the symptoms of abuse.

The differential diagnosis of alcohol abuse/dependence is somewhat complex. The complexity derives from the difficulty in disentangling the mood disorder from the symptoms of alcohol dependence and abuse. If possible, determining whether the alcohol use or the depressive mood began first is the most helpful clue to the differential diagnosis. The relatively sudden onset of significant alcohol problems in an older person who has either been abstinent before late life or has been an infrequent drinker suggests that the mood disorder has precipitated the alcohol problem. Persons recently moved into retirement communities and exposed to alcohol and the "expectation" to drink (to be assimilated into the social group) may be at special risk for developing alcohol problems comorbid with depression (the depression being precipitated by the move and loss of old friends and the previous social network).

Alcohol and drugs can lead to an organic mood disorder. The most frequently abused medications in older persons, the benzodiazepines, also produce depressive symptoms in older adults. Gradual withdrawal from these medications usually determines whether the depression is an organic mood disorder (secondary to the medication) or if the medications are simply used to symptomatically relieve the elder of the depressive mood.

■ TREATMENT

Withdrawal is the first step in the treatment of alcohol abuse/dependence that is comorbid with the depressive symptoms. As noted, alcohol is a depressant and therefore the depressed mood may be a result of alcohol. Outpatient withdrawal is possible in the milder cases of alcohol dependence. To be successful, the patient must be highly motivated and willing to permit open monitoring of the withdrawal program by the family with frequent (often daily) contact with the clinician (Blazer, 1989). The use of nonpharmacologic alcohol detoxification units for a few days is an example of the bridge between outpatient withdrawal and withdrawal within the hospital. In the initial phase of inpatient withdrawal, restoring fluid and electrolyte balance is essential. Yet thirst and complaints of dry mucous membranes must not mislead the clinician, since the older alcoholic may not be dehydrated but rather experiences dryness secondary to the alcohol expired from the lungs. The clinician should therefore begin with 500 to 1000 ml of 5% normal saline while waiting for blood chemistry results to determine the state of the dehydration. Glucose solution should be avoided, since many elderly alcoholics subsist on diets that are high in carbohydrates and do not metabolize carbohydrates as quickly as normal elders. Fluids should be supplemented with parenteral B vitamins, because of the poor dietary intake among older alcoholics. In addition, persons suffering chronic alcoholism may also suffer a magnesium deficiency, which can be corrected by deep intramuscular injections of magnesium at a dose of 0.1 to 0.15 ml/kg.

After stabilization of the older alcoholic's fluid and electrolyte balance, the clinician begins withdrawal. This usually takes place with medications that are cross-tolerant with the alcohol. Chlordiazepoxide has been a drug of choice for many clinicians because of its relatively extended half-life and clear cross-tolerance. Other drugs, such as diazepam, can also be used. Dosage depends on age, weight, and amount of alcohol consumed daily before beginning withdrawal. Once a usual starting dose is selected, doses must be carefully titrated (by observation of behavior) during the first 24 to 48 hours of withdrawal. A usual starting dose is between 50 and 200 mg every 6 to 12 hours until the delirium, agitation, and/or hallucinations improve. Once an adequate dose is instituted, the benzodiazepine can be decreased at a rate of approximately 20% per day.

If an overt delirium emerges, including seizures and hallucinations, diazepam may be a better anticonvulsant because of its more rapid onset and easier adjustability of dose (given its shorter half-life). Excessive medication is reflected by memory problems, dysarthria, and ataxia. If intoxication occurs, the next dose of the drug should be eliminated and the patient observed for a decrease in the toxic symptoms and/or reemergence of the withdrawal symptoms. The benzodiazepine is then reinstituted, depending on the balance of withdrawal and toxic symptoms. Withdrawal of the older person from a sedative hypnotic agent and/or an antianxiety agent (the two drugs most frequently abused by elders) is usually instituted with the drug that is being abused (or multiple drugs if they are used) and withdrawn on a schedule similar to that described for alcohol.

Social withdrawal programs (detoxication centers), as mentioned previously, are not as applicable to the alcoholic elder. The potential for medical complications during the withdrawal process coupled with the unwillingness of most elders to be withdrawn at facilities other than a medical setting decrease the value of these programs.

After detoxication, the major challenge emerges for the clinician and the alcoholic older adult (i.e., remaining drug- or alcohol-free). The clinician should consider the use of the prophylactic agent disulfiram (Antabuse) via an Antabuse "contract" established between the patient and a family member, friend, or a clinical setting (e.g., a physician's office or emergency room). The person or setting in contact with the alcoholic elder is responsible for administering the daily dose of disulfiram and the older alcoholic in turn must take the tablet when offered. The patient and family members are warned of the potential adverse effects of the interaction of disulfiram if alcohol is ingested. Acetaldehyde increases in the blood secondary to this combination and leads to a flushing of the face, tense throbbing in the head and neck, difficulty breathing, nausea, vomiting, sweating, thirst, chest pains, increased blood pressure, dizziness, blurred vision, and confusion. Although disulfiram is not contraindicated in late life, the health of the older alcoholic must be good if the drug is to be used.

Family intervention is usually of more value in treating the late life alcoholic than persons earlier in life (especially if the alcoholic is more dependent on family members and less mobile). First, family should be warned of the severe and potentially irreversible problems that alcohol can create in the older adult, especially memory problems. Family members are usually more concerned with the immediate effects of intoxication rather than the long-term effects of alcohol dependence. Each time the elder visits the clinician after initial withdrawal, family members should be included in the session (usually in combination with the elderly alcoholic).

Self-help groups are essential to the long-term support of abstinence among older alcoholics. Alcoholics Anonymous (AA) is a very effective means of encouraging abstinence for persons throughout life. Such support groups provide social support for abstinence either through pressures applied from peers who have suffered similar problems or from the development of a social network that is free of alcohol. Alcoholics Anonymous may be especially helpful to the alcoholic who is discouraged and lonely secondary to isolation and feelings of uselessness. Older alcoholics should not be forced to join self-help groups, however. Coercion to join such a group may undermine the elder's feeling that he or she is self-sufficient (although a false security and self-sufficiency usually leads to the use of alcohol again).

If the elderly alcoholic, once withdrawn from alcohol, exhibits continued symptoms of depression (and these symptoms may be predominantly endogenous, such as sleep difficulty, agitation, and diurnal variation), then antidepressant medications should be initiated. Lithium can also be used to prevent recurrent depression and treat rapid-cycling depression if needed. Agitation may be controlled with the use of antianxiety agents. There is little evidence that older persons experiencing alcohol problems are likely to abuse these drugs when their use is carefully monitored (although the alcoholic is at greater risk for abuse).

■ SKID-ROW ALCOHOLICS: ARE THEY DEPRESSED?

Every major metropolitan area has a skid-row district (Bouge, 1963). Although private clinicians do not encounter these patients in day-to-day practice, every physician covering the emergency room of a Veterans Administration hospital or a municipal hospital encounters skid-row alcoholics. The first encounters with these individuals often occur when a physician is serving his or her internship. Initial idealism and optimism soon turn to frustration and scorn as much effort is put into withdrawing these patients from alcohol and correcting their physiologic abnormalities only to have them return to the street and begin drinking within hours after discharge. The skid-row alcoholic often returns for treatment within a matter of days or weeks.

Are skid-row alcoholics depressed? If so, then therapeutic optimism and the treatment of these individuals would be appropriate. Observation of skid-row alcoholics initially suggests that mood plays a major role in the clinical picture. They look sad, express a hopeless outlook concerning the future, and appear only to desire the immediate gratification of another drink. Would a comprehensive approach to the treatment of depression in such patients reverse the life-style and drinking patterns they exhibit?

Skid row was first used to describe a street in Seattle. Logs from a nearby saw mill would skid down the street past flop houses, taverns, and gambling halls to the river. Since that time, the concept of skid row is cheap service establishments, inexpensive and poorly maintained housing, and a population of predominantly homeless men. In recent years, these individuals have been more likely to be homeless as opposed to living in poorly maintained housing and make up a sizable proportion of the current homeless population. The elderly are overrepresented in this group compared with the general population (Bahr, 1973; Bouge, 1963). What are the characteristics of these individuals? How do they end up with such a life-style?

Schuckit and Pastor (1979) reviewed in detail the literature on skid row. The residents of skid row often demonstrate physical and psychologic disabilities coupled with downward economic mobility. Most of these individuals have lower class origins, which may contribute to the increased rate of physical and psychologic impairment (Hollingshead and Redlich, 1958). In contrast with young skid-row residents, older residents show the highest rates of degenerative physical disease, such as cardiovascular disease, genitourinary disease, and perceptual problems. The elderly frequently cite unemployment or specific physical disabilities as reasons for being on skid row (Bahr and Caplow, 1973). Two patterns for arriving on skid row have been described. The early pattern is characterized by an onset of heavy drinking between the ages of 20 and 30 years, which is associated with poor occupational and marital adjustment. These persons are frequently arrested for offenses that are unrelated to drunkenness. The late-onset patients are characterized by stable marriages and occupations until approximately 40 years of age, at which time increased drinking occurs associated with an increase in problems related to drinking. It is unlikely that individuals who follow the early pattern often survive to old age.

Obtaining and consuming alcohol, as well as recovering from the effects of alcohol, are the central characteristics of the life-style on skid row (Wiseman, 1970). However, Bouge (1963) suggests that the alcoholic image may be inappropriate for the older skid-row residents, who are less likely to be heavy drinkers than are those at other stages of the life cycle. Psychiatric problems, such as depression, are more likely to be seen among the light-to-moderate drinkers. Skid-row alcoholics experience many conditions that may precipitate depression, including nutritional deficiency, organic brain syndrome, anemia, and psychotic disturbances (Schuckit and Pastor, 1979). Affective disorders are more common in older skid-row residents than in younger ones (Goldfarb, 1970). Goldfarb described these patients as the "patients nobody wants."

Studies of the skid-row population, such as Spradley's anthropologic study *You Owe Yourself A Drunk* (1970), suggest that skid row is a subculture or a way of life. Affective disorders and other psychopathologic conditions therefore do not account for skid-row residents and the skid-row life-style, if this theory is correct. Many clinicians have arrived at similar conclusions after numerous encounters with individuals who repeatedly visit emergency rooms. Yet the homeless population in the United States currently includes many persons other than the skid-row alcoholic. Specifically, many persons who were formally residents at mental hospitals for schizophrenia. Therapeutic optimism should not be totally deflated, however, since some patients with treatable depression will be discovered if the clinician maintains an awareness.

REFERENCES

American Psychiatric Association: *Diagnostic Statistical Manual of Mental Disorders* (3rd Edition-Revised). Washington, DC, American Psychiatric Association, 1987.

Bahr HM: *Skid-Row: Introduction to Dis-affiliation.* New York, Oxford University Press, 1973.

Bahr HM, Caplow T: *Older Men Drunk and Sober.* New York, New York University Press, 1973.

Blazer DG: Alcohol and drug problems in the elderly. In Busse EW, Blazer DG (eds): *Geriatric Psychiatry*. Washington, DC, American Psychiatric Press, 1989, pp. 489-514.

Bouge DJ: *Skid-row in American Cities*. Chicago, Community and Family Studies Center, University of Chicago, 1963.

Callahan D, Cisin IH: Drinking behavior and drinking problems in the United States. In Kissin B, Begleiter H (eds): *The Biology of Alcoholism* (Vol IV). New York, Plenum, 1976.

Finlayson RE, Hurt RD, Davis LJ, Morse RM: Alcoholism in elderly persons: a study of the psychiatric and psychosocial features of 216 inpatients, *Mayo Clinic Proceedings* 63:761-768, 1988.

Goldfarb C: Patients Nobody Wants: Skid-row alcoholics, *Diseases of the Nervous System* 31:274, 1970.

Hollingshead AB, Redlich FC: *Social Class and Mental Illness*. New York, John Wiley and Sons, 1958.

Myers JK, Weissman MM, Tischler GL, Holzer CE, Leaf PJ, et al: Six-month prevalence of psychiatric disorders in three communities, *Archives of General Psychiatry* 41:959-970, 1984.

Schuckit MA: Geriatric alcoholism and drug abuse, *The Gerontologist* 17:168-174, 1977.

Schuckit MA, Pastor PA: Alcohol-related psychopathology in the aged. In Kaplan HI (ed): *Psychopathology of Aging*. New York, Academic Press, 1979, pp. 211-227.

Spradley JP: *You Owe Yourself a Drunk*. Boston, Little, Brown and Company, 1970.

Wiseman JP: *Relations of the Lost: The Treatment of Skid-row Alcoholics*. Inglewood Cliffs, New Jersey, Prentice-Hall, 1970.

16

Depression, Pseudodementia, and Neurologic Disease

Distinguishing between late life depression and neurologic disorders is one of the more perplexing clinical problems confronted by health care professionals treating older adults. Frequently, this problem has been subsumed under the construct "Pseudodementia" (i.e., the differential diagnosis of depression versus dementia). Comorbid depression and dementia, however, is by far the more common clinical problem encountered in practice. After the case presentation, which illustrates comorbid depression and dementia, the emerging data regarding the neurology and neuropathology of depression are reviewed. Next, a review of the signs and symptoms of cognitive impairment in the midst of depression, derived predominantly from psychologic studies are discussed. Then laboratory diagnostic studies (predominantly brain imaging that has been implemented to study cognitive impairment in depression) and comorbidity of depressive symptoms and disorders resulting from structural changes in the brain are reviewed. Although many (if not most) neurologic disorders that affect cortical structures can lead to depressive symptoms, the three most common that are likely to be manifested by comorbid depression and cognitive impairment are dementia of the Alzheimer's type (DAT), cerebral vascular accident (stroke), and Parkinson's disease. A description of the depressive pseudodementia syndrome is presented. At the conclusion of the chapter, recommendations for the diagnosis and treatment of depressive symptoms accompanied by cognitive impairment are discussed.

■ CASE PRESENTATION

Ms. S. was a 70-year-old woman who, according to her primary care physician, was suffering from severe Alzheimer's disease. Care for her had become so difficult at home that her family planned to institutionalize her. Nevertheless, because of the sudden onset of her symptoms (4 months before referral), she was referred for a thorough psychiatric evaluation.

According to the family, the patient had been retired for approximately 4 years from working in a mill. She could have continued to work but found the stress of work increasingly difficult and requested to retire. She cared for an invalid husband (who died 5 months before the psychiatric evaluation) for 2 years before his death. During the last few months of his illness, however, the patient's two daughters were called on to assist in his care, since the patient found the responsibility increasingly difficult.

About 2 or 3 weeks after his death, the patient's condition deteriorated dramatically. She refused to eat or would eat only minimal amounts of food and lost 10 pounds in weight by the time of psychiatric evaluation. She paced at night and would become agitated on occasion. When asked questions regarding the location of her husband's will and other business matters, the patient had great difficulty in answering. She usually would respond by, "I don't know." In addition, she would ruminate frequently that she was worthless and was of "no value to anybody." She often stated that she wanted to die but did not overtly threaten suicide.

On psychiatric evaluation, it was determined that the patient was suffering from a severe major depressive episode with psychotic features. A trial of antidepressant medication was not effective (she was treated with nortriptyline), and she was referred for electroconvulsive therapy (ECT). After six treatments using unilateral nondominant ECT, the patient was much improved. She returned home but still had some difficulty in functioning in her household (not preparing her food and not being able to organize housework). The family subsequently elected to have her move in with one of her daughters (who was more than willing). The patient remained pleasant and cooperative, began to gain weight, and was most helpful around the house, according to the daughter. Nevertheless, her memory continued to be impaired over the next 4 years. In retrospect the family believed that she had suffered some memory difficulties for at least 2 years before her psychiatric hospitalization. These memory problems had rendered care of her invalid husband more stressful.

This patient experienced a severe and psychotic episode of major depression. In addition, however, she also experienced a chronic progressive dementia (although of only mild-to-moderate severity). The severe cognitive impairment that she experienced during the depressive episode was undoubtably complicated by the progressive Alzheimer's disease.

■ COGNITIVE DEFICITS SECONDARY TO DEPRESSIVE DISORDERS

Memory problems are the most frequent cognitive deficits associated with depressive disorders (Sternberg and Jarvik, 1976; Miller and Lewis, 1978). Language and visual/spatial impairments have also been associated with cognitive deficits (Emory and Breslau, 1989). A number of investigators have explored the reason that memory impairments are commonly associated with depressive disorders. Some have examined the severity of depressive disorder as a factor. Others have examined the type of memory impairment. For example, memory tests that require more effort have been found to be more impaired in depressive disorders than memory tasks that require less effort (Weingartner et al, 1981).

Cavanaugh and Wettson (1983) administered the DAT Depression Inventory and the Mini-Mental Status Examination (MMSE) to a randomly selected sample of medical inpatients (n = 289). They found significant association between severity of depression and cognitive dysfunction as measured by these scales overall, although the moderate-to-severe depressed inpatient scored lower on the MMSE than normal. In patients 65 years of age and older, those who were depressed scored significantly lower on the MMSE than those who were not depressed. The authors hypothesize that some cognitive impairment may underlie depression in the elderly and therefore lead to a decrease in reserve capacity. The experience of a depressive disorder would therefore reveal memory problems that would not be evident in the absence of the depressive disorder. In a study of cognitive dysfunction and depression, McHugh and Folstein (1979) found that only patients 60 years of age and older developed cognitive dysfunction when depressed.

A number of studies document the association between depression and selected aspects of memory. Sweeney et al (1989) studied 21 patients with major depression who were not demented (average age 64). Severity of depression was related to attention (but not to age per se), and patient age was related to learning and recall. Verbal learning memory measures did not fall below normal values even in the most severely depressed. On the other hand, facial recognition was significantly impaired relative to test norms. This pattern of cognitive dysfunction in depression differs from the cognitive changes normally associated with aging. Rossi et al (1990) studied 20 patients who received ECT (an average age of 47 treatments) and 20 controls. Before ECT the complex figure test was administered (this test measures visual/spatial impairment). The complex figure test results were abnormal in the depressed, but the MMSE scores were normal. This is consistent with the finding that depressives show impairment on tests of nondominant hemisphere.

Watts and Cooper (1989) compared depressed patients with normal subjects. They found that depressed patients did not exhibit good recall in a test of memory for stories, which in turn suggests that depressed patients do not use structured, organized stories when encoding them compared with normal patients. Golinkoff and Sweeney (1989), in a comparison study of depressed and normal subjects in their twenties, found that depressed subjects have impaired associative memory. These results suggest that there is a memory impairment in depression that appears to be independent of any general cognitive inefficiency or problem allocating cognitive effect. The impairment is evident with both recall and recognition memory tasks and is not restricted to difficult and demanding learning tasks.

LaRue et al (1986) found secondary memory (a common characteristic of dementia) to be more impaired in demented than in depressed subjects, yet the depressed performed more poorly than controls. O'Hara et al (1986) in a large community survey, found that subjects with depressive disorders (defined by Research Diagnostic Criteria [RDC]) did not differ from individuals with high symptom levels of depression but without an RDC diagnosis in terms of memory problems. All subjects with significant depressive symptoms have higher levels of memory complaint than subjects with low symptom levels. Niederehe and Yoder (1989) studied meta-memory in late life depressives. Meta-memory is the individual's knowledge and awareness of memory and the monitoring of information storage and retrieval operations. Depressed subjects, regardless of age, did not appear to be less knowledgeable about memory or to hold different perceptions about the relationship of age and memory. Older subjects were more sensitive than younger subjects to specific areas and issues of memory decline. For example, older adults were as adept at recalling important information but not as adept at retaining information and were aware of these memory difficulties. In general, self-appraisal of one's memory in everyday situations is poorly correlated with objectively assessed memory performance.

Emory and Breslau (1989) compared individuals with major depression, patients with Alzheimer's disease, and control subjects. The depressed elderly performed better than Alzheimer's patients on structured language tasks with repetition, naming, auditory/verbal comprehension, syntax, and reading but worse than controls. Complexity appeared to be the key intervening variable. Although the reason for a language deficit in major depression is unknown, according to these authors, it is not justifiable to rule out an organic explanation for language difficulties. They recognize, however, that the concept of complexity may overlap with the concept of information processing (see below), which involves energy, attentional capacity, and intentionality. The least complex tasks are performed with the most ease in both depressed patients and Alzheimer's patients.

Cohen et al (1982) used motor and memory tasks to assess motivational factors in learning by depressed patients. Depressed patients exhibit impairment in central motivational states. The most severe depression-related impairment was found in cognitive and motor tasks that required substantial effort. They described a "lack of effort" on the part of the depressed patients who exhibited an increased dependency, indecisiveness, and avoidance of responsibility. In other words a type of giving up or learned helplessness may contribute to memory and cognitive dysfunction in the depressed. Weingartener et al (1981) suggest that "effortful" cognition is impaired in the depressed, whereas automatic cognition is not. Depressed patients use weak or incomplete encoding of information. If the depressed patient is provided organization and structure, then learning-memory deficits are not apparent. Disruptions of arousal/activation in depression can account for these cognitive impairments. They studied ten subjects (all less than 59 years of age) to reach these conclusions.

In summary, cognitive problems, especially memory problems, have been long associated with depressive disorders, regardless of age. Some evidence exists that these problems may manifest themselves more frequently in the depressed elderly because of decreased reserve capacity and lack of motivation. The use of standard psychologic tests to distinguish these differences, however, is not helpful in the midst of a depressive episode.

■ LABORATORY TESTS AND THE DISTINCTION OF DEPRESSION AND DEMENTIA

A number of laboratory tests have been hypothesized to enable clinicians to differentiate depression and dementia. Three tests have been studied extensively in the literature; the electroencephalogram (EEG); brain imaging studies (especially magnetic resonance imaging [MRI]); and the Dexamethasone Suppression Test (DST). None of these tests has proven to be useful in routine clinical evaluations, yet differences across disorders do emerge in these tests that may provide additional information to the clinician evaluating the older adult who must distinguish depression and dementia or who must determine the relative contribution of each to the clinical presentation.

Brenner et al (1989) compared mixed depression and dementia, depressive pseudodementia, DAT, controls, and major depression without cognitive dysfunctioning using the EEG. In patients with depression or depressive pseudodementia the EEG was normal or showed only mild abnormality. In contrast, patients with dementia or dementia secondary to depression had abnormal EEG. Both the depressive and pseudodementia groups, however, did show significant slowing of the dominant posterior rhythm. Prinz and Vitello (1989) found that alpha rhythms on the EEG decrease with increased age and also that the mean alpha rhythm is decreased in both Alzheimer's disease and major depression compared with controls. They found the decrease is greater in Alzheimer's disease than major depression, permitting an overall correct discrimination of 72% between Alzheimer's disease and major depression and 77% between Alzheimer's disease and controls. Reynolds et al (1988; 1988a) found that the results of sleep polysomnography in persons with depression and those with normal aging are similar, such as decreased rapid eye movement (REM) latency, increased disruption of sleep, and early-morning awakening, but sleep studies may be helpful in identifying major depression when they are carried out by experienced polysomnographers. Specifically, they found that they could discriminate across normal aging, depression, and dementia by using specialized encephalographic sleep data. In general, however, routine EEG are not useful in discriminating depression from dementia.

In a literature review of various imaging techniques, Morris and Rappaport (1990) conclude from current evidence that cortical atrophy may be an important factor in the genesis of mood disorders of old age. Therefore imaging may be a potentially useful technique for discriminating depression from dementia. Figiel et al (1989), in a study of pre-ECT patients (all of whom were elderly), found a variety of brain changes on MRI, including cortical atrophy, subcortical encephalomalacia, lateral ventricular enlargement, and lesion of the pons. These brain changes did not change with ECT, although the majority of the individuals responded to ECT. Although most of these patients had soft neurologic signs, there were no persistent cognitive changes associated with MRI changes. After ECT, however, these patients performed with much more variability on memory scales than patients after ECT without such changes. Coffey et al (1990) identified subcortical hyperintensities on MRI to be significantly more common and more severe in the elderly depressed patients referred for ECT than in age-matched controls. Pearlson et al (1989) found that individuals with cognitive impairment and major depression had ECT results that were between individuals with pure major depression and patients with Alzheimer's disease without major depression. Most of the patients with depression and cognitive function returned to normal in their cognitive functioning after treatment of the depressive episode.

These findings on MRI scanning must be interpreted with caution, however. Awad et al (1986) suggest that the signal hyperintensities in white matter apparent on these MRI images most likely reflect changes in water content of extracellular space, resulting in increase of the photon signal. Such changes could derive from dilation of the perivascular space or vascular ectasia, resulting in shrinkage or atrophy of brain parynchyma around blood vessels (see Chapter 4 for a more detailed description of the possible pathologic significance of these changes). Nasrella et al (1989) suggest that interpretations must account for pretreatment and posttreatment effects, since both lithium carbonate and tricyclic antidepressants cause fluid shifts that could account for the ventricular enlargement and sulcus widening seen on the MRI scans and CT scans of patients with depression who are treated with medication. Figiel et al (1989) also suggested that these changes are much more frequent in first-onset depression in late life than in elderly depressed persons who had their first-onset depressive episodes earlier in life.

The diagnostic test for depression that has received the most attention during the past decade has been the DST. The DST has not only been suggested as a biologic marker for depression (regardless of age) but also is thought to suggest dysregulation of the hypothalamic-pituitary adrenal axis in depression. The relevance of the DST to the distinction between depression and dementia is complex, however. Steroid intake has been shown to produce cortical atrophy when taken over long periods of time, which may be reversible after discontinuance of the steroid. Therefore atrophy of the cortex (a finding in dementia) may be secondary to chronic cortisol levels in the blood secondary to chronic depressive illness. Certain areas of the brain, particularly the hippocampus, are vulnerable to a neurotoxic effect of prolonged exposure to cortisol (Uno et al, 1989). The correlation between ventricular brain ratio and 24-hour urinary excretion of cortisol has been reported in affective-disorder patients (Kellner et al, 1983).

A number of investigators have studied the role the DST in distinguishing depression and dementia. Rabey et al (1990) found that the DST does not distinguish depression and dementia in Parkinson's disease. Parkinson's disease nonsuppressors show higher basal values of plasma ACTH, beta-endorphine, and cortisol (similar to patients with major depression). Therefore, even when clinically undetected, both Parkinson's disease and major depression may be associated with a dysregulation of the hypothalamic pituitary adrenal (HPA) axis. Krishnan et al (1988) studied patients with Alzheimer's disease with and without major depression. The DST results were not related to the diagnosis of major depression or to the severity of depression. DST nonsuppression was found in 31% of patients with major depression alone and in 25% of patients with major depression and Alzheimer's disease. In a study of 29 elderly depressed subjects, Siegel et al (1989) found plasma cortisol levels before and after administration of 0.5 mg of dexamethasone were positively correlated with the Global Deterioration Scale. They suggest that the increased activity of the HPA axis could contribute to the cognitive impairment observed in major depression.

Although these studies provide interesting areas of inquiry for understanding the pathophysiology of depression, dementia, and the comorbidity of depression and dementia, none of the laboratory tests studied are as yet useful in the clinical differentiation of depression and dementia. When combined with clinical data, they may provide some degree of additional discrimination. For some tests (e.g., sleep EEGs), the conditions required for the test, such as no medications for many days, preclude the routine use of the test in making a differential diagnosis. Other tests, such as the DST and MRI scanning, may reveal results that are associated with both depression and dementia but are neither specific nor sensitive to acute conditions and therefore do not permit discrimination.

■ DEPRESSION IN DEMENTING ILLNESSES

The distinction of depression versus dementia is much less relevant to clinical practice than the comorbidity of depression and the common dementing illnesses affecting older adults. The literature regarding the frequency of comorbid depression with dementing illness is substantial and almost invariably suggests a clear relationship between the two disorders. Given the interest in the neuropathology of depression in the elderly and its relation to the neuropathologic changes found in dementing disorders, this association is expected. Nevertheless, clear neuropathologic explanations for depressive illness in the dementing disorders are not, as yet, forthcoming from clinical investigators.

Alois Alzheimer (1907), in his initial case description of Alzheimer's disease, found depression and delusions to be components of the syndrome. Since that time, many studies have emerged that clearly document the increased likelihood of depression in Alzheimer's disease compared with normal age-matched older adults. In a literature review, Wragg and Jeste (1989) found 30 studies in which depression and psychotic symptoms occurred in 30% to 40% of Alzheimer's disease patients. Symptoms of depression were two to three times as frequent as diagnosable mood or psychotic disorders. In most studies, however, the estimates of prevalence of major depression in Alzheimer's disease are somewhat lower.

Many studies have emerged estimating the prevalence of depression in Alzheimer's disease, a few of which are reviewed next. Virtually all report similar ranges of prevalence. Reifler et al (1989) found that 20% of Alzheimer's disease patients admitted to an outpatient memory disorders clinic experienced major depression. Depression was more severe in the less cognitively impaired. Patterson et al (1990) found that 18% of Alzheimer's patients in an outpatient setting had mild-to-moderate symptoms of depression. Lazarus et al (1987) found mild depression in 40% of the patients compared with 12% of the controls. The main depressive symptoms that distinguished depresesed Alzheimer patients from controls were depressed mood, decline in work and activities, psychomotor retardation, anxiety, obsessive/compulsive symptoms, helplessness, hopelessness, and worthlessness. Guilt, suicidal ideation, late insomnia, and psychomotor agitation were not common in DAT patients. Merrian et al (1988) found depressive disorders in 87% of Alzheimer's disease patients (yet this included all varieties of depressive disorders). As with Reifler et al, they found that severe depressive symptoms were greater in the less cognitively impaired.

Investigators have also addressed the issue of prognosis of individuals with combined depression and dementia. Reynolds et al (1986), in a 2-year follow-up of patients with mixed symptoms of depression and dementia, found that higher MMSE scores (≥ 21), higher Hamilton Depression Rating Scores (≥ 21), and sleep efficiency of less than 75% predicted a better score on the Global Dementia Scale and Hamilton Depression Scale at follow-up. Lopez et al (1990), in a 1-year follow-up of Alzheimer's and major depressed patients versus those with Alzheimer's disease alone, found no difference in the pattern of neuropsychologic deficits between the two groups at outcome. This suggests that depression that is comorbid with Alzheimer's disease does not modify the neuropsychologic features nor rate of progression of the Alzheimer's disease per se.

Some investigators have been interested in the past history and family history of depression in Alzheimer's disease. Pearlson et al (1990), when comparing depressed with nondepressed Alzheimer patients, found that the life-time risk for major depression was greater in the first degree-relatives of an index case of Alzheimer's disease, suggesting that depression in Alzheimer's disease is genetically related to primary mood disorders.

Rovner et al (1989) found that 30% of depressed Alzheimer's patients had a previous history of psychiatric illness and 70% had a history of major depression.

Other investigators have explored the difference in the prevalence of comorbid depression in Alzheimer's disease versus multiinfarct dementia. Cummings et al (1987) found a depressed mood in 7% of Alzheimer's patients and 60% of multiinfarct disease patients. The diagnosis of major depression in this sample was made in none of the Alzheimer's disease subjects but in 27% of the multiinfarct dementia subjects. Prevalence estimates for major depression in this study were significantly different because case finding methods were different.

At least two studies have emerged regarding treatment response. Greenwald et al (1989) found that 11% of dementia patients met criteria for major depression. When compared with nondemented depressed, 70% responded to antidepressant therapy, compared with 73% of the nondemented depressed. After treatment, although cognitive impairment persisted in the demented subjects, cognitive performance did improve. This study did not include a placebo-control group. Reifler et al (1989), in a placebo-control study, found that imipramine led to an improvement of depressive symptoms in individuals with comorbid depression and Alzheimer's disease but did not lead to improved cognitive impairment in Alzheimer's patients. The placebo group responded equally well in terms of improved depressed symptoms.

In summary, these studies suggest that depressive symptoms and the diagnosis of major depression is much more frequent in Alzheimer's patients than in age-matched controls. The etiology of depression in Alzheimer's disease remains undetermined, but a common neuropathologic etiology cannot be ruled out. Nevertheless, major depression may be treated effectively with pharmacologic intervention (although this remains to be demonstrated with placebo-control studies), with an expectation of improvement at least equal to age-matched controls. Nevertheless, treatment of depressive symptoms does not appear to significantly improve the cognitive impairment associated with Alzheimer's disease.

Depression is frequently comorbid with stroke. Wade et al (1987), in a community study of stroke, assessed survivors at 3 weeks, 6 months, and 12 months after stroke. Between 25% to 30% were depressed at each of the three times of assessment. Over 50% of the patients were depressed at the 3-week follow-up and remained so at the 1-year follow-up. Factors associated with depression in stroke included a loss of functional independence, a low level of other activities, low reasoning ability, female gender, and living with someone else. Robinson et al (1983) found 25% of patients with a left-hemispheric lesion met symptom criteria for major depression and 39% criteria for at least minor depression. About 60% of patients with a left-anterior lesion suffered major depression, but only 12% with posterior lesions had depressive symptoms. In addition, 37% of patients with brain-stem lesions were depressed, yet none with right-anterior lesions had major depression and only 17% with the right-posterior lesions had symptoms. In this report, Robinson et al report that usual assessment instruments for depression, such as a structured interview (e.g., the Present State Examination) and self-rating depression scales (e.g., the Zung Scale), were effective screening instruments in stroke victims.

Few investigators dispute the comorbidity of stroke and depression. Robins (1976), however, in a comparison of 18 patients with stroke and 18 age- and gender-matched patients with another chronic disability, found no difference in the levels of depression between the two groups.

The clinician may have difficulty in distinguishing symptoms of depression from symptoms of stroke. For example, vegetative symptoms of depression, such as pain, sleep disturbance, and psychomotor retardation or agitation, may also be part of the stroke syndrome. Poor emotional control (e.g., outbursts of crying) may also occur in stroke and depression. Lipsey et al (1986) found the phenomenology of depression after stroke and nonneurologic-related depression to be similar. The only difference was that cognitive and physical impairment was greater in stroke patients. Bolla-Wilson et al (1989) compared left- and right-hemispheric stroke victims. Persons with left-sided strokes and co-morbid depression exhibited a greater decline in cognitive performance or a "dementia in depression" syndrome, whereas persons with right-sided lesions with concomitant depression did not exhibit such cognitive decline. Patients with right-hemispheric lesions may also have inappropriate cheerfulness (Robinson et al, 1983).

House (1987) studied the frequent clinical observation that emotional lability is characteristic of stroke. He found that emotional expression in stroke, such as crying or laughing, is uncontrollable by the patient. The emotions are socially inappropriate and embarrassing to the patient, for example, crying suddenly at a trivial experience (e.g., receiving a greeting card). Nevertheless, he noted that this symptom is not uncommon with stroke. Robinson et al (1983) found the severity of depression is significantly correlated with the severity of intellectual impairment and physical impairment, as well as the age and quality of social supports of patients.

Robinson et al (1982b) found the duration of untreated depression in 103 outpatients after stroke was 7 to 8 months in two thirds of the patients. In the period from 6 months to 2 years after stroke, there was a significant increase in the prevalence and severity of depression compared with other time periods after a stroke. Parikh et al (1990), in a 2-year follow-up of 63 patients, found that patients with an in-hospital index diagnosis of depression (either major or minor) were significantly more impaired on both physical activity and language function than were nondepressed patients during the index episode. This impairment persisted even if the depression remitted during the outcome interval. These findings suggest that if early motivation for physical recovery is lost (perhaps because of a lack of motivation secondary to depression), then maximum levels of recovery are not achieved.

Lipsey et al (1984) studied the treatment of depression after stroke. They found these depressions responded to nortriptyline in a double-blind study. Redding et al (1986) found depressed patients with a stroke had a greater improvement of activities of daily living when treated with trazeodone compared with placebo. In an older study, Post (1962) found that among 11 of 100 patients with depression associated with stroke, 6 recovered from the depression after ECT.

As with Alzheimer's disease, depression is much more frequent in stroke than would be expected by chance. The evidence is not clear, however, whether the depression associated with stroke is more frequent than would be expected with the physical and psychologic impairment associated with another disorder producing equal disability. As with Alzheimer's disease, depression that is comorbid with stroke can be treated with medication and even ECT. In most studies the symptoms of depression associated with stroke are similar to those symptoms found in classic major depression according to Research Diagnostic Criteria or the Diagnostic and Statistical Manual (DSM-III-R) criteria.

Perhaps no dementing disorder, other than Alzheimer's disease, has been more associated with depressive symptoms by clinical investigators than the subcortical dementia secondary to Parkinson's disease. Many of the symptoms of Parkinson's disease, such as mask facies, paucity of movement, and lack of emotional responsiveness, are symptoms that frequently accompany depression.

Parkinson's disease has long been known to be associated with a dementia syndrome. Korczyn (1986) found that, among a sample of 119 patients suffering Parkinson's disease, 38% suffered mild dementia and 46% suffered severe dementia. The authors conclude that dementia is one of the protean manifestations of Parkinson's disease, together with hyperkinesis, rigid tremor, and loss of postural reflexes. The demented patients were somewhat older than the nondemented and similar to patients suffering senile dementia of the Alzheimer's type with EEG abnormalities and ventricular dilation on CT scan.

At the molecular level, Robins (1983), notes that the brains of patients with Parkinson's disease have markedly decreased levels of dopamine and lower levels of norepinephrine and serotonin. Improvement in neurologic function after treatment of Parkinson's disease does not lead to a corresponding improvement in the depression (Hayes et al, 1966; Marsh et al, 1973). Therefore treatment of Parkinson's disease with dopamine agonists may not reverse the neurochemical abnormalities that predispose the parkinsonian patient to depression.

Santo et al (1989), in a chart review of 339 patients with Parkinson's disease, estimated a 10.9% prevalence of dementia, according to DSM-III criteria, a 51% prevalence of depression (not exclusive of latent depression), and a comorbid diagnosis of depression and dementia in 5.4%. In 115 patients involved in a prospective study, they found patients who were either depressed or demented had lower cerebrospinal fluid serotonin than other parkinsonian patients. This finding suggests a unique neurochemical contribution to depression in Parkinson's disease, since levels of 5-hydroxyindoleacetic acid (5-HIAA) can be reduced in Alzheimer's disease but tend to be even lower in Parkinson's disease. In this study, depressed patients did not differ in age or severity of physical symptoms from the nondepressed patients. Bieliauskas and Glantz (1989) found 70% of 33 patients without a previous psychiatric diagnosis suffering from Parkinson's disease were depressed. The depression was not related to the presence of memory and attention deficits, years of Parkinson's disease, age, or indices of frontal cortex-related functioning.

Starkstein et al (1990) found in 105 patients with Parkinson's disease, 21% met criteria for major depression and 20% met criteria for minor depression. Prevalence by length of illness showed a bimodal distribution with an increased prevalence during the early and late stages and a decreased prevalence during the middle stages of the disorder. Depressed parkinsonian patients in this study had activities of daily living (ADL) impairment and poorer cognitive functioning. In another study (Starkstein et al, 1989), these investigators compared early (younger than 55) and late (older than 55) onset of Parkinson's disease. The early-onset group experienced a higher prevalence of depression than the late-onset group. Tremor, akinesia, and rigidity were more severe in the late-onset group. Depression in the early-onset group was associated with cognitive impairment and duration of the disease. In the late-onset group, depression was associated with ADL impairment.

A number of investigators have focused on the nature of the depressive symptoms in

Parkinson's disease. Huber et al (1990) studied a group of elderly patients suffering Parkinson's disease and found its symptoms related to both mood and self-reproach present in the early stages of Parkinson's disease but did not increase in severity with advancing disease. Somatic complaints, such as the inability to work, fatigue, concern about health, and physical appearance, were evident early and increased as the disease progressed (not unexpected, given the increasing disability associated with Parkinson's disease). Vegetative symptoms, on the other hand, were seen only in the later stages of Parkinson's disease. Brown and McCarthy (1990) compared parkinsonian patients with normal patients and found that the depressive symptoms that were prominent in Parkinson's disease include depressed mood, loss of interest, and poor concentration. Sadness, moodiness, irritability, tension, worry, and pessimism, along with indecision and inability to get started, were also common symptoms in the depressed parkinsonian patient. Huber et al (1988) considered the severity of depressive symptoms in parkinsonian patients. In this study, they conclude that parkinsonian patients can be subtyped by severity of depression. In contrast, patients with more pronounced rigidity and bradykinesia were also more likely to exhibit cognitive deficits and disability.

Many investigators have focused on the degree of disability in parkinsonian patients and the relationships of disability to depressive symptoms. Schiffer et al (1988) compared patients with Parkinson's disease and multiple sclerosis (MS). Although the prevalence of depression in these two disorders was approximately equal, parkinsonian patients were more likely to exhibit anxiety and panic disorder in the midst of their depression than patients with MS. Ehmann et al (1990) compared depressive symptoms of parkinsonian patients and disabled controls. Parkinsonian patients had significantly greater total scores on the Beck Depressive Inventory (i.e., depression in Parkinson's disease was not solely related to disability). Gotham et al (1986) compared patients with Parkinson's disease, normal aging individuals, and patients suffering arthritic conditions. Age, duration of illness, and specific symptoms of parkinsonian patients, (especially rigidity, akinesia, and disability) were not related to depression. Brown et al (1988) found depression to be related to disability in Parkinson's disease over 1 year, however. The rates of change in disability, according to this group, may be the most important factor in long-term parkinsonian patients.

Despite the numerous studies documenting the comorbidity of depression and Parkinson's disease, few treatment studies have been reported. Kuniyoshi et al (1989) reported two cases in which the first manifestation of Parkinson's disease was depression. In both cases the symptoms of depression and Parkinson's disease improved with the administration of L-dopa. The authors conclude that Parkinson's disease should be suspected in cases of persistent and treatment-resistant depression, but these results are preliminary.

In summary the association of both mild and severe depression with Parkinson's disease is at least as great as depression associated with Alzheimer's disease. Few studies have been performed to date and no conclusive studies demonstrate that the treatment of depression in the midst of Parkinson's disease is effective in relieving symptoms of depression or the symptoms of Parkinson's disease in contrast to treatment studies of depression and Alzheimer's disease. On the other hand, treatment of the parkinsonian symptoms is well established and, to some degree, since this treatment improves physical function, an improvement of depressive symptoms should result.

■ PSEUDODEMENTIA AND DEPRESSION

A discussion of depression and pseudodementia must be placed in the context of the comorbidity of depression with the dementing disorder. The term *pseudodementia* was coined by Wernicke (1906) to refer to chronic hysterical states mimicking mental weakness. Wells (1979) described pseudodementia as the syndrome in which dementia is mimicked or caricatured by functional psychiatric disorders, with marked dependency being the most frequent symptom. Most patients with pseudodementia, according to Wells, do suffer a concomitant depressed affect. Barry and Moskowitz (1988), in a literature review, found definitions of treatable dementias, reversible dementias, or pseudodementias vary from study to study. Some exclude depression and some include alcoholic dementia as a so-called pseudodementia. In most studies, depression is the most common cause of reversible dementia, followed by drug toxicity. Kiloh (1962) used the term *pseudodementia* to describe a variety of patients in whom "the diagnosis of dementia is entertained but has to be abandoned because of the subsequent course of the illness . . . in these patients the picture of dementia may very closely be mimicked."

There are few prevalence studies of pseudodementia. Larson et al (1985), in a series of 200 patients referred to a memory disorders clinic, found 5% suffered major depression exclusively. Marsden and Harrison (1972) found 8 out of 106 patients with memory problems suffered from depression and 1 suffered from mania. Haward (1977) found 33% of 49 patients with suspected dementia to have pseudodementia. This figure, however, is much higher than has been found in other studies. Folstein and McHugh (1978) estimate that approximately 50% of elderly depressives suffered some cognitive deficits similar to dementia. Roth (1976) estimated that 15% of depressed patients over 60 years of age have significant cognitive deficits.

Knott and Fleminger (1975), in a study that attempted to identify characteristics that distinguish dementia from pseudodementia, found memory disturbance to be the most prominent symptom in both dementia and nondemented subjects and did not discriminate the subjects. Disorientation was not a distinguishing characteristic either. Dementia patients had problems with naming, writing, calculation, and motor praxis in contrast to pseudodementia patients. Bulbena (1986) suggests, from a meta-analysis that he compared with his own sample of 22 pseudodementia subjects, the possibility of two subtypes of pseudodementia, one with depression and one with delirium. More of the pseudodemented patients had a history of psychiatric illness compared with the truly demented patients.

Other studies have been devoted to differential diagnosis. Emery (1988) found that, in Alzheimer's disease, primary memory is best preserved, whereas in depression and normal aging, tertiary memory is best preserved. For example, problems with orientation and the provision of information are more preserved in depressive pseudodementia than in dementia. The best distinction between depression and senile dementia, however, was in the capacity for remembering old information with the depressed better able to remember. Regarding language, senile dementia of the Alzheimer's type was best discriminated from normal aging by complex tasks (e.g., tests for syntactic complexity and word fluency) and was best discriminated from pseudodementia by the least complex oral language measures, such as responsive speech and sentence completion (i.e., the capacity for implicit speech processing is better preserved in depressive pseudodementia than in senile dementia of the Alzheimer's type). Reynolds (1988), in a study of

14 patients with pseudodementia and 28 with primary degenerative dementia, found patients with pseudodementia showed significantly greater pretreatment early morning awakening, increased ratings of psychologic anxiety, and more impaired libido. Dementia patients showed more disorientation to time, greater difficulty finding their way around, and more impairment in dressing. Reynolds and Hoch (1987) found family history of affective disorder or dementia may assist in the differential diagnosis of depression from dementia. Rabins et al (1984) found reversible dementia to be distinguished from dementia by a higher frequency of previous depression, recurrent depressed mood, delusions, and increased MMSE scores.

Lazarus et al (1987) found patients with primary degenerative dementia have higher scores on items assessing intrapsychic rather than neurovegetative symptoms of depression (e.g., anxiety, helplessness, hopelessness, and worthlessness) and less problems with sleep and weight loss. In a study of 11 patients with pseudodementia, Caine (1981) found patients with pseudodementia can learn new information (e.g., delayed verbal recall is preserved although immediate recall is poor). In addition, these patients had no problems copying a figure (a task that is problematic for demented subjects). Folstein et al (1975) found patients with reversible dementia syndrome frequently score higher on the MMSE, whereas patients with dementia score lower (a cutoff of 22 being the place where dementia can be distinguished from pseudodementia). Wells (1979) notes that near-miss versus do-not-know answers may help differentiate dementia from pseudodementia, although patients with pseudodementia often perform poorly on neuropsychologic tests. For example, pseudodemented patients respond to a question by "I don't know," whereas demented patients attempt to answer questions but answer them incorrectly. Poor performance, however, is inconsistent from one test to another on psychologic testing in pseudodementia, whereas there is a consistent poor performance across tests in dementia patients.

Laboratory studies have been thought to be of value in distinguishing depression from dementia and therefore in assisting in the identification of the patient suffering pseudodementia. These tests have been reviewed previously. Spar (1983) is one of a number of investigators who found that the DST does not distinguish depression from dementia well. Sleep studies (e.g., those performed by Reynolds and Hoch, 1987) and imaging studies have been equally unsuccessful in providing accurate differentiation between these conditions. Although the laboratory may be of value in providing additional diagnostic data, no laboratory test is currently available that identifies pseudodementia. Therefore the workup of the patient suspected of having pseudodementia should that combine the workup of dementia and pseudodementia.

Regarding the routine clinical workup, the National Institutes of Health Consensus Conference on the Assessment of Dementia 1987 concluded that all new patients with the onset of dementia should have the following standard diagnostic studies: a complete blood count, electrolyte panel, screening metabolic panel, thyroid function test, vitamin B12 and folic acid deficiency tests, serologic test for syphilis and, depending on history, a screen for immunodeficiency antibodies, urinalysis, electrocardiogram, and chest x ray. Other ancillary tests suggested to be useful but not necessary were CT of the brain and focal neurologic signs of dementia of brief duration. MRI is an alternative to CT scans. EEGs would be appropriate if altered consciousness or suspected seizures complicate the clinical picture.

Neuropsychologic evaluation is appropriate to obtain baseline information against which to measure changes when diagnosis is in doubt, to document function before and after treatment in cases of exceptionally bright individuals suspected of early dementia and in cases of ambiguous imaging findings that require elucidation, to help distinguish dementia from depression and delirium, and to provide additional information about the extent and nature of impairment after focal or multifocal brain injuries. In cases where language is a major problem, speech and language analysis by a speech pathologist should be requested.

Studies considered experimental by this group included MRI, regional cerebral blood flow and metabolism measurements, lumbar puncture, electrophysiologic probes (e.g., event-related potential), brain biopsy, molecular genetic studies, and ultrasound.

The best means, however, of differentiating dementia from depression is through outcome studies. Reynolds et al (1986) found a favorable outcome in patients with mixed depression and cognitive impairment associated with higher Hamilton Depression score was relatively intact cognitive functioning, and neurovegetative signs of depression (particularly sleep disturbances). Grunhaus et al (1983), in a retrospective study, found a profile for the diagnosis of patients with depressive pseudodementia (i.e., patients with cognitive impairment who improved over time) to include a dysphoric mood, an abnormal DST, normal CT scan, and a tendency to respond to adequate tricyclic antidepressant therapy or ECT. Krall and Emery (1989) followed 44 pseudodemented subjects for 4 to 18 years, all of whom showed initial clearing of depression and improvement of cognitive functioning. Over the follow-up period, 79% developed primary degenerative dementia. The development of dementia appeared to go through the following four steps: (1) recurrent episodes of bipolar/unipolar depression; (2) one or more episodes of depression in which cognitive functioning was impaired; (3) an episode of depression that appeared very much like senile dementia but then remitted; and (4) presentation of dementia without remission. The progression from stage "2" through "4" required an average of more than 9 years. Outcome, in retrospect, assists the clinician to identify patterns of symptom presentation at baseline associated with improvement in cognitive function.

■ CONCLUSION

From this review, a number of recommendations, both general and specific, can be made regarding the diagnostic workup and treatment of persons suffering from depressive disorders that are confused with comorbid or dementing disorders.

First, clinicians must be sensitive to the comorbidity of depressive symptoms and major depression with dementia of the Alzheimer's type, Parkinson's disease, stroke, and other dementing disorders. If the clinician identifies symptoms of both the depressed mood and cognitive impairment, combined workup for depression and dementia is the preferred course. Psychologic tests of cognition during an acute episode of depression with clinically significant cognitive impairment, are of questionable benefit. Testing after an episode, on the other hand, once the depressive episode has remitted, often reveals that the cognitive impairment continues and can be valuable not only in predicting outcome but also for establishing a benchmark of cognitive functioning uncomplicated by depression to be used for future reference.

Neurologic workup of the older adult suffering from a depressive disorder and coexisting cognitive impairment can be most informative in identifying the individual for the potential irreversible dementing disorder (e.g., stroke and Parkinson's disease). Laboratory tests, on the other hand, are of questionable value in differentiating depression from dementing disorders. The DST, sleep studies, and imaging studies are sensitive tests for both depression and dementia but are not specific. Laboratory tests may be used to rule out more rare forms of cerebral pathology (e.g., normal pressure hydrocephalus and tumor). Cerebrospinal fluid studies are of little benefit clinically at present, except where clear indication of their use emerges during the clinical evaluation.

Treatment of depression in the midst of a dementing episode is usually indicated with antidepressant medication, although the clinician must closely monitor potential side effects, especially anticholinergic effects. These anticholinergic effects, however, are usually not significant enough to preclude the use of antidepressant drugs. The medical status of the patient must be considered to determine if antidepressant medication is indicated. There is no documented evidence that psychotherapy is beneficial during an acute episode of depression and concomitant cognitive impairment. On the other hand, once the depression remits and cognitive function improves, psychotherapy may be of value in preventing the recurrence of a depressive episode with subsequent cognitive difficulties. Treatment of the underlying disorder that produces cognitive impairment (e.g., in the case of Parkinson's disease) is indicated and may lead to an improvement of the depressive symptoms. For most of the dementing disorders, however, no definitive treatment is readily available, and therefore improvement of functional status is the goal of the treatment with the hope that improvement in functional status may improve depressive symptomatology.

REFERENCES

Alzheimer A: Uber eine eigenartige Erkrankung der Hirnrinde, *Algmeine Zeitsrift fur Psychitrie und Psychiatrish-Gerentliche Medizin* 64:146-148, 1907.

Awad IA, Johnson PC, Spetzler RF, Hodak JA: Incidental subcortical lesions identified on magnetic resonance imaging in the elderly, II. Postmortem Pathologic Correlations, *Stroke* 17:1090-1097, 1986.

Barry PT, Moskowitz MA: The diagnosis of reversible dementia in the elderly: a critical review, *Archives of Internal Medicine* 148:1914-1918, 1988.

Bieliauskas LA, Glantz RH: Depression type in Parkinson's disease, *Journal of Clinical and Experimental Neuropsychology* 11:597-604, 1989.

Bleuler E: *Textbook of Psychiatry.* New York, Macmillan, 1924, p. 175.

Bolla-Wilson K, Robinson RG, Starkstein SE, Boston J, Price TR: Lateralization of dementia of depression in stroke patients, *American Journal of Psychiatry* 146:627-634, 1989.

Brenner RP, Reynolds CF, Vulrich RF: EEG findings in depressive pseudodementia and dementia with secondary depression, *Electroencephalography in Clinical Neurophysiology* 72:298-304, 1989.

Brown RG, MacCarthy B: Psychiatric morbidity in patients with Parkinson's disease, *Psychological Medicine* 20:77-87, 1990.

Brown RG, MacCarthy B, Gatham AM, Der GJ, Marsden CD: Depression and disability in Parkinson's disease: the follow-up of 132 cases, *Psychological Medicine,* 18:49-55, 1988.

Bulbena A, Berriose GE: Pseudodementia: facts and figures, *British Journal of Psychiatry* 148:87-94, 1986.

Caine E: Pseudodementia, *Archives of General Psychiatry* 38:1359-1364, 1981.

Cavanaugh SVA, Wettson R: The relationship between severity of depression, cognitive dysfunction and age in medical inpatients, *American Journal of Psychiatry* 140:495-496, 1983.

Cohen RM, Weingartner H, Smallberg SA, Picker D, Murphy DL: Effort and cognition in depression, *Archives of General Psychiatry* 39:593-597, 1982.

Coffey CE, Figiel GS, Djang WT, Weiner RD: Subcortical hyperintensity on magnetic resonance imaging. A comparison of normal and depressed elderly subjects, *American Journal of Psychiatry* 147:187-189, 1990.

Cummings JL, Miller B, Hill MA, Neshkes R: Neuropsychiatric aspects of multi-infarct dementia and dementia of the Alzheimer type, *Archives of Neurology* 44:389-393, 1987.

Ehmann TS, Beninger RJ, Gawel MJ, Riopelle RJ: Coping, social support, and depressive symptoms in Parkinson's disease, *Journal of Geriatric Psychiatry and Neurology* 3:85-90, 1990.

Emery VOB: Pseudodementia: a theoretical and empirical discussion, *Cleveland Western Reserve Geriatric Education Center Interdisciplinary Monograph Series*, 1988.

Emory OB, Breslau LD: Language deficits in depression: comparisons with SDAT in normal aging, *Journal of Gerontology: Medical Sciences* 44:M85-M92, 1989.

Figiel GS, Coffey CE, Weiner RD: Brain magnetic resonance imaging in elderly depressed patients receiving electroconvulsive therapy, *Convulsive Therapy* 5:26-34, 1989.

Folstein MF, Folstein SE, McHugh PR: "Mini-Mental State": a practical method for grading the cognitive state, *Journal of Psychiatric Research* 12:189-193, 1975.

Folstein M, McHugh P: Dementia syndrome of depression, *Aging* 7:87-93, 1978.

Golinkoff M, Sweeney JA: Cognitive impairments in depression, *Journal of Affective Disorders* 17:105-112, 1989.

Gotham AM, Brown RG, Marshden CD: Depression in Parkinson's disease: a quantitative and qualitative analysis, *Journal of Neurology, Neurosurgery and Psychiatry* 49:381-389, 1986.

Greenwald BS, Kramer-Ginsberg E, Marin DB, Laitman LB, Hermann CK, et al: Dementia with co-existant major depression, *American Journal of Psychiatry* 146:1472-1478, 1989.

Grunhaus L, Dilsaver S, Greden JF, Carroll BJ: Depressive pseudodementia: a suggested diagnostic profile, *Biological Psychiatry* 18(2):215-225, 1983.

Haward L: Cognition in dementia presenilis. In Smith W, Kinsbourne M (eds): *Aging and Dementia*. New York, Spectrum, 1977.

Hayes P, Krikler B, Walsh LS: Psychological changes following surgical treatment of Parkinsonism, *American Journal of Psychiatry* 123:657-662, 1966.

Horne A: Mood disorders after stroke: a review of the evidence, *International Journal of Geriatric Psychiatry* 2:211-221, 1987.

Huber SJ, Freidenberg DL, Paulson GW, Shuttleworth EC, Christy JA: The pattern of depressive symptoms varies with progression of Parkinson's disease, *Journal of Neurology, Neurosurgery and Psychiatry* 53:275-278, 1990.

Huber SJ, Paulson GW, Shuttleworth EC: Depression in Parkinson's disease, *Neuropsychiatry, Neuropsychology and Behavioral Neurology* 1:47-51, 1988.

Kellner CH, Rubinow DR, Gold PW, Post RM: Relationship of cortisol hypersecretion to brain CT scan alters in depressed patients. *Psychiatry Research* 8:191-197, 1983.

Kiloh L: Pseudo-dementia, *Acta Psychiatrica Scandinavica* 37:336-351, 1962.

Knott P, Fleminger J: Presenile dementia: the difficulties of early diagnosis, *Acta Psychiatrica Scandinavia* 51:210-217, 1975.

Korczyn AD: Dementia in Parkinson's disease. In Fisher A, Hanin I, Lachman C (eds): *Alzheimer's and Parkinson's Disease: Strategies for Research and Development*. New York, Plenum Press, 1986, pp. 177-189.

Krall VA, Emery OB: Long-term follow-up of depressive pseudodementia of the aged, *Canadian Journal of Psychiatry* 34:445-446, 1989.

Krishnan KR, Goli V, Ellinwood EH: Gluckencephalopathy in patients diagnosed as major depressive, *Biological Psychiatry* 23:519-522, 1988.

Krishnan KRR, Hayman A, Ritchie JC: Depression in early-onset Alzheimer's disease: clinical and neuroendocrine correlates, *Biological Psychiatry* 24:937-940, 1988.

Kuniyoshi M, Arikawa K, Miura C, Inanga K: Parkinsonism manifesting depression as the first sign, *The Japanese Journal of Psychiatry and Neurology* 43:37-43, 1989.

Larson EB, Reifler BV, Sumi SM, et al: Diagnostic evaluation of 200 elderly outpatients with suspected dementia, *Journal of Gerontology* 40:536-543, 1985.

LaRue A, D'Elia LF, Clark EO, Spar JE, Jarvik LF: Clinical tests of memory in dementia, depression and healthy aging, *Journal of Psychology and Aging* 1:69-77, 1986.

Lazarus LW, Newton N, Cohler B, Lesser J, et al: Frequency in presentation of depressive symptoms in patients with primary degenerative dementia, *American Journal of Psychiatry* 144:41-45, 1987.

Lipsey JR, Robinson RG, Pearlson GD, Raok, Price TR: Nortriptyline treatment of post-stroke depression: a double-blind study, Lancet 1:297-300, 1984.

Lipsey JR, Spencer WC, Rabins PV, Robinson RG: Phenomenological comparison of post-stroke depression and functional depression, American Journal of Psychiatry 143:527-529, 1986.

Lopez OL, Boller F, Becker JT, Miller M, Reynolds CF, III: Alzheimer's disease and depression: neuropsychological impairment in progression of illness, American Journal of Psychiatry 147:855, 860, 1990.

Marsden C, Harrison MJ: Outcome of investigations of patients with presenile dementia, British Medical Journal 2:249-252, 1972.

Marsh GG, Markham CH: Does levodopa alter depression and psychopathology in Parkinsonian patients? Journal of Neurology, Neurosurgery and Psychiatry 36:925-935, 1973.

McHugh, PR, Folstein M: Psychopathology of dementia: implications for neuropathology. In Katzman R (ed): Congential and Acquired Cognitive Disorders. New York, Ravin Press, 1979.

Merrian AE, Aronson MK, Gaston P, Wey SL, Katz I: The psychiatric symptoms of Alzheimer's disease, Journal of the American Geriatrics Society 27:7-12, 1988.

Miller E, Lewis P: Recognition memory in elderly patients with depression and dementia: a signal detection analysis, Journal of Abnormal Psychology 86:84-86, 1978.

Morris P, Rapport SI: Neuroimaging and affective disorder in late life: a review, Canadian Journal of Psychiatry 35:347-354, 1990.

Nasrella HA, Coffman JA, Olson SC: Structural brain imaging findings in affective disorders: an overview, Journal of Neuropsychiatry 1:22-26, 1989.

National Institutes of Health: Differential Diagnosis of Dementing Diseases. Consensus Development Conference Statement, (vol 6, no 11), 1987.

Niederehe G, Yoder C: Meta memory perceptions in depressions of young and older adults, Journal of Nervous and Mental Diseases 177:4-14, 1989.

O'Hara MW, Hinrichs JV, Kohout FJ, Wallace RB, Lemke JH: Memory complaint and memory performance in the depressed elderly, Psychology and Aging 1:208-214, 1986.

Parikh RM, Robinson RG, Lipsey JR, Starkstein SE, Fedoroff JP, et al: The impact of post-stroke depression on recovery in activities of daily living over a two-year follow-up, Archives of Neurology 47:785-789, 1990.

Patterson MB, Schnell AH, Martin RJ, Mendez MF, Smyth KA, et al: Assessment of behavioral and affective symptoms in Alzheimer's disease, Journal of Geriatric Psychiatry and Neurology 3:21-30, 1990.

Pearlson GD, Rabins PV, Kim WS, Speedle LJ, Moberg PJ, et al: Structural brain CT changes and cognitive deficits in elderly depressives with and without reversible dementia (pseudodementia), Psychological Medicine 19:573-584, 1989.

Pearlson GD, Ross CA, Lohr WD, et al: Association between family history of affective disorder and the depressive syndromes of Alzheimer's disease, American Journal of Psychiatry 147:452-456, 1990.

Post F: The significance of affective symptoms and old age, Maudsley Monograph 10. London, Oxford University Press, 1962.

Prinz PN, Vitello MV: Dominant occipital (alpha) rhythm frequency in early stage Alzheimer's disease and depression, Electroencephalogy and Clinical Neurophysiology 73:427-432, 1989.

Rabey JM, Scharf M, Oberman Z, Zohar M, Graff E: Cortisol, ACTH, and beta-endorphin after dexamethasone administration in Parkinson's dementia, Biological Psychiatry 27:581-591, 1990.

Rabins PV, Merchant A, Nestadt G: Criteria for diagnosing reversible dementia caused by depression, British Journal of Psychiatry 144:488-492, 1984.

Reding MJ, Orto LA, Winter SW, Fortuna IM, DiPonte P, et al: Antidepressant therapy after stroke, Archives of Neurology 43:763-765, 1986.

Reifler BV, Teri L, Raskind M, Veith R, Barnes R, et al: Double-blind trial of imipramine in Alzheimer's disease patients with and without depression, American Journal of Psychiatry 146:45-49, 1989.

Reynolds CF, III, Hoch CL, Kupfer D, Buysse DJ, Houck PR, et al: Bedside differentiation of depressive pseudodementia from dementia, American Journal of Psychiatry

Reynolds CF, III, Hoch CC: Differential diagnosis of depressive pseudodementia and primary degenerative dementia, Psychiatric Annals 17:743-748, 1987. 145:1099-1103, 1988.

Reynolds CF, III, Kupfer DJ, Hoch CC, Stack JA, Houck PR, et al: Two-year follow-up of elderly patients with mixed depression and dementia: clinical electroencephalographic sleep findings, Journal of American Geriatrics Society 34:793-799, 1986.

Reynolds CF, III, Kupfer DJ, Houck PR, Hoch CC, Stack JA, et al: Reliable discrimination of elderly depressed and demented patients by electroencephalographic sleep data, *Archives of General Psychiatry* 45:258-264, 1988.

Robins AH: Are stroke patients more depressed than other disabled subjects? *Journal of Chronic Diseases* 29:479-482, 1976.

Robins AH: Prevalence and management of depression in patients with Parkinsonism, *Geriatric Medicine Today* 2:69-73, 1983.

Robinson RG, Kubos KL, Starr LB, Rao K, Price TR: Mood changes in stroke patients: relationship to lesion location, *Comprehensive Psychiatry* 24:555-556, 1983.

Robinson RG, Price TR: Post-stroke depressive disorders: a follow-up study of 103 patients, *Stroke* 13:635-641, 1982.

Robinson RG, Starr LB, Kubos KL, et al: A two-year longitudinal study of post-stroke mood disorders: findings during the initial evaluation, *Stroke* 14:736-741, 1983.

Rossi A, Stratta P, Nisticho R: Visuo-spatial impairment in depression. A controlled ECT study, *Acta Psychiatrica Scandinavica* 81:245-249, 1990.

Roth M: The psychiatric disorders of later life, *Psychiatric Annuals* 6:417-445, 1976.

Rovner BW, Broadhead J, Spencer M, Carson K, Folstein MF: Depression and Alzheimer's disease, *American Journal of Psychiatry* 146:350-353, 1989.

Sano M, Stern Y, Williams J, Cote L, Rosenstein R, et al: Coexisting dementia and depression in Parkinson's disease, *Archives of Neurology* 46:1284-1286, 1989.

Schiffer RB, Kurlan R, Rubin A, Buer S: Evidence for a typical depression in Parkinson's disease, *American Journal of Psychiatry* 145:1020-1022, 1988.

Siegel B, Gurevich D, Oxenkrug GF: Cognitive impairment in cortisol resistence to dexamethasone suppression test in elderly depression, *Biological Psychiatry* 25:229-234, 1989.

Spar JE, LaRue A: Major depression in the elderly—DSM-III criteria and the dexamethasone suppression test as predictors of treatment response, *American Journal of Psychiatry* 140:844-847, 1983.

Starkstein SE, Berthier ML, Bolduck PL, Preziosi TJ, Robinson RG: Depression in patients with early vs. late onset Parkinson's disease, *Neurology* 39:441-445, 1989.

Starkstein SE, Preziosi TJ, Bolduck, PL Robinson RG: Depression in Parkinson's disease, *Journal of Nervous and Mental Diseases* 178:27-31, 1990.

Sternberg DF, Jarvik ME: Memory functions in depression, *Archives of General Psychiatry* 33:219-224, 1976.

Sweeney JA, Wetzler S, Stokes P, Kocsis J: Cognitive functioning in depression, *Journal of Clinical Psychology* 45:836-842, 1989.

Uno H, Tarara R, Else JG, Suleman MA, Sapolsky RM: Hippocampal damage associated with prolonged and fatal stress in primates, *Journal of Neurosciences* 9:1705-1711, 1989.

Wade DT, Lagh Smith J, Hewer RA: Depressed mood after stroke: a community study of its frequency, *British Journal of Psychiatry* 151:200-205, 1987.

Watts FN, Cooper Z: The effects of depression on structural aspects of the recall of prose, *Journal of Abnormal Psychology* 98:150-153, 1989.

Weingartner H, Cohen RM, Murphy DL, Martello J, Gerdt C: Cognitive processes in depression, *Archives of General Psychiatry* 38:42-47, 1981.

Wells C: Pseudodementia, *American Journal of Psychiatry* 136:895-900, 1979.

Wernicke K: *Fundamentals of Psychiatry.* Leipzig, Thime, 1906.

Wragg RE, Jeste DJ: Overview of depression and psychosis in Alzheimer's disease, *American Journal of Psychiatry* 146:577-587, 1989.

The Treatment of Late Life Depression

17

Psychotherapy for Depression in Late Life

Although it has received less attention in the literature on treatment of late life depression than pharmacotherapy, psychotherapy nonetheless is central to the treatment of the depressed elder. Psychotherapy, especially the ongoing relationship between the patient experiencing late life depression and the therapist, is critical to successfully implementing the overall package of therapies prescribed for the depressed older adult. After a discussion of the historical perspectives of psychotherapy with older adults, general psychotherapeutic principles are described in this chapter. Then the process of psychotherapy in the elderly is reviewed, with attention directed toward issues such as transference, countertransference, resistance, regression, and the role of reminiscence. Common themes of therapy in depressed elders are discussed next. Although each older adult has a unique story to tell, common themes can be extracted from these stories that reflect issues raised by the impact of depression on the process of aging. Finally, the different types of psychotherapy that have been suggested for treating depressed elders are reviewed, including dynamic psychotherapy, supportive therapy, brief therapy, cognitive therapy, interpersonal therapy, bibliotherapy, behavioral therapy, and group therapy.

■ HISTORICAL PERSPECTIVES

Early investigators of psychotherapy in late life, regardless of the psychiatric disorder being treated, sought to determine if psychotherapy was effective in older adults. Freud (1924) believed psychoanalytic therapy was contraindicated in the elderly (he defined elderly as individuals 40 or more years of age). The elasticity of mental processes was, according to Freud, lacking and the mass of material that accumulated by mid-life to late life would prolong treatment interminably. In addition, the future decline in health and well-being of older adults would negate the accomplishments of psychotherapy. Freud also believed that neuroses were less important and less disabling among older persons compared with the young. Freud, however, engaged in self-analysis until he died in his eighties, reflecting especially on his beliefs and his role in society.

Jellife (1925), although he reported some successes in psychoanalytic therapy with older adults, noted that "neurosis or psychosis is a better solution of their (older adults) life difficulties than any that I, as an agent of reality, can offer." In other words, neurosis was an acceptable solution to the problems of late life. Finischel (1945) suggested the difficult living situations, which he considered typical of older persons, and/or the physical illnesses they suffer, may lend the neurosis suffered by the elder the best type of adjustment.

Not all early psychoanalytic therapists were as negative regarding psychotherapy among the elderly, however. Abraham (1949) believes the age of onset of the neurosis was more important in determining the outcome of therapy than the age of the patient. Jung (1963) views the age of 40 (or thereabout) as an opportunity for fundamental change in personality (i.e., the "noon of life"). "Individuation" begins in the forties and extends over the remainder of the life cycle. Jungian analysis seeks to help the individual in mid-life and late life to become an individual and generate new levels of meaning, awareness, and understanding. Some have suggested that one learns to enter life through a Freudian analysis and to leave life through a Jungian analysis. Erikson (1959) proposes the developmental task of later life as resolving the conflict of integration versus despair, a task that could be addressed and facilitated through psychotherapy.

Although the attitude toward psychotherapy with the elderly has improved in recent years, the debate continues. Meerloo (1973) suggests that the elderly are less resistant than the young to psychotherapy because of the nearness of death, making them more willing to engage in the life review necessary for psychotherapy. Hollander (1952) reinforces Freud's belief that older persons are not suitable for psychoanalytic psychotherapy. He suggests that when a person has turned to the past or delayed specific ways of adjustment, it is best not to tamper with these defenses. Older persons, according to Hollander, are rigid in general and interested in maintaining an established self-concept. Chaisson-Stewart (1985) believes the elderly have decreased capacity for mental abstraction, rigidity of defenses, style or personality characteristics, and reduced opportunity to make the choices in life that are necessary if psychotherapy is to motivate change in the individual's behavior.

■ APPROACH TO THE PATIENT

The initial goal of psychotherapy, regardless of age, is to develop a therapeutic alliance. In a study of the relationship between the process and outcome in psychotherapy, Gurman and Razin (1977) found the climate of the therapeutic relationship (i.e., the therapeutic alliance) to be the most robust predictor of outcome. Marmar et al (1989), however, found no agreement between therapist's and patient's judgment of alliance. Only patient commitment to therapy was found to be associated with outcome among alliance factors.

Marzilia et al (1981) suggest a series of factors essential in developing a therapeutic alliance (see box on p. 271). Therapeutic understanding and involvement have received

---

Factors Essential for Developing a Therapeutic Alliance

The capacity of the patient to work in therapy (e.g., focusing on self-disclosure and willingness to explore one's own contributions to the problems leading to therapy).

Patient commitment (the extent to which the patient values coming to treatment and optimizes time in therapy).

Goal consensus (the degree to which the patient and therapist are in agreement regarding goals of therapy).

A working strategy consensus (the extent to which the patient and therapist are in agreement regarding strategies in therapy).

Therapist understanding and involvement (empathy, respectfulness, nonjudgmental acceptance, and involvement in the treatment process).

Adapted from Marzilia E, et al: *American Journal of Psychiatry,* 138:361-364, 1981.

the most attention by therapists treating older persons as being somewhat different in late life psychotherapy compared with early stages of the life cycle. Gotesman (1980) suggests that, to develop empathy with the older adult, the young therapist must learn what it is to be old. The younger therapist must be able to empathize with physical disabilities, the loss of social opportunities, and the changing role faced by older adults.

A number of authors have commented on the relationship between the age of the therapist and the age of the patient. Garetz (1975) found that older psychiatrists tend to see a higher proportion of older patients and find them more interesting and gratifying than younger psychiatrists. Karasu et al (1979) explored the effects of therapist and patient age as factors in the evaluation and treatment of adult psychiatric outpatients. Therapists view older patients as sicker and less treatable than young patients (i.e., patients of the same age group as the therapist). Both older and younger patients were significantly less likely to remain in treatment with a therapist than patients near the age of the therapist. Therefore the age of the therapist in relation to the patient may be more important than the actual age of the patient. Gallagher et al (1965) found 66% of psychiatric patients at a public hospital between the ages of 15 and 29 in active psychotherapy compared with only 15% of those between the ages of 40 and 65. Psychiatrists at this hospital tended to be young.

Other investigators have suggested approaches to older patients that improve the therapeutic alliance and increase the likelihood of successful therapy. Bienenfeld (1990) suggests that the younger therapist, to work effectively with the older adult, must have both confidence in his or her skills and be relaxed in the therapeutic encounter. Busse and Pfeiffer (1973) found that the elderly respond better to therapy when specific goals are stated and the therapist plays a more active role in therapy than with the young. One way to be more active is to advocate for the patient (perhaps with another physician). Another way is to take a more educated or informative approach (i.e., be willing to provide information to the older patient). Orne and Wendon (1968) suggest that, especially for older adults, there needs to be a socialization to psychotherapy. The older patient should be introduced to what is going to happen in psychotherapy. For example, one of the stated goals may be that through therapy the older adult is to learn new ways of coping with problems.

Weinberg (1975) suggests that the therapist should allow elderly patients enough time for self-expression, to allay their anxiety and insecurity, and to permit patients to gratify their dependency needs through therapy. In addition, the therapist should play an active role in assisting patients to find activities that will make them more physically and socially attractive, as well as to help them plan their daily activities. Burnside (1978) suggests that the therapist should touch and stroke the geriatric patient. Sexual inhibition to touch is less frequent in late life. The therapist, however, must beware lest he or she give the message that the older patient is "sexless" through inappropriate familiarity.

In summary the therapist working with the older adult can be more relaxed and sociable and take more the role of a teacher than is generally accepted for the treatment of younger adults. Yet the therapist must maintain those behaviors essential to alliance-building, regardless of age. For example, confidentiality of the older patient must always be respected (even if the older person is cognitively impaired and the initiative for treatment comes from the family). The therapist must be consistent in his or her approach and available to the older person between therapy sessions. Most older persons do not abuse the telephone, and the willingness of the therapist to be available by telephone can be of great reassurance to the depressed older adult. The therapist can also share more of his or her own life with the older person, even information regarding family and common interests (e.g., sports or religion). The tension and uneasiness that many elders experience when they first encounter a therapist can be overcome by friendly confidence exhibited by the therapist. Humor may also be beneficial to easing tension.

If therapy is to be successful with the older adult, the therapist must be certain that the older person understands the therapist and is understood by the therapist. Perceptual problems, such as problems in hearing and vision, as well as problems with dysarthria or anomia, may interfere with the therapeutic process. Ensuring adequate lighting within the office of the therapist and positioning oneself near enough to the patient for easy communication (and possibly touch) are essential for communication with the visually and hearing impaired elderly.

■ THE PROCESS OF PSYCHOTHERAPY IN THE ELDERLY

Regardless of the type of psychotherapy used to treat the depressed older adult, the therapist must be aware of certain factors that emerge in the process of therapy. Transference (i.e., feelings or thoughts about the therapist arising from previous experience) may be associated with the elderly patient's relationship with siblings, parents, or even children (Wheeler and Bienenfeld, 1990). The younger therapist must be especially aware of the possibility that the older adult may transfer feelings toward his or her child to the therapist (Gotjahn, 1955). The transference may be protective and paternal (the elder may express much concern about the therapist's health and well-being, as well as display curiousness regarding the therapist's personal and family life). At other times, transference may be negative, with a sense that the therapist does not care for the older adult because the children have not shown care.

Countertransference (i.e., feelings of the therapist toward the patient that arise from experiences before and beyond therapy) also may play a significant role in the treatment of the depressed elder. Wayne (1952) suggests that problems may emerge when younger therapists treat older adults from the effects of unresolved conflicts with the therapist's own parents. On other occasions, the therapist, having developed exaggerated dependency on his or her parents, may transfer those feelings to the patient (Reichtschaffen, 1959). The therapist's own views about aging may impact the therapeutic process as well. For example, if the therapist has developed negative views about intelligence and aging, then he or she may be more sympathetic than empathetic toward the elderly person and more pessimistic than optimistic about change (Weinberg, 1975). For therapy to be successful, therapists should have a genuine liking for older adults and a realistic understanding of the aging process.

Transference and countertransference are inevitable in the therapeutic process. In more dynamic forms of therapy, therapists are called on to interpret the transference. Meerloo (1955) deemphasizes, however, the need to interpret or solve the transference in treating older adults. There is no problem in the therapist serving as a substitute social contact or even family member for the older patient.

Regardless of specific feelings toward the therapist, many older persons are resistant to therapy itself (Wheeler and Bienenfeld, 1990). This opposition to treatment may be conscious or unconscious. Resistance should be interpreted or at least verbalized by the therapist. At times, family involvement may decrease the resistance. At other times, the older person may interpret the therapist as allying with the family, and therefore resistance will increase. Steuer (1982) emphasizes that many elders believe only the "crazy" should see a psychiatrist. They belong to a "do-it-yourself" birth cohort in that they have been taught, since childhood, that one should solve one's own problems and should not reveal weakness to others. If an elder cannot maintain self-reliance, then the elder believes that he or she suffers some type of moral weakness, as opposed to a mental illness.

Resistance may derive from rigidity. Lawton (1952) classifies the rigidity of older persons into the following four types: (1) diminished capacity for new learning (based on irreversible biologic changes); (2) rut formation, which develops through the continued practice of old habits; (3) protective rigidity against change as a defense against fear; and (4) compulsive rigidity of the perfectionistic elder. Steuer (1982) suggests that behavior is conditioned more slowly in older persons and extinguished more quickly when compared with young adults. Yet this perceived increased rigidity in elders may not derive from the aging process itself but rather the cognitive functioning and socioeconomic environment of older adults. Yeseavage and Karasu (1982) found that older persons actually have a diminished resistance to change and increased motivation for therapy based on perception of a shorter life span and the perspectives gained from a lifetime of experiences.

Rigidity may not be so much a part of the aging process as it is a life-long personality style (or at least a reflection of overall personality composition). In an analysis of the Stanford Psychotherapy Outcome Studies, Thompson et al (1988) found the presence of a preexisting personality disorder predicted a lack of response to psychiatric treatment. Rigidity and other personality characteristics that obstruct the process of psychotherapy must not be assumed, however, to be primarily due to aging rather than age-associated factors. For example, Gotesman (1980) suggests that the primary factor predicting success in psychotherapy is the motivation for therapy. Within the restrictive environment experience by some elders, motivation may not be as great and therefore rigidity perceived by the therapist may in fact be the elder's reaction to realistic circumstances.

Older persons in therapy often exhibit a desire to reminisce (Wheeler and Bienenfeld, 1990). According to Erikson (1950), integration of one's life is the essential psychologic task to be accomplished in late life. Therefore reminiscence should be encouraged in therapy (Butler, 1963). The "life review," characterized by the progressive return to consciousness of past experiences including unresolved conflicts, permits the older adult to review, rework, and reintegrate past experiences. Reminiscence may also be an escape from a boring, bleak, or pessimistic view of the present and future. Life review often takes the form of storytelling, but if the elder repeats himself or herself too often, it can be maladaptive to the therapeutic process.

Zarit (1980) suggests that the central goal of therapy in the elderly and the process by which the goal is achieved is restitution. The therapist must encourage the older adult to take a more active control of his or her life. The experience of uncontrollable events leads to passivity and withdrawal, which are cardinal symptoms of depression (Seligman, 1975). The process of restitution may come through finding meaning to one's life or exploring religious and ethical values. On other occasions, teaching new behavioral skills or encouraging increased social relations facilitates the process of restitution in therapy.

Gotesman (1980) summarized the following characteristics of psychotherapy for the elderly that facilitate improvement: (1) development of insight through interpretation; (2) symptom-relief through catharsis; (3) relief to strained relations through the availability of another contact; (4) delayed deterioration through the development of adaptive skills; (5) adaptation to the present situation through a more rational appraisal of that situation; (6) development of self-care and social skills that enable the older adult to be more active in engaging his or her environment; (7) increased activity through overcoming resistance to new experiences; and (8) increased independence as evidenced by fewer demands on one's environment. These characteristics of therapy apply regardless of the type of psychotherapy for the depressed elder.

■ TYPES OF PSYCHOTHERAPY FOR THE DEPRESSED ELDERLY

Dynamic Psychotherapy

Many authors have commented on adapting psychodynamic theory and therapy to depression in late life. Mosely and Lazarus (1990) suggest that, in the first session, the therapist actively works through the patient's negative sterotypes of therapy, taking an active, warm, and energizing role. Issues that the therapist should address include the following: (1) adapting to and maintaining dignity and self-esteem in the face of losses and stresses associated with aging; (2) resolving prior intrapsychic conflicts and interpersonal conflicts reawakened by the losses and stresses of aging; and (3) reviewing one's life and its meaning. In the process of addressing these issues the depressed elder may despair, become hopeless, and degrade himself or herself. An idealized transference may develop in which the therapist is perceived as omnipotent and benevolent in contrast to the depleted elder (Lazarus, 1980). Techniques for working through the transference and reestablishing the self-esteem of the depressed elder include communicating empathically how the patient experienced losses and their meaning, working through the grief for losses, encouraging the patient to rediscover old and discover new relationships, and clarifying the origins of the transference.

Cath (1966) conceptualizes the dynamics of depression in the elderly as deriving from an early narcissistic wound in the absence of love. Depression is precipitated by losses experienced by the elderly and eventually leads to an ego state beyond depression, (i.e., depletion) (see Chapter 5 on psychologic causes of depression in the elderly). Such an older person lives in an empty world and feels a shrinkage of sense of self. Therapy, therefore, is directed to increasing activity and socialization of the patient and to involvement of the patient in meaningful human contacts. The therapist consciously establishes himself or herself as the desirable object to facilitate socialization.

Verwoerdt (1976) suggests a cause of depression in the elderly as attack and restraint (i.e., external forces that produce pain, which restricts activity to satisfy drives). Another cause postulated by Verwoerdt is threat, which comes from anticipating losses in the future. Loss equivalents are a form of envy in which another person's gain is thought of as a loss for the older patient. Older persons may overvalue meaningful objects and therefore loss of the object becomes catastrophic. The patient expands this thinking such that he or she believes everything is bad everywhere. Hostility also plays a role in depression and leads to a turning of anger against self and protest at the loss of the overvalued object. The task of therapy, according to Verwoerdt, is to enable the patient to recognize these negative patterns of thinking (patterns that are similar to those of Beck's cognitive psychotherapy, according to Steuer [1982]).

Steuer (1982) suggests extending the process of reminiscence (Butler, 1963). Reminiscence or life review is encouraged by awareness of approaching death. The life review can take two forms: mild and accompanied by nostalgic and vague regrets or severe and associated with anxiety, guilt, and depression (a depression that can lead to suicide attempts if the person reviewing his or her life is not supported by an understanding therapist). If the older person can be encouraged to pursue a life review with a supportive therapist, then maintenance and strengthening of self-concept can be attained (Boylin et al, 1976).

Grunes (1987) recommends brief dynamic psychotherapy for older adults and suggests using the approach by Ferenczi (1952). First, the therapist confronts both passivity and regression in the patient. The problem of termination is obviated by having a specific number of predetermined sessions agreed on in advance, with a set termination date. Emphasis is placed on affective expression rather than the intellectual (or more cognitive) evaluation of symptoms. Early, rapid diagnosis and elucidation of the basic conflict becomes the focus of therapy. Goldfarb (1974) believed that brief dynamic therapy, as described previously, could be of value in older adults. He deemphasized the need to interpret the transference. Since older persons suffer from ego weaknesses, they can be supported by an alliance with a powerful person (i.e., the elder feels strong through the therapist). The older person will work to appear worthwhile to the therapist and therefore will improve symptomatically.

Myers (1984) describes a number of cases of dynamic psychotherapy with older adults where depression was the primary symptom, one of the few monographs on dynamic therapy in the elderly. In a later publication, Myers (1989) discusses the specific contribution of loss of the physically athletic part of the self in late life depression. Myers' work is unique in the application of traditional dynamic psychotherapy to older adults.

Most of his work, however, is with persons in their fifties and sixties who are in good physical health and who financially can participate in traditional dynamic psychotherapy. Given physical and financial constraints, traditional dynamic therapy is probably not especially applicable to the treatment of late life depression. Nevertheless, principles from investigators such as Lazarus, Cath, Verwoerdt, and Myers are valuable in the psychodynamic formulation of late life depression and the application of modified dynamic therapy.

Supportive Therapy

Wayne (1952, 1953) suggests a number of techniques for supportive therapy. Supportive therapy derives from dynamic therapy in that the conceptualization of the disorder is based on dynamic principles. The therapist, however, takes a different role than in traditional dynamic therapy. First, the therapist has a much more active role in directing therapy. He or she does not hesitate to intervene in the patient's life, to give guidance and reassurance, and to actively minimize dependency by focusing on current problems and their solutions. The therapist also encourages the patient to take an active role in solving his or her own problems. Education regarding the origin of problems and ways in which they may be approached are central. Supportive therapy should be flexible in terms of scheduling and termination should not be a major barrier to the process of therapy. Rather, the older person should be allowed to gradually decrease the number of sessions in which he or she participates. A key to supportive therapy is focus on limited and circumstantial problems, especially a focus on the current problems. No attempt is made to rekindle old conflicts.

Alexander (1944) suggests that, when the ego is weak, it is unreasonable to encourage the older adult to release old unconscious conflicts. Guidance is used to assist patients through difficult times, reassurance counteracts feelings of inferiority, and a protective environment is provided to decrease the contribution of anxiety. A primary consideration in the treatment of older persons should be the evaluation of "ego strength." Alexander, like other dynamic psychotherapists, believes that older persons are not capable of usual dynamic treatment. In addition, he believes, as did Freud, that older persons were not capable of change and therefore less adaptive to insight therapy.

In actuality, most therapists working with older adults combine supportive approaches in therapy, such as those suggested by Wayne and Alexander, with whatever therapeutic modalities are instituted. Supportive therapy does not usually interfere with other forms of therapy and supportive techniques, as described previously, are most valuable in establishing the therapeutic alliance.

Brief Psychotherapy

Brief psychotherapy is not to be confused with supportive therapy. Approaches to brief therapy include both dynamic and cognitive/behavioral confrontation. Brief therapy has been accepted as a useful psychotherapy for older adults because of the lack of long-term time commitments and the flexibility and logistical ease of the therapy. Lazarus and Groves (1980) suggest that brief therapy can be of value in treating older persons because of the following reasons (1) it takes into account the finitude of the older person's life; (2) it conveys an expectation that the patient can master current stress and see that he or she was capable of doing so in the past with only short-term intervention; (3) it reduces the patient's fear of protracted dependency on the therapist; and (4) and it brings into focus the therapy's inevitable termination, thereby reducing the financial burden of therapy.

Reichtschaffen (1959), in a review of psychotherapy with older adults, applies the brief therapeutic approach developed by Martin (1944) to treating depressed older adults. The elements of the method include the following:

1. The patient is asked to relate his or her life history in detail from earliest memory to the present. Interpretation of dreams is not stressed but rather the elder is asked to report relevant thoughts or images that might come to his or her mind through the life review.
2. Brief 20-minute sessions are complemented by tests and other tools to obtain as much historical information as possible.
3. The patient is encouraged to take a "will do" perspective to the therapy (i.e., the patient is asked openly to abandon attempts to resist therapy).
4. The therapist, early in therapy, appraises the maladjustive reactions in the patient.
5. The patient is given a slogan or summary statement after each session, such as "Don't let your daughter aggravate you."
6. Exercises are prescribed between sessions. For example, the elder is asked to try to solve a specific problem between sessions rather than forgetting or ignoring therapy between sessions.
7. Subsequent interviews are devoted to filling out charts and regulating daily activities.

This brief therapeutic approach is similar to cognitive therapy for depression in the elderly (see next section). Reichtschaffen suggests the method may have "therapeutic effects of overcoming pessimistic inertia and of convincing the client that he had his maladjustment corrected."

Goldfarb (1955, 1956; Goldfarb and Turner, 1953; Goldfarb and Berinis, 1974) pioneered brief therapy for treating older adults. He suggests that therapy could be accomplished through five- to 15-minute sessions once a week, with gradual increase of time between sessions. He recommends brief therapy especially for treating the psychologic difficulties associated with acute and chronic physical illnesses that accompany aging. Goldfarb emphasizes the therapist as a parent figure and attempts to increase the patient's self-esteem by providing emotional gratification to the patient. He believes the patient should leave each session convinced of "having the therapist or at least of having some control over the therapist." For example, the therapist may apologize to the patient or admire the patient for some skill or thought. That is to say, patients gain a sense that they are able to effect the thoughts and behavior of the therapist. The therapist also emphasizes that he or she looks forward to the visits by the patient each week. Goldfarb believes brief therapy was especially useful in treating older adults with depressive symptoms in nursing homes.

Busse and Pfeiffer (1977) encourage therapists, during brief therapy, to take an active role in identifying and clarifying the patient's problem. Limited goals should be set in therapy, such as symptom relief, support for adaptation to changing life circumstances, acceptance or increased dependency as a normal aspect of the aging process, and renewed or continued involvement in meaningful activity. They also recommend "symbolic giving" (i.e., encouraging social conversation during a part of the session to enhance the patient's belief of being a part of a meaningful relationship in therapy).

Cognitive Therapy

Cognitive therapy derives directly from Beck's theory of the cognitive contribution to depression (Beck et al, 1979). (See Chapter 5.) Gallagher and Thompson (1983) have modified traditional cognitive therapy for treating depression in the elderly. Their approach to cognitive therapy in the elderly follows.

The aim of cognitive therapy for depression in the elderly is to reverse negative cognitive sets in the older adult by the following: (1) monitoring negative thoughts; (2) recognizing the connection between negative thoughts and feelings of depression; (3) examining the evidence for and against specific autonomic thoughts; (4) developing more reality-oriented or realistic interpretations of reality; and (5) identifying and altering dysfunctional beliefs (schemas) that predispose to developing negative cognitions. One tool for reversing negative cognitive sets is to use a daily record of dysfunctional thoughts. An example of such a record is exhibited in Table 17-1. Logging a daily record is a tedious process but gradually leads to improved feelings when the elder logically considers the origin of these dysfunctional thoughts.

Another approach to confronting negative cognitive sets is to identify the underlying dysfunctional beliefs or schemas. Cognitive therapists believe the identification of such schemas requires several therapy sessions. For example, the older person may, during the initial therapy sessions, seek the attention and approval of the therapist. Seeking approval may be a means to establish his or her own self-worth in a depressed elder who has poor self-worth. The therapist, once the pattern is identified, can ask the patient how much it "costs" to seek attention and approval. Much valuable time in therapy may be consumed by working through such dysfunctional beliefs.

Gallagher and Thompson (1983) suggest some modifications of the usual cognitive therapy techniques for older adults. First, they suggest the need of socialization to treatment. Older persons, as described previously, may be inherently suspicious of any form

TABLE 17-1. Daily Record of Dysfunctional Thoughts

Date	Situation	Emotion	Automatic thoughts	Rational response
November 10	At home Sunday night waiting for son to call. It's 10 PM and he doesn't call.	Sad, miserable, abandoned, and lonely.	Why didn't he call? Why is he rejecting me? I feel so lonely, I don't know what to do. Why are *my* children the ones who don't care about their mother when other children care about their parents?	My son may have had some business problems that precluded him from calling. He may, as he does many times, call tomorrow night.

of psychotherapy. Therefore the therapist initially confronts the patient's attitudes and expectations regarding therapy. For example, the therapist asks, "Do you think this treatment is for you?" Parallel to listening to the expectations of the patient, the therapist explains the process of cognitive therapy and what the patient can and cannot expect the therapy to accomplish. For example, cognitive therapy will not change underlying personality function. Therapists should emphasize that cognitive therapy is a learning process that can change automatic thoughts and behaviors. Patients and therapists do not just "discuss" problems and feelings. Rather, they identify negative thoughts and develop means for modifying these thoughts.

The therapist working with the older adult must also enhance the learning capabilities of the elder. Material should be presented through multimodal processes. The use of the chart of dysfunctional attitudes (Table 17-2) is a means to visually represent cognitive material. The use of visual material in group cognitive therapy (see later section) is another means to enhance learning. Age-specific examples should be used, such as issues surrounding retirement, role changes experienced by persons, declining physical health, and perceived abandonment by children and friends. Therapists must be patient, since older adults may not progress in therapy as quickly as younger persons. Cognitive therapy encourages changes in behavior, yet older persons may have difficulty making changes for they are inherently more cautious. Recognition and support of the difficulty elders may experience in taking risks facilitates the therapy.

The therapist should recognize the specific cognitive distortions that older persons bring to therapy. Some elders believe they are too old to change. Others believe their problems reside totally in the environment ("If only Mary would change, I wouldn't be depressed"). Elders may also degrade the inexperience of a younger therapist ("You're too young to help me"). Each of these beliefs should be confronted as a negative thought contributing to the depressive process.

Finally, Gallagher and Thompson emphasize a graduated process of termination. There is rarely a need to terminate therapy abruptly. Patients can benefit from periodic sessions, so-called booster sessions, of cognitive therapy. Termination too quickly may reinforce the cognitive distortion that, once again, the elder is being abandoned.

Cognitive therapy has been demonstrated to be effective in treating depression in older adults, especially depression not associated with melancholic symptoms. In a volunteer study, Jarvik et al (1982) compared antidepressant medications, cognitive therapy, psychodynamic therapy, and placebo. After 26 weeks, the Hamilton Depression Scale scores improved most for medications, intermediate for both psychotherapy groups, and the least for placebo. Most persons randomized to the psychotherapy groups were improved but not fully remitted of symptoms at the 26-week follow-up. Cognitive therapy, in this study, did not lead to more improvement than psychodynamic therapy. Butler et al (1987), in a study of group cognitive therapy, placebo, alprazolam, and supportive therapy over 20 weeks, found that depressive symptoms had improved in the cognitive therapy group only. The cognitive therapy group also experienced fewer dropouts than the medication group. Thompson et al (1987), in a study of 91 depressed elders assigned to one of three psychotherapy groups (behavior therapy, cognitive therapy, and psychodynamic therapy) and followed for 16 to 20 sessions, found all treatment groups demonstrated significant reduction in self-report and observer-rated measures of depression. About 52% achieved a remission of the depression. At the 2-year follow-up (Gallagher-Thompson et al, 1990), 77% of those not depressed at the follow-up after treatment continued free of depression. In a later study, Thompson et al (1987) found that the combination of cognitive/behavioral therapy and desipramine in depressed elderly outpatients was superior to desipramine alone.

Interpersonal Therapy

Interpersonal therapy (Klerman et al, 1984; Haynes, in press) views depression as occurring within, but not necessarily caused by, an interpersonal context that may be accessible to treatment. Older persons who become depressed at first receive support and attention from their social network. As time progresses, however, they become more withdrawn, irritable, and self-deprecating. Social network members withdraw or become critical of the depressed elder. Therapy is designed to interrupt this negative interaction between the depressed elder and the social support network by restoring realistic expectations regarding the network and facilitating effective communication. Interpersonal therapy is similar to cognitive therapy in its goals and includes interpersonal skill training, clarifying and modifying expectations, and role-play.

Sholomskas et al (1983) report a series of cases of older persons treated with interpersonal therapy, supporting the usefulness of the interpersonal therapy for treating depressed older adults. They suggest therapeutic strategies that focus on the following four problem areas:

- Grief—Grief often accompanies role transition, such as the transition to widowhood or unemployment. Goals of therapy are to facilitate the mourning process and help the patient reestablish interests in relationships that can substitute for the loss.
- Interpersonal role disputes—The patient and at least one other significant person, in this situation, have nonreciprocal expectations about their relationship. For example, an elderly woman takes an apartment near her daughter and becomes angry with the daughter because the daughter does not meet her expectations regarding assistance. She expects her daughter to shop with her, provide transportation, and visit her often. The goals of therapy are to help the patient identify the dispute, assist the patient in making choices about a plan of action, and encourage the patient to modify maladaptive communicative patterns. One aspect of interpersonal therapy is to assist the elder in recognizing varied personalities and life-styles among social network members.
- Role transition—For example, the older adult retires from a social role, such as playing golf, because of a change in physical status. One therapeutic goal is to consciously link the role transition with the depression for the patient. Another goal is to enable the patient to regard the new role in a more positive, less restrictive manner. In other words the older adult may substitute one role for another and even grow into the new role by developing a sense of mastery vis-à-vis demands of the new role.
- Interpersonal deficits—Older adults often develop inadequate or unsustaining interpersonal relationships. The following three types may emerge: social isolation (long-standing deficiencies in social relationships); deficits in the quality of the social relation (the social contacts are adequate, but the older adult cannot enjoy them); and deficits in social skills (a preexisting personality pattern disrupts the social re-

lationship). The goal of treatment, in this case, is to decrease the patient's social isolation. The focus must be on past relationships (because of a lack of current relationships), and the relationship with the therapist provides an opportunity to practice developing relationships.

Bibliotherapy

Scoggin et al (1987) describe a form of therapy similar to cognitive and interpersonal therapy (i.e., self-help through bibliotherapy). Bibliotherapy is actually a variant in the process of therapy as opposed to the goals of therapy. Self-help via bibliotherapy has a number of advantages. For example, bibliotherapy does not require as much travel, is cost-effective and individualized, improves self-reliance, and takes advantage of the fact that older adults tend to perform cognitive tasks optimally under self-paced conditions. In a study of 29 persons 60 years of age and older with a minimum of a high school education, these investigators found that, by instructing the depressed elder to read a book, such as Victor Frankl's *Man's Search for Meaning* or David Burns' *Feeling Good*, dysfunctional thinking was significantly reduced. The treatment is of little benefit for elders who are severely depressed, who do not enjoy reading, or who read poorly.

Behavior Therapy

Haynes (in press) suggests that behavior therapy views depression as a state in which there is a relative shift toward the negative in the balance of negative and positive reinforcers or less predictability in the ability to obtain positive reinforcements. For example, the older person who changes residence experiences many negative reinforcements when leaving home, such as fear of the new neighborhood, fewer social contacts, and few positive reinforcements. The goal of behavior therapy is the restitution of positive reinforcers (both their availability and predictability). For example, scheduling pleasant events and training in certain skills to obtain mastery over the new environment, especially in social interactions, are components of behavior therapy. Behavior therapy is therefore similar to cognitive and interpersonal therapy.

Cautela and Mansfield (1977) reviewed the advantages of behavior therapy for the older adult. Behavior is the target for change as opposed to emphasizing a "review" of the past or current feelings and therefore is accepted more readily by older adults. Behavioral techniques often are of short duration as well. The therapist is active, providing direction, structure, and explicit goals. The elder is assumed to be the agent of change and has control over his or her environment, thus counteracting perceptions of hopelessness and helplessness. The therapist demonstrates, whenever possible, the relationship between mood and activity, as well as helping the patient monitor activities and concomitant mood changes. Activity scheduling is then initiated to counteract periods during the day when moods tend to decline or to avoid experiences that precipitate a depressed mood. The patient is instructed to distribute enjoyable and interesting activities throughout the week. Behavior therapists also assist patients to become more self-sufficient and ultimately to take control of their own scheduling. Behavioral techniques have been shown to be effective in treating stress, anxiety, and depression in late life (Fry, 1986).

Group Therapy

Group therapy for depressed elders enhances socialization, encourages attitudinal changes, and assists the older adult in personal development. Interaction with older adults or with younger persons in groups tends to counteract myths and societal stereotypes of aging. Behavioral modification and reality orientation are strengths of groups (Moberg and Lazarus, 1990).

From the factors identified by Yalom (1970) as linked to therapeutic change in group therapy, the following five were selected by Moberg and Lazarus as applicable to the elderly: (1) imparting information, such as helpful advice; (2) resocialization and remotivation, such as counteracting loneliness through group participation; (3) enhancement of self-esteem through recognizing that the problems experienced by the depressed elder are not unique; (4) emotional catharsis that permits isolated older persons to express their feelings of frustration and sense of failure; and (5) expression of existential concerns, such as anxiety about death and a wish to find a meaning in existence. Steuer (1982) suggests additional curative factors, such as encouraging appropriate goal-setting behavior and altruism.

There has been a debate in the literature about whether age should be mixed in therapeutic groups (Steuer, 1982). Butler (1975) and Yalom (1975) recommend age integration but cautioned against too wide an age gap. Gotjahn (1978) recommends age homogeneity, so that the patient could focus on issues specific to the elderly. Steuer (1982) suggests more attention be directed to differences between the young-old and the old-old as opposed to simply dichotomizing the old and the young. In other words the problems faced by the older person are more important than age in determining the makeup of a therapeutic group.

Linden (1953) suggests that it is important to provide immediate social satisfaction in therapeutic groups (i.e., an "opportunistic" orientation). Therefore every activity need not always be a serious effort. The therapist should seek opportunities for lighthearted fun and stimulating experiences, such as didactic talks, praising or joining with individual members, and questioning them about past experiences.

A number of investigators (Mintz et al, 1981; Salvendy, 1989) have found group therapy to be effective in the treatment of older adults. Salvendy (1989) describes the use of brief group psychotherapy as a method to treat the psychologic effects of retirement. Factors associated with maladjustment in retirement amenable to group therapy include the following: no interest in outside work; isolation (especially among the single, separated, and divorced); painful physical illnesses; financial worries; and forced or induced early retirement. The goal of group therapy is to encourage group members to reflect on and come to grips with one's life in the work force without bitterness or disappointment. Groups also encourage retirees to adapt to changing roles. The leader of the group, according to Salvendy, must instill a sense of hope.

REFERENCES

Abraham K: The applicability of psychoanalytic treatment to patients of an advanced age. In Abraham K: *Selected Papers of Psychoanalysis.* London, Hogarth Press, 1949, pp. 312-317.

Alexander FG: The indications for psychoanalytic therapy, *Bulletin to the New York Academy of Medicine* 20:319-334, 1944.

Beck AT, Rush AJ, Shaw BF, Emery G: *Cognitive Therapy of Depression.* New York, Guilford Press, 1979.

Bienenfeld D (ed): *Verwoerdt's Clinical Journal of Psychiatry,* ed 3. Baltimore, Williams and Wikins, 1990.

Boylin W, Gorden SK, Nehrke MF: Reminiscing and ego integrity in institutionalized elderly males, *The Gerontologist* 16:118-124, 1976.

Burns DD: *Feeling Good: The New Mood Therapy.* New York, The New American Library, 1980.

Burnside IM: Group work with the mentally impaired elderly. In Burnside IM (ed): *Working with the Elderly: Group Process and Techniques.* North Scituate, Massachusetts, Duxberry Press, 1978.

Busse EW, Pfeiffer E: *Behavior and Adaptation in Late Life* (ed 2). Boston, Little, Brown and Company, 1977.

Busse EW, Pfeiffer E: *Mental Illness in Later Life.* Washington, DC, The American Psychiatric Association, 1973.

Butler LE, Scoggin F, Kirkish P, Schretlen D, Corbishley A, et al: Group cognitive therapy and alprazolam in the treatment of depressed older adults, *Journal of Consulting and Clinical Psychology* 55:550-556, 1987.

Butler RN: The life review: an interpretation of reminiscence in the aged, *Psychiatry* 26:65, 1963.

Butler RN: Psychotherapy in older age. In Aereti S (ed): *American Handbook of Psychiatry,* ed 2, (vol 5). New York, Basic Books, 1975, pp. 807-828.

Cath S: Beyond depression: the depleted state. A study in ecopsychology in the aged, *Canadian Psychiatric Association Journal* 11 (special supplement):S329-S339, 1966.

Cautuela JP, Mansfield L: A behavioral approach to geriatrics. In Gentry WP (ed): *Geropsychology.* Cambridge, Massachusetts, Ballinger, 1977, pp. 21-42.

Chaisson-Stewart GM: Psychotherapy. In Chaisson-Stewart GM (ed): *Depression in the Elderly: An Interdisciplinary Approach.* New York, John Wiley and Sons, 1985, pp. 263-287.

Erikson EH: *Childhood and Society.* New York, Norton, 1950.

Erikson E: Identity and the life cycle, *Psychological Issues* 1:1-171, 1959.

Ferenczi S: The future development of an active therapy in psychoanalysis. In Rickman J (ed): *Further Contributions to the Theory and Technique of Psychoanalysis* (vol 2). New York, Basic Books, 1952, pp. 198-216.

Finischel O: *The Psychoanalytic Theory of Neurosis.* New York, WW Norton, 1945.

Frankl VE: *Man's Search for Meaning.* New York, Pocket Books, 1939.

Freud S: On Psychotherapy. In Freud S: *Collected Papers (vol I).* London, Hogarth Press, 1924, 249-263.

Fry TS: *Depression, Stress, and Adaptation in the Elderly: Psychological Assessment and Intervention.* Rockville, Maryland, Aspen, 1986.

Gallagher DE, Thompson LW: Effectiveness of psychotherapy for both endogenous and non-endogenous depression in older adults, *Journal of Gerontology* 18:707-712, 1983.

Gallagher EB, Sharraf MR, Levinson DJ: The influence of patient and therapist in determining the use of psychotherapy in a hospital setting, *Psychiatry* 28:297-310, 1965.

Gallagher-Thompson D, Henley-Peterson P, Thompson LW:Maintenance of gains *versus* relapse following brief psychotherapy for depression, *Journal of Consulting and Clinical Psychology* 58:371-374, 1990.

Garetz FK: The psychiatrists involvement with aged patients, *American Journal of Psychiatry* 132:63-65, 1975.

Goldfarb AI: Masked depression in the elderly. In Lesse S (ed): *Masked Depression.* New York, Jason Aronson, 1974, pp. 236-250.

Goldfarb AI: Psychotherapy with aged persons: patterns of adjustment in a home for the aged, *Mental Hygiene* 39:608-621, 1955.

Goldfarb AI: The rationale for psychotherapy with older persons, *The American Journal of Medical Science* 232:181-185, 1956.

Goldfarb AI, Berinis JS: Brief psychotherapy in the treatment of emotional disorders in physically-ill geriatric patients, *The Gerontologist* 14:143-153, 1974.

Goldfarb AI, Turner H: Psychotherapy of aged persons. II: Utilization and effectiveness of "brief" therapy, *American Journal of Psychiatry* 109:916-921, 1953.

Gotesman KG: Behavioral and dynamic psychotherapy with the elderly. In Birin J, Sloane RB (eds): *Handbook of Mental Health and Aging.* New York, Academic Press, 1980, pp. 775-805.

Gotjahn M: Analytic psychotherapy with the elderly, *Psychoanalysis Review* 42:419-427, 1955.

Gotjahn M: Group communication and group therapy with the aged: A promising project. In Jarvik L F (ed): *Aging in the Twenty-First Century.* New York, Gardner Press, 1978, pp. 113-122.

Grunes JM: The aged in psychotherapy: psychodynamic contributions to the treatment process. In Sadavoy J, Leszcz M (eds): *Treating the Elderly With Psychotherapy: The Scope for Change in Late Life.* Madison, CT, International Universities Press, 1987.

Gurman AS, Razin AM (eds): *Effective Psychotherapy: A Handbook of Research.* New York, Pergamon, 1977.

Haynes C: Psychotherapy of depression and dysthymia. In Copeland JR, Abou-Saleh M, Blazer DG (eds): *Psychiatry of Old Age: An International Textbook*. London, John Wiley and Sons, (in press).

Hollander MH: Individualizing the aged, *Social Case Work* 33:337-342, 1952.

Jarvik LF, Mintz J, Steuer J, Gurner R: Treating geriatric depression: A twenty-six-week interim analysis, *Journal of the American Geriatrics Society* 30:713-717, 1982.

Jellife SE: The old age factor in psychoanalytic therapy, *The Medical Journal of Records* 121:7-12, 1925.

Jung K: *Memories, Dreams, Reflections*. New York, Pantheon, 1963.

Karasu TB, Stein SP, Charles ES: Age factors in patient-therapist relationship, *Journal of Nervous and Mental Diseases* 167:100-104, 1979.

Klerman GL, Weissman MM, Rounsaville BJ, Chevron ES: *Interpersonal Psychotherapy of Depression* New York, Basic Books, 1984.

Lawton G: Psychotherapy with older persons, *Psychoanalysis* 1:27-41, 1952.

Lazarus LW: Self-psychology in psychotherapy with the elderly: theory and practice, *Journal of Geriatric Psychiatry* 13:69-82, 1980.

Lazarus LW, Groves L: Brief psychotherapy with the elderly: a study of process and outcome. In Sadavoy J, Leszcz M (eds): *Treating the Elderly With Psychotherapy: The Scope for Change in Late Life*. Madison, CT, International Universities Press, 1987.

Levinson DJ: *The Seasons of a Man's Life*. New York, Alfred A. Knopf, 1978, pp. 4-5, 33.

Linden ME: Group psychotherapy with institutionalized senile women: Study in gerontologic human relations, *International Journal of Group Psychotherapy* 3:150-170, 1953.

Marmar CR, Gaston L, Gallagher D, Thompson L: Alliance and outcome in late-life depression, *Journal of Nervous and Mental Diseases* 77:464-471, 1989.

Martin LJ: *A Handbook for Old Age Counselors*. San Francisco, Geurtz, 1944.

Marzilia E, Marmar CR, Krupnik J: Therapeutic alliance scales: Development and relationship to psychotherapy outcome, *American Journal of Psychiatry* 138:361-364, 1981.

Meerloo JAM: Contribution to psychoanalysis to the problem of the aged. In Heiman M (ed): *Psychoanalysis and Social Work*. New York, International Universities Press, 1973. pp. 321-337.

Meerloo JAM: Psychotherapy with elderly people, *Geriatrics* 10:583-587, 1955.

Mintz J, Steuer J, Jarvik L: Psychotherapy with depressed elderly patients: Research considerations, *Journal of Consulting and Clinical Psychology* 49:542-548, 1981.

Moberg PJ, Lazarus LW: Psychotherapy of depression in the elderly, *Psychiatric Annals* 20:92-96, 1990.

Myers WA: *Dynamic Therapy of the Older Patient*. New York, Aronson, 1984.

Myers WA: I can't play ball anymore, *Journal of Geriatric Psychiatry* 22:121-139, 1989.

Orne MT, Wendon PH: Anticipatory socialization for psychotherapy: method and rationale, *American Journal of Psychiatry* 124:1202-1212, 1968.

Reichtschaffen A: Psychotherapy with geriatric patients: a review of the literature, *Journal of Gerontology* 14:73-84, 1959.

Salvendy JT: Brief group psychotherapy and retirement, *Group* 13:43-57, 1989.

Scoggin F, Hamblin D, Butler L: Bibliotherapy for depressed older adults: A self-help alternative, *The Gerontologist* 27:383-387, 1987.

Seligman MEP: Depression and learned helplessness. In Friedman RJ, Katz MM (eds): *The Psychology of Depression: Contemporary Theory and Research*. Washington, DC, VH Winston, 1974.

Sholomskas AJ, Chevron ES, Prusoff BA, Berry C: Short-term interpersonal therapy (IPT) with the depressed elderly: case reports and discussions, *American Journal of Psychotherapy* 37:552-565, 1983.

Steuer J: Psychotherapy for depressed elders. In Blazer DG (ed): *Depression in Late Life*. St. Louis, Mosby, 1982.

Thompson LW, Gallagher D, Breckenridge JS: Comparative effectiveness for psychotherapies for depressed elders, *Journal of Consulting and Clinical Psychology* 55:385-390, 1987.

Thompson LW, Gallagher D, Czirr R: Personality disorder and outcome in the treatment of late-life depression, *Journal of Geriatric Psychiatry* 21:133-146, 1988.

Verwoerdt E: *Clinical Geropsychiatry*. Baltimore, Williams and Wilkins, 1976.

Wayne GJ: Modified psychoanalytic therapy in senescence, *Psychoanalytic Reviews* 40:99-116, 1953.

Wayne GJ: Psychotherapy in late life, *Annals of Investigations in Medicine and Surgery* 6:88-91, 1952.

Weinberg J: Geriatric psychiatry. In Freedman AM, Kaplan HI, Saddock BJ (eds): *Comprehensive Textbook of Psychiatry* (vol II). Baltimore, Williams and Wilkins, 1975.

Wheeler BG, Bienenfeld D: Principles of individual psychotherapy. In Bienenfeld D (ed): *Verwoerdt's Clinical Journal of Psychiatry*, (ed3). Baltimore, Williams and Wilkins, 1990, pp. 204-222.

Yalom ID: *The Theory and Practice of Group Psychotherapy*. New York, Basic Books, 1975.

Yesavage JA, Karasu TB: Psychotherapy with elderly patients. *American Journal of Psychotherapy* 36:41-55, 1982.

Zarit SH: *Aging and Mental Disorders: Psychological Approaches to Assessment and Treatment*. New York, Free Press, 1980.

18

Family Therapy with the Depressed Older Adult

When the clinician encounters a physical dysfunction in a patient, a diagnostic workup to determine the cause of that dysfunction is initiated. In a similar matter the clinician must undertake the evaluation of dysfunction in the families of the depressed older adult. Such an evaluation requires the acquisition of information along a number of separate parameters. Just as a white blood cell count alone is not pathognomonic of a staphylococcal pneumonia, the complaint by an elderly patient that his or her family "no longer cares" does not reveal the specific problem within the family.

The family may be viewed as a system analogous to an organ system, such as the cardiovascular system (Miller and Miller, 1979). Difficulty at a given time within the system, such as the onset of depressive symptoms in an older family member, affects other parts of the system. Although the clinician may have occasion to evaluate the family of the older adult for a variety of problems, a common family problem is distress placed on the family by a depressed older member. However, the guidelines for evaluation presented in this chapter are applicable for the evaluation of other problems. Three types of information are required to evaluate the family system for therapeutic intervention. First, the clinician must determine the nature of the system. Evaluation of the nature of the system requires knowledge of families, how they operate, specific knowledge of particular family members, and especially knowledge regarding the elderly patient. Second, the clinician must determine if a crisis actually exists within the family (i.e., whether the family has been disrupted). The clinician frequently encounters the family of an older depressed patient, which appears to be disrupted and dysfunctional,

This chapter is abstracted from Blazer DG and Siegler I: Evaluating the family of the elderly patient with depressive disorders. In Blazer DG, Siegler I (eds): *Working with the Family of the Older Adult*. Menlo Park, California: Addison Welsey, 1981 and revised from the chapter by the same title from the first edition of Blazer DG: *Depression in Late Life*. St Louis, Mosby, 1982, pp. 221-235.

only to learn that the family has interacted and functioned in this manner for years. The dysfunctional family may cause, in part, the depressive syndrome in the older adult. What appears to be a crisis in family functions may in fact be usual, although not optimal, family functioning. Third, if a depression creates family dysfunction or exaggerates existing function, the clinician must determine the nature of that crisis (i.e., the way in which the crisis has disrupted the family). Family therapists have learned that the presenting symptom, such as the complaint by a child that "Mom is depressed," does not always represent the actual problem, since the presenting complaint may well provide the excuse for the family seeking help to correct its dysfunction.

This chapter is devoted to the evaluation of the family system and intervention techniques. Information considered optimal in determining the nature of the family the presence or absences of a crisis within the family, and the nature of that crisis can be obtained by assessing certain areas of family structure and functioning. As with all psychiatric assessment, there is the potential for both underutilization and overutilization of diagnostic procedures. The values of the family may be quite complex. Therefore the goal for this chapter is to present the clinician a useful framework for family evaluation that will provide adequate but not detailed guidelines. Time constraints experienced by the busy clinician also limit the breadth and depth of family assessment.

■ EVALUATION OF THE FAMILY SYSTEM

The elements of a optimal evaluation procedure for assessing the family system in the primary care physician's office are outlined in the box on p. 288. The evaluation includes a consideration of individual family members and family structure, interactions, atmosphere, values, support and tolerance, and finally stressors and rewards. Each element is described in some detail, and the types of questions to include in the assessment of these elements are suggested. The following case illustrates evaluation of the family system.

■ CASE PRESENTATION

A 70-year-old recently retired business owner was taken to an outpatient clinic by his wife and two sons. The patient stated that he was depressed and had been so for about 15 months. Significant events that he associated with the depression included the death of his first wife and subsequent retirement from his business 4 years before being brought to the clinic. The family stated that the patient had been agitated, discouraged, and refused to become involved in any activities for over a year. His continued despondency, physical complaints, and pessimism had been especially burdensome to the second wife. The patient expressed concern about his behavior during his first wife's terminal illness but little remorse for her death. He noted, "I have so much to live for and to enjoy, but I cannot enjoy things." Changes in the patient's life had undoubtedly played a significant role in the onset of symptoms. These changes included the death of his first wife, his remarriage, and his decision to transfer controlling interest of the family business to his youngest son.

The patient was a strong-willed and independent man most of his life and had suffered a number of crises in his early life. He had never been treated psychiatrically before being brought to the outpatient clinic. Nevertheless, he reported difficulty with alcohol and although he had ceased drinking, he was currently taking a number of psychotropic medications, in

Elements of Family Evaluation for the Family of the Older Adult

Family Members and Family Structure

Definition of the Family
Individual characteristics of family
  members
Physical location of family members
Roles and role relationships

Family Interaction

Frequency of family interaction
Quality of family interaction
  Compatible versus conflictual
  Cohesive versus fragmented
  Productive versus nonproductive
  Fragile versus stable
  Rigid versus flexible

Family Atmosphere

Tense versus relaxed
Hopeful versus resigned

Family Values

Values concerning health and health
  care
Values concerning the elderly

Family Support and Tolerance

Availability
Tangible supportive services (i.e., ge-
  neric services)
Perception of intangible support
  Dependability
  Interaction
  Belongingness
  Intimacy
  Usefulness
Family tolerance of disturbing behav-
  iors

Family stressors and rewards

cluding flurazepam, meprobamate, and secobarbital, which were prescribed by his primary care physician. He experienced no improvement with the use of these medications.

No members of his immediate family had suffered from psychiatric illness, mood swings, or alcohol/drug abuse. The patient stated that he had an aunt who had been taken to a mental institution early in life but could not remember the reason for her hospitalization. He was financially secure and physically independent, and therefore required little tangible support from his family. However, he demanded much of his wife's attention. During the day, he would continually ask her questions about finances, his health, and medical appointments and would complain to her of his feelings of depression. Although he did not require actual supervision, the family members were concerned enough about his behavior that they felt uncomfortable leaving him alone for extended periods of time.

The patient felt that he was of little use to the family, given his current state of "depression" and was especially concerned that he no longer had a role in the family business. Although he maintained frequent interaction with both of his sons, this interaction was usually marked by conflicts and angry outbursts secondary to his demanding behavior. The reason for seeking psychiatric help at the time of the initial evaluation was not an acute change in his mood but reaching the limit of the family's tolerance for his continued physical and emotional complaints and demands. His active resistance to any suggestions made by the family concerning the use of his time was especially frustrating to family members.

The patient's oldest son, a prominent business man in another city, took control of family matters after his father's disability. Only at his suggestion had the patient agreed to seek medical attention, and at this son's insistence the family managed to get the patient to the outpatient clinic. The older son was rational yet disengaged throughout the evaluation and usually allied with the physician in determining the appropriate therapeutic intervention for his father. The patient's wife was the most stressed of the family members. She stated frequently that she did not know how much longer she could tolerate his continuous somatic complaints, his unwillingness to leave the house, and his unreasonable demands. She complied with almost every demand that the patient made and, in essence, was his sole caretaker during the depressive illness. Although the younger son would occasionally take the father on a short business trip, there was little rest for the wife from her caretaking responsibilities.

The younger son expressed much anger about his father. He viewed his father's suffering as deserved, given his authoritative and demanding behavior in the past. The father had made life for his mother "hell," according to the son. He expressed great frustration at his attempts to interact with his father, most of which ended up in a uproar. The younger son had taken sole responsibility for the family business after his father's retirement and had little desire to give his father increased responsibility or even a role in the business. Not only did the son cite technical changes in the business that rendered the father's advice less valuable, but he also noted that the father was disruptive when he visited the office.

■ FAMILY MEMBERS AND FAMILY STRUCTURE

What is a family? For the purposes of this discussion, the family consist of individuals who are genetically related, who have developed relationships, or who are living together as if they were related (Miller and Miller, 1979). In recent years the term *nuclear family*, as opposed to *extended family*, has become popular. The nuclear family consists of spouses plus children, usually living in the same household. The extended family consists of other kin such as grandchildren, siblings living outside the family, and cousins. Working with older adults generally entails working with the nuclear family plus the extended family, although the absolute number of individuals with whom the clinician comes in contact may be limited.

The first concerns of the clinician evaluating the family of an older depressed patient are the individual characteristics of family members that may aid in the diagnosis or therapy of the patient. If the patient has an acute, severe mood disorder or if the condition has been recurrent, there is a possibility that other family members may have similar problems. The older adult with a chronic depressive disorder that has lasted for years is less likely to have a positive family history of depression than the older adult with episodic depression. Inquiries should assess whether family members have experienced the following: severe mood swings, suicide attempts or actual suicides, episodic alcohol abuse, periods of social withdrawal, the use of nerve medicines (especially antidepressants), previous psychiatric hospitalizations, treatment with electroconvulsive therapy, or periods of elation or excited behavior. Elderly depressed patients who have recurrent episodes may have children or grandchildren who suffer from bipolar illness. These elders may respond well to prophylaxis with lithium carbonate. History of a family member who responded to a particular antidepressant agent should assist the physician in choosing the appropriate agent for the elderly depressed patient.

The physical location of the family is less important today than in previous years, since children living at great distances can interact daily by telephone and arrive within a day by air travel if an emergency occurs. The quality and quantity of family interactions are more important indicators of family functioning. The presence of a depressive disorder in a previously active older adult requires family members to take on specific roles in coping with the crisis. The roles taken by family members should enable the family to actively intervene, adequately cope, and appropriately support the older person during the depressive disorder. Unfortunately, family members, through their individual roles, may perpetuate psychiatric symptoms in the older person. Garetz (1979) has suggested a number of roles that family members may take on when interacting with the mentally or physically ill older person. A modification of these roles is presented in the box on p. 291.

In the case presentation, the roles of facilitator, manager, and victim are clear. The younger son is a facilitator of the depression, the older son is the manager, and the wife is the victim. Depressed patients of any age appear to be asking for help, and therefore the appearance of a manager in the family is usual. If the depressed older adult has previously been problematic to other family members, they may perceive (either consciously or unconsciously) the depressive symptoms as retribution for previous behavior. Depressed patients can place a considerable burden on the family leading to the emergence of a victim among the family roles who subjectively experiences the burden more than other family members.

Roles within the family may shift, and individuals may assume more than one role at the same time. The roles described in the box provide a useful framework for understanding function in the family of the depressed older adult. However, the depressed older adult may play other roles within the family and should not be considered the patient alone. When interacting with family members over time, the clinician may join the family (i.e., take on roles within the family—especially the role of a manager). When such a role is taken consciously, the benefits may be significant. However, if the clinician inadvertently plays another familial role of which he or she is not aware, difficulty in managing the patient and family usually emerges. Clinicians practicing in small towns, where there is a high probability that the families they treat are also seen socially, are at great risk for unwittingly taken on familial roles. The clinician perceptions in such situations include anger at the family for their demands and a sense of responsibility so great that the clinical problems are "taken home" by the clinician. Referral to another clinician, usually in another city, is the best alternative in such cases.

Family roles do not only compose an overall system, but subsystems as well. For example, in the case described the patient, elder son, and younger son form a subsystem related to the control and operation of the family business. The clinician during the assessment of the family, should seek to identify coalitions, alignments, and triangles in the family (i.e., subsystems that impart overall family structure and function).

■ FAMILY INTERACTION

Frequency of Interaction

An important characteristic of the family of the older depressed patient is the frequency of the older adult interaction with other family members. Interaction can be assessed by asking the following questions:

- How often do your son and daughter (and so forth) visit you in your home?
- How often do you visit other family members in their homes?
- How frequently do you contact family members by telephone?
- How many of your family members live within 30 minutes driving distance?
- How often do you visit your closest friends either by phone or in person?

Roles of Family Members Caring for an Impaired Elder

Facilitator

The facilitator is an individual in the family who resists medical or psychiatric compliance to maintain the stablity achieved with the family secondary to the long-term effects of a dysfunctional older person. The illness is thereby facilitated. This individual may present many obstacles to therapeutic intervention to maintain a perceived equilibrium within the family system. In other words, such an individual believes (consciously or unconsciously) that he or she or the family is better served with the older person in a sick or dependent role than in a more healthy role.

Victim

The victim is an individual in the family who perceives the illness of the older person as a direct threat to herself and himself. This is more likely to be the individual who has the most frequent contact with the family and therefore with the physician. The person may in turn criticize the physician for not being able to accomplish anything with the patient.

Manager

The manager is the family member who takes charge of the family during a crisis. He or she is calm, cool, and somewhat overly intellectual in contact with the physician. The manager can be very helpful to the practitioner in arranging tangible supports but has less ability to provide emotional support for the older patient or other family members. Frequently, the manager lives some distance from the family members who are most intimately involved in caring for the older person.

Caretaker

The caretaker is the individual who has an innate need to care for the sick. He or she may provide inexhaustable help to the severely disabled older person, sometimes maintaining an older adult in the home for beyond the point at which institutionalization is appropriate. Avoiding opportunities for respite, the individual is frequently worn out to the point that he or she can find no useful or meaningful activity outside of caretaking. When the older person dies, the caretaker may suffer a tremendous void, which manifests itself in a severe and prolonged grief reaction. This caretaking activity can be manipulative when it is motivated by guilt or when it prevents the older person from achieving a greater sense of independence.

Escapee

The escapee is the family member who is withdrawn from the usual interactions within the family and who is often blamed for not showing more care and concern for the older person. Typically a son or daughter who has moved a good distance from the family, the escapee often becomes involved in some other altruistic endeavor (e.g., religious or civic activity) and therefore does not desire to devote time to caring for the older adult. Families fraught with conflict frequently have escapees. Whether consciously or unconsciously, the escapee recognizes the toxic nature of family interactions and withdraws out of self-defense. The individual may function well outside the family but is very resistant to being drawn back into the stressed and conflicted family.

Continued.

Roles of Family Members Caring for an Impaired Elder—cont'd

Patient

   The patient is the older person who is identified as having the problem that precipitated the family crisis or who has required considerable physical and emotional
output from other family members. For years family therapists have reported that the
identified patient (or problem) in the family may only be a "ticket" to enter a helping
relationship. Yet the actual problem leading to family discord may only be periph-
erally related to the illness of an older adult.

Telephone contact between the older depressed patient and family members is an
important indicator of social ties. Many older persons prefer to visit over the phone
rather than in person. If elders experience a hearing impairment (see Chapter 8), bone
conduction via the receiver facilitates their ability to hear and they are thus able to
communicate more effectively.

Depressed older persons may withdraw, decreasing their interactions with members
of the family, or they may increase significantly the amount of interaction through demanding dependence. The older person's perception of not understanding what is going
on or of not participating in important decision-making activities (generally exacerbated
by feelings of insecurity) can be frustrating to the spouse who attempts to manage affairs. If the spouse attempts to distance himself or herself, the depressed elder may per-
cieve a lack of interest or withdrawal. Children are often turned to via increasing phone
calls or actual visits.

Quality of Interaction

Of greater importance than frequency of interaction is the quality of interaction between the older person and family members and the interaction of family members among
themselves. Interaction can be considered both in terms of individual dyads and collectively. The quality of interaction can be assessed along the five parameters described
next.

Compatible versus Conflictual

Do family members usually agree? Do frequent conflicts and differences arise during
conversation even concerning minor issues? Have old conflicts, especially between the
older parent and his or her middle-aged children, been brought to the surface after dor-
mancy? The development of health problems in an older adult that requires the intervention of children who have been detached emotionally and physically from their parents during most of their adult years provides an environment for the resurgence of old
conflicts. The ability of middle-aged children to resolve their conflicts with the aging
parents has been termed *filial maturity* and plays a critical role in the ability of that child
to provide both emotional and physical support to the depressed older person. Mature
children resolve their conflicts or do not allow them to interfere with their ability to
respond effectively during a time of need.

Depressed older adults often belong to one of two categories. Each has the potential
for resurrecting or creating conflict within the family when the depressive symptoms

arise. First, many depressed elders, especially men, have been dominant figures within the family. The dominance and control by these elders over many years has led to considerable repressed hostility and covert rebellion on the part of other family members, especially children. When such an elder exhibits depressive symptoms (and appears weak or vulnerable), these old conflicts are often brought to the surface. Yet children also empathize with their parents and experience considerable guilt about their anger. When conflict is coupled with a need to take responsibility for the care of the depressed elder, the problem is magnified.

Second, many depressed elders have been quiet caretakers of the family for years. These elders, frequently women, have regularly prepared meals, served as willing babysitters for children, buffered the ups and downs of their children and spouses (either emotional or financial), and held the family together. The onset of a depressive reaction in such a person immediately precipitates family conflict. Family members wish to aid the depressive older adult but lack the ability to work together in management of the problem because the family peacemaker becomes the problem. The family conflict increases the anxiety of individual family members and angry outbursts often ensue. When other individuals in the family seek to assume the caretaking role, conflict and competition often arise, especially between children.

Cohesive versus Fragmented

Does the family stick together even in times of crisis? Does the family usually present as a unit as opposed to isolated individualism? Do individual family members express interest in and concern about the positions or views of other family members? Even families that are in conflict may be cohesive. Certain families tend to hold together and withstand both internal and external stress to a remarkable degree. When the clinician encounters such a family, it is imperative to involve the family as a unit in treating the depressed elder. A cohesive family that opposes the clinician easily undermines most attempts at therapeutic intervention.

Productive versus Nonproductive

Can the family work together to accomplish certain tasks necessary to aid the depressed older adult? Has the family demonstrated the ability to work productively in other endeavors, such as a family business or in planning a family vacation? If the older patient resisted coming to the clinician's office or into the hospital, was the family successful in motivating the patient to seek medical attention? Family members accompany older persons to the clinician's office in at least one third of the cases. On many occasions, an individual family member has undertaken the responsibility for care of the older person to the exclusion of but agreement from the remainder of the family. However, on other occasions the family has worked as a unit to pursue medical care. A productive family is a most valuable ally to the clinician working with a depressed older adult.

Fragile versus Stable

Has the family remained stable both in its members and interactions over time? Is the family capable of providing support over an extended period of time? Have relationships within the family been maintained? Is divorce a frequent pattern? Do children, adolescents, and young adults maintain contact with older family members? Fragile families usually provide little support to the older depressed patient, especially when one member has undertaken the role of caretaker or manager. If previous family crises have disturbed family equilibrium and have rendered the family incapable of maintaining significant interaction and productivity, the onset of depression in an older adult is likely to reap the same consequences.

Rigid versus Flexible

How fluent are the roles within the family? If the manager or identified leader of a family becomes incapacitated or dies, are other members ready, willing, and able to take on this role? Will family members accept the leadership of another member of the family? Are the usual family procedures for working through a problem flexible? The illness of an older person who has previously been in excellent health and has provided leadership, wisdom, and stability to the family necessitates that the family adapt a new mode of operation. The flexibility of the family in such a situation to adapt by regrouping and developing new hierarchical patterns is critical to the family's ability to support and care for the older depressed member.

■ FAMILY ATMOSPHERE

Clinicians who have worked with families quickly recognize certain characteristics that can be described as family atmosphere. The dimensions of family atmosphere can be assessed as outlined next.

Anxious versus Relaxed

The clinician can easily detect the relative degree of tension within the family setting by noting his or her own feelings during the family interview. Tension perceived by the clinician is usually associated with family conflict and is often, although not always, associated with the tendency of families to be fragmented or even fragile. However, the level of tension within a family may also indicate the level of energy available for productive work in aiding the older depressed adult. A relaxed family may be a family that is passive and nonproductive, allowing each family member to be tossed on the waves of circumstances without concern.

Hopeful versus Resigned

The hopeful family is most often the productive and supportive family. When a clinician encounters an older patient with a condition that is potentially correctable, such as a depressive disorder, it is important for the family to realize the potential for improvement and to be ready to make the appropriate changes in living arrangements and personal relationships necessary to effect optimal care. A family resigned to keeping an older person in a depressed or dependent state, such as residence in a long-term facility, can be a persistent obstacle to the clinician who advises a change in living arrangements or structure within the family to improve the elder's mental health. In fact, family resistance to change is among the most difficult factors hindering the transfer of patients from long-term care facilities back to independent or semiindependent living in the community. Yet clinicians must recognize that the responsibilities placed on the family when the partially impaired older person lives in the community may be extremely disruptive to the family. A resigned or pessimistic attitude in a family is often associated with a lack of flexibility and a low energy within the family setting.

Unfortunately, certain families maintain idealistic and unrealistic expectations of their older members. These hopeful families continually search for magical cures and for a clinician who will promise reversals of chronic illness. They often do not carry out practical suggestions for rehabilitation and restructuring of the family setting that can improve the emotional state and life satisfaction of the depressed older adult, rather expecting some instantaneous improvement through the miracle of modern medicine. Such families are potential victims of charlatans who peddle medications and treatments at exorbitant prices. Idealistic families may place great faith in the clinician. When their expectations are not met, the clinician may be subject to criticism, abuse, or even a malpractice suit. In working with such a family the clinician should advise the family of the realistic expectations of treatment from the outset without quelling the hope that is always necessary for families to be productive in caring for their older loved one.

■ FAMILY VALUES

What are the family values concerning mental health? Optimal mental health and a positive outlook may be the norm in certain families, and the family members may therefore be intolerant of any member who does not maintain such a positive outlook. Such families do not accept the depression of an older member or the fact that a family member—the depressed elder—requires mental health care. Other families expect their older members to be depressed or dissatisfied. Every complaint from the elder is considered a sign of physical and psychologic decline, which is expected along with diminished activity and increased contact with the health care system (i.e., the "sick role"). Physicians and nurses play important long-term roles within the structure and dynamics of these families. If by chance the family loses contact with the health care system over time, family dynamics may be seriously altered. Health is a family affair.

What are the family values about late life? These values generally relate to the family's larger cultural framework. For example, the Mormon culture respects older persons to a greater degree than most other cultures within the United States. Therefore a Mormon family would be expected to have a greater respect for the elder and to maintain important roles for elders in family and community life. Families that no longer allow the older person to maintain an active role are probably at greater risk for older members' becoming physically and mentally impaired.

The clinician must also determine the perception of responsibility by the family toward the older depressed patient. Mutual aid is generally the norm. Older persons may provide services, such as babysitting or housework, information and advice, support for children's decisions, and even gifts of money (Troll, Miller, and Atchley, 1979). Gifts to the children may be indirect, such as generous allowances and gifts to grandchildren. Children in turn provide services, such as shopping, housework, and financial and administrative help. Yet in one study (Laurie, 1978), only 15% of the elders received help from their children. In fact the proportion of older people who regularly help their children tends to exceed the proportion who receive help from their children.

The more vulnerable the older depressed person, the more likely he or she is to expect aid from children (i.e., filial responsibility) (Seelback, 1978). These expectations are usually realized, since when the elderly living at home become impaired, their families are likely to provide aid (regardless of race or socioeconomic status). Family members occasionally do not perceive filial responsibility. Elaborate plans presented by a health care team to an unmotivated family may then be a waste of time. Yet the family that has a sense of responsibility for its older members can provide a most beneficial adjunct to the health of the elderly.

■ FAMILY SUPPORT AND TOLERANCE

Four areas of support are of importance to the clinician in planning to involve families in the care of the depressed older adult. These include the availability of the family for support to the older person over time, the actual tangible services provided by the family to the older person, the older person's perception of the support of the family, and family tolerance of particular behaviors by the older person. The first question to ask an older depressed patient concerning family support is, "If you become ill, is there a family member to take care of you for a short period of time?" The second question is, "If you become disabled and must be cared for indefinitely, do you have a family member who will care for you over an extended period of time?" The perception of long-term support from the family by an older person is one of the most important factors in the older person's adaptation to chronic physical and mental illness. Most older patients are capable of answering these questions accurately despite their depressed affect.

The next step in evaluating the family of the depressed older adult is to assess the services provided to the older adult by the family. Although social and economic environments and, to a significant extent, the physical health capacity of the older adult determine the services required, certain services are needed more when depression is present. The family often feels the responsibility to encourage and facilitate social and recreational activities. They may go so far as to plan activities or classes and to take the depressed elder to these activities. Unfortunately, the older person who harbors anger toward family members will resist these attempts to increase social and recreational activities. If the depressed elder increasingly withdraws from the social environment, the family may increase the interaction via telephone calls or visits. The family often becomes emotionally drained after frequent attempts to dislodge the depressed elder from self-imposed isolation. If depressive symptoms significantly interfere with the elder's ability to maintain self-care, families often provide services, such as meal preparation, shopping, transportation to medical appointments, homemaker and household services, and even personal care services. Family members may become frustrated when faced with delivering such services when they know the older person is physically capable of his or her own care. When family members fear suicide or gross self-neglect, they often feel responsible for providing continuous supervision for the depressed elder. This supervision, often by a spouse or a child who lives with the elder, places a tremendous strain by isolating the caretaker from other family and social endeavors and occasionally depletes the family economic resources.

Regardless of the actual service provision by a family, the older person develops certain perceptions of support that he or she receives from the family. Perception of support may be as important as the actual delivery of services in determining not only family interactions but the health outcomes of the older person over time. Particularly important for older people are four "intangible supports" (Blazer, 1980), which can be described as follows:

1. *A dependable social network.* Does the older person perceive the family as available in case of severe illness over an extended period of time? Can the older person "count on" the family to assist in times of major or even minor crises? Is the family capable of helping the older person in times of crisis?

2. *Social participation or interaction.* Does the older person understand what is going on in the family at a given point in time? Does the family understand the older person and appreciate the significance of his or her concerns? Is open communication a norm between the older person and other family members?

3. *Belongingness.* Does the older person continue to fit into the family and have a role within the family? Does the elder feel at ease in family gatherings?

4. *Intimacy.* Can deep emotional feelings be expressed to family members without ridicule or disinterest? Is the family perceived as being emphatic and sharing of its emotions with the older person?

The depressed elder's view of his or her relationship with the family may be that of being a useless burden. The perception of not being able to contribute to the family, either because his or her services are no longer required or because the depression disorder has interfered with the ability to provide services, significantly decreases the self-esteem of the depressed elder. Such an individual may also feel a lack of belongingness in the family, as if the individual and the family no longer have common interests and activities; the patient may feel most insecure when he or she is not present or at least close to family gatherings.

Regardless of the actual supportive services provided by family members and the perceived support by the older person, every family has its level of tolerance. The clinician must be aware of the behaviors that are particularly difficult for family members to tolerate and must aid families confronted with these behaviors. Different families have more or less tolerance for different behaviors associated with depression in late life. The continued somatic complaints and pessimism expressed by depressed elders may be unbearable to some family members but easily tolerated by others. The refusal of a previously dominant and controlling individual to take responsibility may be very difficult for the spouse and children to tolerate. Other families may resent the increased demand placed on them for tangible support via services, such as supervision and housekeeping. Most families have difficulty hearing and responding to the depressed elder's talk of suicide. The clinician must assess each family for its tolerance of the depressed older person's behavior.

■ FAMILY STRESSORS AND REWARDS

The disability of an older depressed family member may threaten the living arrangements of the individual and be quite stressful to the family. The onset of depression in the older person may occur after recent changes have taken place within the family. These changes may be closely related to the depressed elder, such as the death of a spouse. On the other hand, the changes may be more remote, such as a change in family business (i.e., either a boom or a recession) or the marriage or divorce of a grandchild or child. Most events that precipitate depressive symptoms in older persons are losses of one type or another.

Stress within the family also derives from the stress of caring for the depressed older persons. The burden may exhibit itself in a number of ways. For example, the changing mood states and expressions of fear and anxiety by the depressed elder may place strains on family members, especially caretakers. Behavioral symptoms may also contribute to stress, including the decreased activity and interest of the elder combined with demands and complaints, negativity, hostility, agitation, refusal to eat, and difficulty with sleep. As noted previously, suicidal ideation and delusions can be especially disturbing to family members. The caregiver may find that attempts to motivate the depressed elder are frustrated as the elder rejects the activities of the caregiver. Therefore the clinician must account for not only the emotional status of the depressed elder but the emotional status of family members associated with the depressed elder, especially the identified caretaker.

The clinician should recognize, however, that the emergence of a mood disorder in an older adult may not be a totally negative experience for the family. In some cases the onset of a depressed affect may improve the relationship between the depressed elder and family members. Previous conflictual relationships may change to an appreciation for the difficulties faced by the patient and empathy for the patient. Families may also take pleasure in seeing the depressed elder improve in mood and reintegrate into previous activities.

Caregivers may feel that they have been given much by the elder over many years and the occasion of a mood disorder therefore provides an opportunity to return to the patient some of the care received. Caregivers may also experience a sense of growth during the process of caring for the depressed elder, finding that, during the stress of an episode of depression, he or she has become more selfless than previously thought. Caregivers also may enjoy the relationship with the clinician and the sense of empowerment in being a colleague of the physician in the mutual care of the depressed elder.

Depression in an elder may not always be stressful to the family as a system but may enable other members of the family to function more effectively in their roles. If so, then the elderly depressed patient may become "trapped" in the depression, since the family organizes to keep the patient depressed. In the case described, if the elder's depression keeps him from meddling in the family business, then the elder son just may subconsciously wish for the elder to remain depressed.

■ TREATING THE FAMILY OF THE DEPRESSED OLDER ADULT

Treating the family of the depressed elderly patient involves a number of steps. First, the family should be informed of the nature of the depressive disorders in late life and then be alerted to the potential risks, especially suicide. Family members are instructed to look for changes in behavior, such as an increase in discomfort (either physical or emotional) in the depressed elder, increased withdrawal and decreased verbalization of complaints and feelings, changes in long-range plans, increased consumption of alcohol or medications, preoccupation with a gun or knife, and increased expressions of grief over a loved one who died months or years before. Weapons should be removed from easy access, and the family should take responsibility for administering medications if the potential for suicide is high. Families can tolerate the risk of suicide in the elderly for only short periods of time, however. The suicidal elder should be hospitalized as soon as possible.

What if the depressed elder commits suicide? The family members may suffer tremendous guilt if they are alerted to the need to watch for potential suicide and the depressed elder completes the act of suicide. In addition, the family may express considerable anger toward the clinician. If such a situation arises, the clinician should meet with family members to help them express their feelings, which usually range from grief over the loss of a loved one to guilt about not being able to prevent the act to anger at the clinician for not caring for the patient properly. Early intervention and open discussion with all parties involved, may prevent future problems. Nevertheless, as our society becomes more litigious, the clinician should work closely with risk managers because he or she determines the appropriate approach to the family of an elder who commits suicide.

The clinician must attempt to balance the responsibilities he or she takes and the responsibility delegated to the family when treating the potentially suicidal patient who does not require hospitalization. There may be a point at which a patient should no longer be hospitalized for a physical or emotional problem but a remote possibility of suicide exists. The clinician may say to the family that the risk exists but that the best psychiatric knowledge suggests that the patient can be cared for in the home setting. In this way the family and clinician work together as a team, with the clinician taking the responsibility for the decision but with the full knowledge of the family (and even the patient). If a suicide occurs under these conditions, the family members are better able to accept the loss and rarely blame the clinician. When clinicians attempt to predict the unpredictable (i.e., suicide), they are at great risk for angry attacks from family members. Yet dealing with the issue of suicide is only the beginning of work with families of depressed older adults.

The clinician can alleviate many family concerns by explaining the nature of the depressive illness, since comments made by the depressed elder to family members are then no longer taken personally. The covert meaning of many of the symptoms of depression is, "I am unhappy because you have disappointed me" or "You are not treating me as you should." "I am so lonely" suggests to the family that the elder should be visited more often. "I am of no use to anyone" suggests the family has excluded the elder from all useful activities. As noted in Chapter 2, older persons tend to externalize their depression and therefore such comments may be frequent.

The family can benefit from simple instructions about communication with the depressed patient. Methods of responding to expressions of low self-esteem and pessimism, such as paraphrase and expressions of understanding without a sense of responsibility to intervene, can be most effective. Paraphrase is a technique of responding to the thoughts and feelings of another by expressing an understanding of the thoughts and feelings, as if to say, "I hear what you are saying . . . I understand." Behavioral techniques for dealing with demanding or overly dependent patients are also beneficial. For example, to deal with a patient's demand for constant attention, a family member can learn to gradually "wean" the patient, staying away from the patient for a progressively longer period of time each day until a desired level of interaction is reached.

A major decision with the onset of acute depression is whether or not to hospitalize the older adult. Family members are resistant to hospitalizing their elder members, especially when the older person vehemently opposes hospitalization. If is often necessary for the clinician either to take the responsibility for saying that hospitalization is essential (i.e., that the family has no choice in the matter or the clinician should empower the family to make the decision). In such a situation the clinician can inform the patient of the necessity of hospitalization in the presence of the family, who in turn can support the clinician's position. Rarely does a patient refuse hospitalization when faced with the united front of physician and family. The family may be hesitant to take a depressed elder to a psychiatrist or psychologist. The primary care physician, social worker, or other first-line clinician can be of help by recommending a psychiatrist or psychologist and by assuring the family that the primary care clinician and the mental health specialist will work together to help the depressed elder.

Qualls (1988) suggests that the therapist can facilitate family decision making, such as hospitalization, by providing information, teaching decision-making skills, and clarifying family rules (common beliefs) about the process of making good decisions. There are many paradigms for decision making, such as the one by D'Zurilla and Nezu (1982). The steps in this process include the following: defining the problem in behavioral terms, reviewing previously attempted decisions, generating a list of possible solutions, evaluating the potential outcome of each potential solution, choosing the "best" solution, developing a plan for implementing the choice, implementing the plan, evaluating its effectiveness, and making appropriate modifications in the decision over time. Although self-evident, this approach to making decisions is difficult for family members. Decision making and empowering the family members to chose often requires revising family rules. For example, Qualls (1988) suggests that only a few members be "allowed" to have the final say, and one of those may be the depressed elder. Some members criticize all options. By directly confronting families with the covert rules of decision making, families often are freed of anxiety regarding the need to make necessary decisions. Objectively, the family recognizes the need to effect decision making but have difficulty in doing so.

Encouraging family members, especially those assuming the roles of victim and caretaker, to discuss their feelings is essential in a therapeutic process. It is often important for the victim to express his or her frustration in the presence of other family members and for the clinician to acknowledge and not underestimate these feelings. If the entire family can empathize with the caretaker, the family can often be mobilized to do whatever is needed to manage the patient.

REFERENCES

Blazer DG: *Social Support and Mortality in a Community Population of Older Adults.* Ph.D. dissertation, University of North Carolina, Chapel Hill, 1980.

D'Zurilla TJ, Nezu A: Social problem-solving in adults. In Kendall PC (ed): *Advances in Cognitive-Behavioral Research and Therapy.* (vol 1). New York, Academic Press, 1982 pp. 201-274.

Garetz FR: *Responses of Families to Health Problems in the Elderly.* Paper presented at the thirty-sixth annual meeting of the American Geriatrics Society, April, 1979, Washington, DC.

Laurie WF: The Cleveland experience: functional status and services use. In OARS *Multidemensional Functional Assessment.* Durham, North Carolina, Center for the Study of Aging, Duke University, 1978, pp. 89-99.

Miller KT, Miller JL:The Family as a System. Paper presented at the annual meeting of the American College of Psychiatrists, Costa Mesa, California, February, 1979.

Qualls SH: Problems in families of older adults. In Epstein N, Schlesinger S, Dryden W (eds): *Cognitive-Behavioral Therapy with Families.* New York, Brunner-Mazel, 1988.

Seelback WC: Correlates of aged parents and filial responsibility: expectations and realizations. *Family Coordinator* 27:341, 1978.

Troll LE, Miller SJ, Atchley RC: *Families and Later Life.* Belmont, California: Wadsworth, 1979.

19

Psychopharmacology

The elderly consume more drugs than any other age group in the United States. Although persons 65 years of age and older make up only 12% of the population, they account for 30% of all drugs prescribed in the United States (Vestal and Cusak, 1990). The annual cost of medication for older people approaches five billion dollars for prescription drugs each year. In a community survey of persons 65 and older in rural Iowa, 88% of the respondents took at least one prescription or over-the-counter drug (Helling et al, 1987). The average number of drugs taken by each respondent was 2.9, and the average increased with age for both men and women. Over 93% of persons 85 years of age and older took medications. Cardiovascular drugs were the most commonly prescribed (55%) followed by central nervous system agents (11%) and analgesics (9%).

Pharmacologic therapy has significantly improved the prognosis of mood disorders in older adults. Tricyclic antidepressants not only shorten the duration of depressive episodes but also decrease the remission rates from depressive disorders in all age groups. The aging process, however, and the possibility of mutliple drug use by the elderly handicap the clinician's task of prescribing appropriate pharmacotherapy. As described previously (see Chapter 13), certain prescription medications may actually induce depressive illness in late life. Therefore as antidepressant medications are prescribed, other drugs should be eliminated when possible.

Older persons are at risk for potential toxic effects of medications for a number of reasons. First, altered physiologic, pathophysiologic, and social factors render usual prescribing practices inadequate for the elderly. Normal physiologic changes with aging, such as the decreased proportion of muscle tissue and increased proportion of fat tissue, change the usual distribution of medications within the body. Older persons also experience more physical disorders than do younger persons. The majority of the elderly experience at least one chronic condition that augments the normal aging changes and is managed by drug therapy. An example of a pathologic change that alters physiology is chronic renal failure, which may reduce excretion of many medications (Rowe et al, 1976). Social changes, such as loss of a spouse and social isolation, may also lead to altered physiologic processes secondary to progressive inactivity and changing dietary habits.

Second, the elderly are at much greater risk for medication errors. In one study of 50 individuals of 65 years of age and older, 66% were taking prescription drugs without adequate instructions, and 25% were not taking the prescription medication as labeled and directed by the physician. A breakdown of these medication errors reveal that 47% were errors of omission, 20% were errors of inadequate knowledge, 17% were self-medication errors, 10% were incorrect dosages, and 6% were errors of improper timing and frequency of drug intake (Lundin, 1978).

A third reason that older persons are at greater risk for adverse drug reaction is the potential for drug interactions. Studies from Great Britian and Scandinavia reveal that older persons take an average of three to six drugs while in the hospital, with a median of five medications. At times the effect of one drug is significantly altered by the addition of a second agent, which renders the first drug toxic rather than therapeutic. At other times the interaction blocks the action of one of the medications. An example of an interaction quite common in older persons is the additive anticholinergic side effects of phenothiazines, antihistamines, antiparkinsonian agents, and tricyclic antidepressants. Most potiential interactions can be predicted by a knowledge of the pharmacokinetic properties of the drug (absorption, distribution, metabolism, excretion, and tissue deposits) and pharmacodynamics (pharmacologic effects).

■ PHARMACOKINETICS

Just as aging is a dynamic process that not only changes through time but displays its diversity in different structures and functions within the body, drug therapy of the elderly must be considered within the same dynamic framework. The term *pharmacokinetics* refers to the process concerned with the distribution of drugs in the body, their absorption, excretion, and metabolism. In other words, pharmacokinetics is concerned with the process that determines the concentration of different therapeutic agents at their site of action (Burgen and Mitchell, 1978). What are the basic principles of pharmacokinetics that are of importance to the clinician?

Absorption

Therapeutic agents administered to depressed older persons are taken by mouth. They are broken down in intestinal canal and are absorbed into the blood stream. The rate at which a drug is absorbed and the site at which it is absorbed depends on the changes within the gastrointestinal tract as individuals age and the chemical and physical properties of the drug. Alteration in gastric pH, gastric emptying, gastrointestinal absorption surfaces, and motility influences drug absorption (Vestal and Cusak, 1990). The changes that are most common in older persons are an elevated gastric pH secondary to a decrease in hydrocholoric acid, a decreased absorptive surface, a decreased blood flow to the GI tract, and a decrease in gastric motility. The clinical importance of these changes in late life has not been sufficiently studied and is probably not great, since most oral pharmacologic agents taken by older adults are absorbed completely. One agent, clorazepate, requires a low gastric pH for proper absorption because of its chemical structure and therefore would be expected to be less absorbed by older persons compared with other benzodiazepines.

Distribution and Tissue Deposits

Most agents prescribed for older persons for the treatment of depression are stored in body fat. The proportion of body fat to the total body weight increases with age as the proportion of muscle tissue decreases. Other changes include a reduced amount of body water, reduced serum albumin, and increased alpha$_1$-acid glycoprotein. Drugs prescribed for depressed older people would therefore tend to be found in relatively higher concentrations in body fat, to have a longer duration of action secondary to their fat deposit, and, for protein-bound agents, to have a higher proportion of free drug (Vestal and Cussek, 1990).

Of a special importance may be the age differences in protein binding of medications, especially for medications that are highly protein bound. Yet age is only one of a number factors that can change protein binding. For example, drugs that have a greater affinity for alpha$_1$-acid glycoprotein than albumin would be more bound to plasma protein with less free drug in later life, compared with drugs that bind predominately to albumin, which would have a greater proportion of the free drug in the plasma. Tricyclic antidepressants tend to exhibit a decrease in plasma binding with a proportionate increase of free drug.

Metabolism

Aging is associated with reduced numbers of hepatic cells and a reduced hepatic blood flow. Evidence also exists that enzymatic activity in elderly persons is reduced. Since most therapeutic agents prescribed for the treatment of late life depression are metabolized by the liver (e.g., the tricyclic antidepressants and fluoxetine), the slower biotransformation causes drugs to remain in the body for a longer period of time in their active state.

Yet the variation in the capability of the liver to metabolize drugs may be much greater between individuals of the same age than the variation by age because of factors such as smoking (which stimulates demethylation) and the use of phenobarbital (which also stimulates demethylation). These factors account for the large variability in metabolism among the elderly. In contrast to the age-related decrease in demethylation, there appears to be little change in conjugation with age. Both the benzodiazepines and tricyclic antidepressants have been demonstrated to be cleared less quickly by the liver in late life. In general the most common changes in liver metabolism with aging are changes in the oxidation, which affects the hydroxylation of the antidepressant agents imipramine, desipramine, and nortriptyline and the dealkylation of other antidepressants, such as amitriptyline.

Excretion

Aging is associated with a decreased glomerular filtration rate, reduced renal blood flow, and some alteration in tubular functioning (Rowe et al, 1976). Decreased renal function is one of the most consistent biologic changes with increased age. Nevertheless, determination of serum creatinine concentration may not provide the clinician with an accurate estimate of renal functioning. Since lithium carbonate is excreted almost exclusively by the kidneys and has the potential for significant toxic effects at dose levels near the levels required for a therapeutic response, an accurate assessment of clearance is essential. The clinician should obtain a 24-hour creatinine clearance rather than rely on serum creatinine alone.

As with liver function, the variation in renal function is great within a given age group, and therefore each patient must be approached as an individual in regards to his or her potential to excrete specific drugs. In general, however, diminished renal function is common and easily assessed in the elderly by determining creatinine clearance (Vestal and Cusack, 1990). Therefore drugs such as lithium should be prescribed in a lower dose in older persons than to persons in earlier stages of the life cycle.

■ PHARMACODYNAMICS

Pharmacodynamics refers to the physiologic or psychologic response to a drug or a combination of drugs (Vestal and Cusack, 1990). Few psychotropic drugs have been studied from the perspective of pharmacodynamics, yet the benzodiazepines and tricylic antidepressants are beginning to receive more attention in terms of their pharmacodynamic actions. The importance of pharmacodynamics is clear. O'Hanlon et al (1988) found signficiant impairment of "on the road" driving by older persons taking antidepressant medications compared with younger persons. These antidepressants impair driving capabilities and skills, such as visual, perceptual, cognitive, and psychomotor abilities. The benzodiazepines have been studied far more frequently and have been shown to create increased postural sway, decreased reaction time, and increased sedation in older persons, compared with younger persons. The effect of tricyclic antidepressant agents on cardiovascular function illustrates the importance of the study of pharmacodynamics and is discussed in a later section.

Drug interactions are perhaps the most frequent occasion for clinicians to address the issue of pharmacodynamics in the pharmacotherapy of depressed older adults. The potential for drug interactions includes the additive interactions of over-the-counter and prescribed agents that have anticholinergic effects, such as the antihistamines and tricyclic antidepressants. Diuretics that cause sodium depletion, when combined with lithium carbonate for recurrent depressions in late life or the control of manic episodes, may lead to sodium depletion. Selective excretion of sodium leads to an increased reabsorption of lithium, which increases the potential for toxic effects from lithium.

Some typical interactions in the pharmacotherapy of depression in late life are presented in Table 19-1.

■ PRINCIPLES OF PRESCRIBING FOR GERIATRIC PATIENTS

Since depression in older persons is often multidetermined, the physician may often have to initiate more than one treatment. The use of a number of treatment methods

TABLE 19-1. Drug Interactions with Medications used to Treat Late Life
Depression

Drug	Interactive Drug	Interaction Effect	Mechanism of the Interaction
Tricyclic Antidepressant	Barbiturates (such as chloride)	Decreases the antidepressant effect	Lowers the tricyclic antidepressant concentration
	Sympathomimetics	Hypertension and arrhythmias	Inhibits the reuptake mechanism of the neurons
	Stimulant (such as methylphenidate)	Increases the antidepressant effect/ agitation and psychosis	Relative increase in stimulant concentration and tricyclic antidepressant concentration
	Anticonvulsants	Decreases effect of the antidepressant	Increase in metabolism of tricyclic antidepressant
	Monoamine-oxidase inhibitors	Increases the antidepressant effect and may precipitate a hypertensive crisis	Blockade of reuptake with monoamine-oxidase inhibition
	Alcohol	Decreases the tricyclic antidepressant effect	Increases in tricyclic antidepressant
	Phenothiazines	Augmentation of both medications	Decreases rate of metabolism of each drug
	Anticholinergics	Confusion, delirium, tachycardia, urinary retention, and constipation	Additive cholinergic effects
Monoamine Oxidase	Meperidine	Agitation and excitement	Serotonin levels are elevated in the brain
	Tyramine-rich foods	Hypertensive crisis	Impairment of the gastrointestinal breakdown of tyramine, leading to a release of catecholamines
	L-Dopa	Stimulation and hypertension	Increase in catecholamine synthesis
Lithium Carbonate	Thiazide diuretics	Relative increase in lithium concentration	Increased lithium reabsorption with increased sodium and potassium excretion
	Carbamazepine	Augmentation of lithium effect	Mechanism unknown
	Succinylcholine	Prolonged muscle relaxation	Effect at the neuromuscular junction

concurrently has proven to be successful in the management of depression in late life. Pharmacologic therapy is an essential component of this multitherapeutic approach, especially if the patient exhibits the criteria of a major depressive episode with melancholia. The principles of pharmacologic treatment that should be followed are outlined next.

Medication History

Patients often are incapable of relating an accurate history of their drug intake. Therefore at least three procedures may be of benefit in determining current drug use. First, the patient should be encouraged to bring all medications to the physician's office on the first visit. Each medication should be reviewed in detail with the patient, including when it was prescribed, how often the patient takes the medication (i.e., whether the medication is taken continuously, intermittently, or rarely), and what effects the patient perceives from the use of the drug. Second, the patient may not be able to identify certain medications that he or she is taking. The use of a picture chart of the typical prescribed medications (e.g., those available in the *Physician's Desk Reference* [1992]) can help patients identify medications. Third, and probably the most valuable means of getting an accurate drug history, the physician should question a close family member to determine how well the drug-intake perceptions of the patient and family members correspond. Documenting drug use is time-consuming but essential in the treatment of the depressed older adult. The task may be delegated to paraprofessionals within the physician's office, but the task must be accomplished one way or another.

Identification of Target Behaviors for Intervention

Whenever a drug is prescribed for treating depression or manic behavior, the physician must be aware of the symptoms likely to respond to the medication. A depressed affect may not be the primary symptom to be monitored. Most antidepressant medications are more likely to correct sleep disturbances, appetite disturbances, agitation, and retardation rather than to reduce or reverse the depressed affect, at least initially. Symptoms during the diagnostic workup should be documented, and antidepressant therapy should be evaluated periodically to determine whether reversal of symptoms has been effected by given medication. The use of symptom scales, such as the Hamilton Depression Rating Scale and the Montgomery-Asberg Depression Scale, are useful to monitor the progress of drug therapy (see Chapter 2). Increased activity and social interaction are important target symptoms for antidepressant effect.

Smaller Doses of Medications with Increase in Dosage at a Slower Rate

Most tricyclic antidepressants are prescribed for adults at an intial dose of 75 to 150 mg (e.g., imipramine), usually given at bedtime. When prescribing for an older adult, especially one with significant health problems, the starting dose should be cut to one half or one third of the suggested adult dose. Usually medications should be increased from 25% to 50% of the initial dose every 3 to 5 days. The slower metabolism of the tricyclic antidepressants may lead to a toxic reaction from these medications up to 1 or 2 weeks after a particular dose level is achieved. The potential harm from elevated levels of tricyclic antidepressants can be avoided by gradual, stepwise increase in their dosage.

Simplification of the Therapeutic Regimen

To avoid potential noncompliance with a suggested therapeutic regimen, the physician should inform both the patient and a relative or friend of the dose schedule for a particular medication. This is especially true when the older adult exhibits any kind of memory disturbance or is considered to be at risk for poor compliance with prescribed medication regimens. Compliance may be enhanced by the use of memory aids, such as a medication calendar or diary. These aids range from a partitioned container for each day of the week to more complicated dispensers, such as those used to dispense birth control pills. Compliance can often be facilitated by prescribing the medication as infrequently during the day as possible. Compliance decreases in proportion to the number of times per day a given medication is prescribed. With many of the antidepressant drugs, especially the tricyclic antidepressants, the usual practice of prescribing the entire dose at night may not be feasible because of potential for side effects the following morning. If dosage must be divided, giving the drug in the morning and evening is the best alternative. On the other hand, patients often complain of drowsiness in the morning when they receive medication at that time.

Although physicians are not responsible for dispensing medications, it is essential that the physician coordinate his or her activities with the local pharmacist. Pill containers should be labeled so that they can be read by the older adult. In addition, it is difficult if not impossible for the frail or arthritic older person to open child-safe pill bottles. Both the physician and pharamcist should encourage patients to destroy or return all medications that are not currently being used, except for prescriptions taken "as needed." For the patient who may be more seriously depressed, the physician can coordinate with the pharmacist to dispense only a 1-week supply at a time (so that the potential for an overdose is reduced). Once a patient is admitted to the hospital, the physician should urge family members to bring all medications to the hospital. All expired prescriptions should be destroyed with the permission of patient.

Regular Review of Compliance and Plasma Level Determination

Each time the depressed patient returns to the physician's office, a careful review of both medication compliance and change in symptoms should be initiated. A significant breakthrough in the past 20 years has been the availability of therapeutic blood levels for the tricyclic antidepressants. A number of factors contribute to the plasma concentration of the tricyclic antidepressants, such as the half-life of the drug. For example, desipramine has a half-life of 17 hours, whereas desmethyl-doxepin (a metabolite of doxepin) has a half-life of 51 hours, which may increase to even higher levels in the elderly. Other factors include liver metabolism, plasma binding, and even genetic factors (e.g., blood levels are frequently similar in twins and race—blacks may have higher levels per dose than whites) (Amsterdam et al, 1980). Steady-state plasma levels in adults, when input equals output, can be calculated by multiplying the half-life of the drug by five. Older patients show higher steady-state plasma levels of tricyclic antidepressants than do persons at other stages of life and older persons may respond at lower plasma levels. Prescription of lithium carbonate without regular checks of blood levels is ill-advised.

The availability of laboratory testing for plasma levels should not be abused, however. Generally, a check of the level should not take place until the patient has been on a fixed oral dose of the mediation for 5 to 7 days (except when a test dose is given, as described in a later section). Unfortunately, many physicians are reluctant to check plasma levels because of complaints that venipuncture is painful and may leave a disfiguring hematoma in a frail elder. An experienced technician who has worked frequently with the older adult can usually avoid these difficulties. Physicians are often not the best persons to perform the venipuncture.

Monitoring for Side Effects

The most common side effects of medications used to treat depression are the anticholinergic effects, which include mouth dryness, constipation, urinary retention, tachycardia, blurred vision, exacerbation of acute narrow-angle glaucoma, inhibition of sweating, and impotence. More serious side effects include confusion, increased agitation, and the precipitation of a bundle branch block (see discussion later in this section). The central anticholinergic syndromes consist of psychotic thoughts accompanied by symptoms of confusion and agitation, flushing, and dryness of the skin. Recognizing the side effects of anticholinergic overdose is important, especially in the emergency room, since the injection of physostigmine (1 or 2 mg im every 30 minutes) quickly reverses the effects.

Patients with psychotic depressive disorders in late life may be treated concurrently with tricyclic antidepressants and neuroleptics. Therefore clinicians must be aware of the potential for the older adult to develop parkinsonian side effects, mainly manifested by akathisia and dyskinesia. A more consequential adverse effect of all neuroleptics is the development of tardive dyskinesia. Amoxapine, an antidepressant occasionally used in older adults, may lead to phenothiazine-like side effects given its similarity in structure to the phenothiazines.

Although symptoms of withdrawal of tricyclic antidepressants have received less attention in the literature than the potentially dangerous consequences of withdrawal of other agents, such as phenobarbital or the benzodiazepines, they must not be neglected. Abrupt withdrawal of drugs with significant anticholinergic properties can lead to a cholinergic rebound. Symptoms include diffuse sweating, diarrhea, agitation, and occasional confusion. These symptoms may be mistaken for a worsening of the underlying psychiatric condition, which in turn leads to continued use of the pharmacologic agents—a use that may not be indicated.

■ MEDICATION USED TO TREAT DEPRESSIVE DISORDERS

Tricyclic Antidepressants

The tricyclic antidepressants have been the first-line pharmacologic treatment of major depressive disorders since their discovery in the late 1950s. Even with the advent of newer agents, the tricyclic antidepressants remain the drugs of choice. Gershon et al (1988) identified 20 control studies in the literature that document the efficacy of the tricyclic antidepressants in treating depression in late life. Yet older persons tolerate the tricyclic antidepressants poorly. They have a high incidence of side effects, such as hypotension, urinary retention, confusion, constipation, and glaucoma. Plasma levels of the antidepressant medications have been demonstrated to predict response to treatment in older persons (Nelson et al, 1985).

Schneider et al (1987) found that the use of a single dose of nortriptyline in depressed elderly outpatients could help identify the optimum dosage of the medication. Physicians should start with a 25-mg test dose, draw a therapeutic plasma level the next morning, and then begin 75 mg daily, adjusting the dose when the results of the plasma level return. They suggest a range of dosage from less than 50 mg to 125 mg daily. In another study (Schneider et al, 1986), investigators found that pretreatment orthostatic change in systolic blood pressure among older subjects suffering unipolar depression was correlated with improvement in depression. Despite the blood pressure response to a single dose of nortriptyline, no episodes of symptomatic orthostatic hypertension occurred when the subjects were treated with nortriptyline.

Few investigators have examined the long-term effects of tricyclic antidepressants in preventing the recurrence of depression in older adults. Georgotas et al (1988) followed a group of older persons treated with either nortriptyline or phenelzine in a double-blind study from 4 to 8 months. Over this period, 72% remained well, 18% suffered a relapse, 5% dropped out of the study because of side effects to the medication, and 5% were prematurely terminated in a good condition. There was no difference in the therapeutic outcome in these studies by drug, except that all patients who dropped out were on phenelzine and the phenelzine group was more likely to require dose reduction. In a follow-up to this study, Georgotas et al (1988) blindly discontinued the nortriptyline and phenelzine for 1 year after the subjects were on the drugs for a number of months. Patients on phenelzine had a 13% recurrence rate, whereas patients on nortriptyline and placebo had a 54% and 65% recurrence rates, respectively. These findings suggest that giving a tricyclic antidepressant for longer than 8 months may not be as helpful in preventing a recurrence of late life depression as a monomine-oxidase inhibitor (MAOI). One possible reason for the lack of efficacy of nortriptyline in preventing a recurrence is the accumulation of the metabolite 10-OH-nortriptyline, which increases with age. This metabolite at high levels may reduce the antidepressant effect.

Nortriptyline and desipramine are the tricyclic antidepressants most frequently used in the treatment of older adults. As noted previously, these drugs are prescribed because of a more favorable side-effect profile rather than having any greater therapeutic efficacy than other tricyclic antidepressants. The anticholinergic side effects of amitriptyline and imipramine are the primary reasons these drugs are used less frequently in the treatment of older adults. Doxepin hydrochloride has also been popular for treating older patients with depression. The antianxiety activity, decreased anticholinergic properties, and relative absence of electrocardiographic changes render this drug an attractive alternative (Burrows et al, 1976).

Other than anticholinergic effects, the side effect of most concern when using cyclic antidepressants is cardiovascular effects. Glassman et al (1983) studied in detail the effects of imipramine on cardiovascular function. They found the ejection fraction unchanged in depressed patients with left ventricular disease who were treated with imipramine, but these patients were at increased risk for experiencing orthostasis. Roose et al (1986) found nortriptyline to be a relatively safe treatment for depression in patients with left ventricular impairment. The ejection fraction was unchanged by nortriptyline and orthostasis was less prevalent than in patients treated with imipramine. Left ventricular impairment in both studies was defined by a history of congestive heart failure or an enlarged heart on x-ray film.

Rodstein and Oei (1979) investigated the long-term side effects of the tricyclic antidepressants in older patients. They found, in 32 patients studied for an average of 37 weeks, that T-wave inversion was present in two patients and some subjects experienced intermittent left bundle branch block. One subject experienced tachycardia. Hayes et al (1983) also found that heart rate can increase with imipramine and that conduction time can increase as well. Veith et al (1982) confirmed the findings of Glassman and

Roose and also found that premature ventricular contractions were reduced by imipramine but not by doxepin.

Another side effect that receives less attention in the literature but nevertheless is of great importance is the effect of antidepressants on human performance (Deptula and Pomara, 1990). As a rule, older persons are more sensitive to the adverse effects on performance by antidepressant medications. Friedman et al (1966) studied the effects of a single dose of imipramine on a battery of psychomotor tests on older adults. They conclude that imipramine did not consistently affect performance, yet note a trend for imipramine to improve performance on some psychomotor perceptual tasks while impairing performance on abstraction and vigilance tasks. The relevance of singledose studies to the use of medications over time must be questioned, however. Seppala and Linnoila (1983) suggest that tolerance to antidepressant-induced psychomotor impairment might follow multiple doses of the drug over time. Single-dose studies also must take into account that the potential problems inherent in the medications themselves may be balanced by improvement in performance resulting from the treatment of the illness in clinical populations.

Anticholinergic effects from taking these medications are well known and include dry mouth, urinary retention, constipation, confusion, and impaired visual accommodation. If the effects become severe, they may lead to memory loss, psychotic thoughts, hyperthermia, and exacerbation of narrow-angle glaucoma. Antiadrenergic effects are predominantly those of orthostatic hypotension, and the primary antihistaminic effect is sedation. Other side effects that have been reported include weight gain, fine motor tremor, liver toxicity, decreased libido, impaired sexual functioning, and a lowered seizure threshold. In older adult outpatients treated with tricyclic antidepressants, Stein et al (1985) report that 38% reported a decrease of appetite and 34% had a craving for sweets.

Clinicians must also be aware of the side effects that occur with withdrawal from tricyclic antidepressants (Dilsaver and Greden, 1983). The most common syndrome is general somatic or gastrointestinal distress, with or without anxiety and agitation, excessive and vivid dreaming, initial and middle insomnia, movement disorder, and behavioral activation. A "cholinergic overdrive hypothesis" explains most of the phenomena witnessed with the withdrawal of tricyclic antidepressant medications.

Two other cyclic (but not tricyclic antidepressants can be used to treat depressed older adults. Maprotiline was compared with doxepin in a double-blind study among 49 elderly patients (Ahles et al, 1984). Maprotiline was associated with a decrease in periventricular contractions (PVCs) in subjects with a high baseline rate in comparison with doxepin, which was associated with an increase in PVCs. There was no difference between the two drugs in orthostatic blood pressure changes. The authors therefore conclude that maprotiline, similar to imipramine, may have an antiarrhythmic effect that could be beneficial in the treatment of depression when the patient is suffering concomitant periventricular contractions. Maprotiline is a tetracyclic antidepressant and may have an increased risk of seizures compared with other cyclic antidepressants.

Amoxapine is a dibenzoxazepine tricyclic that blocks both norepinephrine and dopamine and therefore exhibits antipsychotic activity, which is unique to the tricyclic antidepressants (Hayes and Kristoff, 1986). The drug, unfortunately, also has a number of side effects not typical of the tricyclic antidepressants, such as hyperprolactemia, galactorrhea, parkinsonian symptoms, dystonias, and even dyskinesia. Amoxapine is thought to have an earlier onset of therapeutic effects. Given that the relative prevalence of psychotic depression in older persons has increased, amoxapine would appear to be a reasonable antidepressant choice in this depressive subtype. The drug, however, has not been demonstrated to be more effective than other antidepressants in treating the depression in older adults. Antidepressants in general are not as effective in treating psychotic depression.

Clomipramine, although only recently introduced in the United States, has been used worldwide for a number of years. In a number of studies the drug has been shown to be effective in treating obsessive-compulsive disorders. Clomipramine is also an antidepressant agent (although it is not approved for marketing as an antidepressant). Clomipramine has significant anticholinergic effects and can lead to postural hypotension and therefore has many of the adverse side effects that are especially troublesome in older persons. The older person with significant obsessive thinking who is otherwise healthy and experiences depressed mood may be a candidate for clomipramine. Dosage is in the range of imipramine.

Monoamine-Oxidase Inhibitors

Phenelzine sulfate, tranylcypromine sulfate, and isocarboxazid are the most commonly used monoamine-oxidase inhibitors (MAOI) in the United States. As described previously (see Chapter 4), the increased monoamine-oxidase activity that accompanies the aging process suggests that these agents may be useful in treating depression in the elderly (Robinson et al, 1972). These agents, however, are a second choice to the tricyclic antidepressants because of their propensity to interact with other drugs, their ability to produce a hypertensive crisis when combined with foods with a high tyramine content, and their rare production of acute hepatic insufficiency. Drugs with which the MAOI can interact adversely include ephedrine, methylphenidate, phenylephrine, and other sympathomimetic medications. If a hypertensive crisis results from MAOI, it should be treated with an alpha blocker, such as phentolamine or with a calcium-channel blocker, such as nifedipine, which should be crushed in the mouth before being swallowed. Earlier reports suggest that adverse reactions, including a hypertensive crisis, may result if MAOI are used in conjunction with the tricyclic antidepressants (Spiker and Pugh, 1976).

Other problems arise with the use of MAOI as well. Salzman (1986) suggests that MAOI should not be used in the elderly who are depressed and have moderate or severe cognitive impairment because these drugs tend to lead to increased agitation, confusion, and restlessness and may lead to paranoid thoughts. In addition, MAOI should not be used in a severe depression that may require electroconvulsive therapy (ECT). The interaction of the MAOI with the short-acting anesthetic agents and neuromuscular blockers (Nardil) inhibits cholinesterase required for ECT, at least 10 days are required off the medication before ECT; 10 days that not only add to increased hospital expense but also to the risk of an adverse outcome from the depression. (Parnate has been cleared for use with ECT.)

Jenike (1984) suggests that tranylcypromine is preferrable to phenelzine because it is a reversible enzyme blocker. When discontinued, tranylcypromine is out of the system within 24 hours. The usual dose of tranylcypromine is 10 mg bid, compared with 15 mg bid for phenelzine. A newer agent, not currently on the market, is moclobemide, a reversible MAOI. Few dietary restrictions are necessary. The drug also leads to fewer side effects, especially agitation and insomnia. This drug has not been demonstrated to be an effective antidepressant in late life. L-deprenyl is a MAOI that is used to delay the onset of disability in Parkinson's disease.

The use of MAOI by elderly persons has been scanty and little evidence exists to either confirm or refute therapeutic efficacy in the elderly. MAOIs should therefore not be the first or even second choice antidepressants selected but may be prescribed if the tricyclic drugs and new generative nontricyclic drugs are ineffective. Ashford and Ford (1979) treated 14 elderly patients with tranylcypromine or phenelzine. Patients with depression associated with dementia showed significant remission of depressive symptoms. Of the nine nondemented patients, three with unipolar depressive symptoms responded as well, whereas those with bipolar symptoms responded poorly. Yet, as with other tricyclic antidepressant trials, demented patients demonstrated little change in their cognitive functioning. Using MAOI has been proposed as the treatment of a typical depression with concomitant symptoms of hysteric or somatization disorder (Quitken et al, 1979). The atypical symptom complex (a depression associated with increased sleep and increased appetite) is relatively uncommon in older adults.

The therapeutic effectiveness of some MAOI is believed to be directly related to the ability of these agents to inhibit monoamine oxidase. The degree of inhibition can be determined by obtaining platelet monoamine-oxidase levels before and after the institution of MAOI. A blood sample should be drawn for platelet monoamine oxidase before institution of the drug. After the patient has been on the medication from 10 days to 2 weeks, a second blood draw is performed. Proper dose levels should lead to an 80% to 90% inhibition of baseline monoamine-oxidase levels.

New Generation Antidepressants

A number of new antidepressant agents have been introduced during the past 10 years. More than one has been thought to be especially applicable to treating older adults, primarily because of a decreased side-effect profile. The first to be introduced was trazodone, a triazolo-pyridone antidepressant with very little anticholinergic activity and a low level of cardiotoxicity. Obvious advantages to such a drug would be the decreased possibility for exacerbation of glaucoma, arrhythmias, and protostatic hypertrophy in the elderly. Although the specific mechanism of action of trazodone is not known, it may be related to the formation of active metabolites, such as M-chlorophenylpiperazine (CPP). Trazodone is also a selective serotonin reuptake inhibitor. Steady-state plasma levels per dose are higher than traditional tricyclic antidepressants. In 11 elderly depressed patients, Montleone et al (1989) found that the steady-state plasma concentration of 650 ng/ml was identified as a threshold value for good antidepressant response. Usual dose in these patients was 150 mg per day, and there was no correlation between side effects and the plasma levels.

Gerner et al (1980), in a double-blind study of 60 elderly patients compared trazodone with imipramine. They found similar therapeutic efficacy and fewer side effects with the trazodone group (specifically cardiovascular and anticholinergic side effects). Klein and Muller (1985), however, found trazodone to be not as effective in treating endogenous depression but as effective in nonendogenous depression as the tricyclics.

Trazodone is not without its adverse effects. The main cardiovascular effects are orthostatic hypotension and dizziness. The drug produces minimal effects on cardiac conduction and does not produce significant EKG changes but does not have the antiarrhythmic effect of imipramine. Priapism is a unique adverse effect of this drug compared with the other antidepressants and may be so severe as to require surgery. Perhaps the most troublesome side effect of trazodone for older adults is sedation. When all of the drug is taken at night, older persons often experience a considerable hangover when arising in the morning. The drug is relatively safe for suicidal elders, however, in that limited symptoms are associated with even a significant overdose of the drug.

Among the new generative antidepressants, fluoxetine has received the most attention. The easy dosing of the drug (20 mg per day, usually given in the morning), the relative absence of anticholinergic and antihistaminic side effects, the lack of a propensity to lead to weight gain (as is typical of tricyclic antidepressants), and a significant initial therapeutic effect has led to widespread use of this medication. The significant therapeutic effect has often been described by patients, regardless of age, as a "wow" effect. Patients described a dramatic benefit much more clearly with fluoxetine than with other antidepressant agents.

Fluoxetine, however, is associated with a number of problems that may be especially troublesome for older persons. The drug leads to significant agitation in selected patients (perhaps as many as 20% to 30% of individuals taking the drug). This agitation probably accounts for the episodic reports of suicide and even homicides by individuals taking the medication. There is no objective evidence, however, suggesting that suicides and/or aggressive behavior are more common with fluoxetine than other antidepressant agents.

A major concern in prescribing fluoxetine to older persons is the extremely long half-life and the availability (as of this writing) of only one dose form (20 mg). If the drug leads to the onset of described side effects, then discontinuation does not lead to remission of the side effects for as long as 7 to 10 days. Because of the long half-life, the steady-state plasma level in older adults may not be achieved for 2 to 3 weeks after initial prescription of the medication and therefore side effects may not be attributed to the medication initially. These problems can in part be avoided by either spacing the dosing of the drug more infrequently (i.e., giving the drug every other day or every third day). In addition, the capsule can be opened and the contents placed in fruit juice and stored in the refrigerator. The patient can then take one half or one third of the dose daily, depending on the therapeutic needs. A liquid form is now available as well. One study (Feighrer et al, 1985) documents the effectiveness of fluoxetine in older depressed persons, but it has not been demonstrated to be more effective than the tricyclic antidepressants.

Bupropion is a unique antidepressant agent, a unicyclic phenylaminoketone. The drug produces few anticholinergic effects and virtually no sedation or effects on blood pressure. It does not inhibit monoamine oxidase nor the reuptake of norepinephrine and serotonin and does not appear to down-regulate to the beta-adrenergic receptor system. It does down-regulate the locus ceruleus and leads to decreased catecholamine turnover. The effect also may be related to its action as a relatively weak presynaptic dopamine-reuptake blocker. As with fluoxetine, bupropion does produce more agitation and excitement than the tricyclic antidepressants and does not lead to weight gain. The most serious side effect of the medication is a dose-related seizure although the drug may also produce psychoses in persons with a previous history of psychosis. Usual dose begins with 75 mg twice a day, increasing to a maximum of 450 mg per day.

Branconnier et al (1983) studied 63 elders on bupropion versus imipramine (the dose being 150 mg to 450 mg a day). Bupropion was as effective as imipramine, and the higher the dose, the more rapid the onset of the antidepressant and anxiolitic activity. Sedation and anticholinergic effects were not observed. Kane et al (1983) also studied 38 patients in a double-blind study, 55 years of age and older, on bupropion versus imipramine. Similar results were found. One practical difficulty in prescribing bupropion is the requirement of multiple daily doses, which reduces compliance.

■ ADJUNCTS TO ANTIDEPRESSANT THERAPY

The pharmacologic activity of drugs such as amphetamine and dextroamphetamine would suggest that these drugs should be beneficial for treating the depressed. The agents cause an outpouring of catecholamine from the presynaptic terminal into the synaptic cleft. Unfortunately, the general and almost uncontrollable excitement precipitated by excess use of these agents make their clinical use problematic. Nevertheless, a number of clinicians have reported the therapeutic efficacy of methylphenidate for reversing apathetic behavior in depressed elders (Crook, 1979). Data on prescribing from the National Disease and Therapeutic Index a few years ago suggest that more than 20% of the outpatients with prescriptions for methylphenidate are persons 65 of age and older. Used in low dosage, methylphenidate may provide an alternative therapeutic agent in patients susceptible to the anticholinergic side effects of tricyclics and for other reasons cannot be treated with antidepressant medication (Katon and Raskind, 1980). Methylphenidate may be especially useful for apathetic depressed elders in nursing homes. Despite the high risk for addiction in some younger persons, doses of 5 to 10 mg given once a day to elders rarely lead to adverse side effects or addiction.

Prange et al (1971) report that the addition of low doses of triiodothyronine (T3) to the tricyclic antidepressants potentiates the therapeutic response of these agents in women. Referring to a number of their laboratory studies, they document a significant connection between thyroid functioning, catecholamines, and the hypothalamus. Although thyroid function does change with age, there have been no studies suggesting the unique therapeutic efficacy of triiodothyronine for treating the depressed elderly. Patients with depressive mood secondary to subclinical hypothyroidism, however, are best treated by correcting the thyroid dysfunction.

Still further studies suggest that the benzodiazepine antianxiety agent alprazolam may be effective in treating persons with reactive or neurotic depression. Pitts et al (1983) studied alprazolam in an open trial of persons 56 to 78 years of age. Two thirds of these depressed inpatients showed a 50% or more increase on the Hamilton Depression Rating Scale with alprazolam therapy. Initial drowsiness was the only side effect observed. In general, however, for more severe depressions, alprazolam would not be considered the drug of choice for treating depression in older adults, not only because of a paucity of studies documenting its therapeutic efficacy but also because of the potential for addiction and the masking of certain symptoms of depression that respond to traditional antidepressant therapy, such as agitation.

■ MOOD-STABILIZING AGENTS

A significant breakthrough in the therapy of manic-depressive illness occurred with the introduction of lithium carbonate. Lithium is proven to be of benefit in both the treatment and prevention of manic attacks in bipolar mood disorders and has been demonstrated, to a lesser degree, to be effective in preventing recurrent attacks of depression in unipolar mood disorders (Coppen et al, 1971). Many late life depressive episodes are recurrent episodes and therefore, lithium has become a popular means of therapeutic management. In addition, the inability to distinguish dysphoric and agitated manic episodes from agitated depressive episodes in some older adults renders a therapeutic trial on lithium in such circumstances a useful diagnostic test. Coppen et al (1983) found lithium carbonate as effective a prophylactic in elderly patients as they originally demonstrated in younger patients. In contrast to the usual recommended therapeutic plasma level of 0.8 to 1.2 μmol/L, they found an excellent response to lithium in patients 70 years of age and older with plasma levels of 0.5 to 0.7 μmol/L.

The major concern with lithium treatment is toxic side effects. There is a narrow margin of safety between the therapeutic range and the toxic range that requires the physician to monitor older patients taking lithium carbonate carefully. Roose et al (1979) found that, among patients older than 60 years who were receiving maintenance lithium therapy, 13% developed lithium toxicity during an 18-month follow-up. This was significantly greater than for younger patients. In addition, 16% had abnormal electrocardiographic tracings, consisting of arrhythmias, such as sinus bradycardia, sinus tacycardia, and frequent premature atrial contractions. The cause of these adverse effects is not known but may result from the increased sensitivity to lithium and/or the decreased renal clearance of lithium leading to higher plasma levels. Slater et al (1984) did not find, in 66 outpatients, that age was associated with higher blood levels of lithium when persons were given similar doses based on their weight. On the other hand, Shulman et al (1987) found the elderly, compared with younger persons, showed a 45% reduction in the mean renal clearance and 25% prolongation of the elimination half-life of lithium. They suspected this was due to the reduction in the mean volume of distribution (a reduction of 23% in older persons).

Less severe adverse side effects of lithium carbonate include epigastric discomfort, fine hand tremor, fatigue, drowsiness, polyuria, and polydipsia. Lithium may exacerbate the essential tremor associated with aging. The tremor, however, can be treated with propanolol. Weight gain is a long-term side effect. The most serious side effects, suggesting a toxic reaction to lithium, are nausea and vomiting, cogwheel rigidity, aphasia, delirium, impaired cognitive functioning, an unsteady gate, muscle twitching, slurred speech, and seizures. Once lithium toxicity appears, a vicious cycle may occur with lithium affecting renal function, thus decreasing clearance. The appropriate treatment of severe lithium toxicity is renal dialysis.

Thyroid dysfunction is another side effect with lithium carbonate and may be more common in women than in men, especially those with a history of thyrotoxicosis. The result is a nontoxic goiter and hypothyroidism, which can be treated with replacement thyroid.

Lithium may interact with other drugs. The most significant interaction is with diuretics that decrease the volume of distribution and therefore increase the risk of toxicity. The mixture of lithium and haloperidol may lead to an exacerbation of extrapyramidal effects and delirium has been reported in isolated cases (Miller et al, 1986).

In treating older adults, renal clearance should be estimated before the administration of lithium carbonate, especially in the frail elderly (Rosenbaum, 1985; Shulman et al, 1987). Lithium clearance can be estimated by a obtaining plasma creatinine level and a 24-hour urine creatinine and calculating clearance through usual formulas. Once the individual on lithium has reached a steady-state plasma concentration and exhibits no adverse effects, lithium levels should be checked initially every 3 weeks and later every 3 to 6 months. Thyroid function should be checked every 6 months initially and thereafter every year. An EKG should be obtained before and after institution of lithium therapy to determine whether the individual suffers from a sick sinus syndrome (an absolute contraindication to lithium therapy) and the effects of lithium on the electrocardiograph.

In recent studies, investigators have explored the use of lithium as an augmentation to antidepressant therapy (Heninger et al, 1983). VanMarwijk et al (1990) performed a retrospective review of 51 geriatric patients in a Dutch psychiatric hospital who were prescribed lithium in addition to the cyclic antidepressants. A response was seen in 65% of the patients. For patients with recurrent depressive episodes, a statistical trend was found toward more responders with more complete responses, compared with patients with first-episode depressions. About 20% of these patients, however, experienced severe side effects from the combination. Kushner (1986) studied the combination of low-dose lithium therapy and antidepressant drugs in physically ill geriatric inpatients (five case reports). He found that lasting remissions of depression could be obtained through this combination of medications, especially when serum levels were kept low (between 0.15 and 0.4 μmol/L).

In rapidly cycling recurrent depressive disorders and other treatment-resistant disorders a number of additional combinations have been suggested. Most of these studies have not focused specifically on the elderly. Kramlinger and Post (1989) studied the addition of lithium to carbamazepine in individuals who were treatmentresistant major depressives. Approximately 53% responded with a moderate to marked improvement.

Lithium carbonate is the primary drug used to control manic episodes regardless of age, yet other drugs have been increasingly used to treat manic episodes in recent years. These drugs are used alone or are used in combination with lithium carbonate. Post et al (1987) studied the use of carbamazepine in doses averaging over 1200 mg per day and blood levels averaging 10.4 mg/dl. Clinical improvement in mood and psychomotor components of the manic syndrome was rapid in onset and generally paralleled improvement observed in patients previously treated with neuroleptics (the standard treatment for acute manic episodes). These data, according to the authors, suggest that many of the predictors of poor response to lithium carbonate (e.g., manic severity, anxiety and dysphoria, rapid cycling, and a negative family history) may be associated with a good response to carbamazepine.

Valproate acid or valproate is another drug that has been used to treat acute manic episodes. Pope et al (1991) conducted a placebo-controlled, double-blind study of valproate in patients with acute manic episodes. Patients treated with valproate reported a 54% mean decrease in their manic symptoms compared with a 5% decrease in controls. Valproate has been especially suggested as being effective in treating so-called organic mood syndromes with manic symptoms. The drug is a simple-branched chain carboxylic acid that is primarily used in the treatment of epilepsy. Valproate is generally well tolerated with the most common side effects being gastrointestinal symptoms, sedation, increased appetite and weight gain, hair loss, tremor, and ataxia.

Hepatic amino transferase enzymes can be elevated with use of valproate, but after the studies, patients generally are medically asymptomatic when such elevations occur. Nevertheless, hepatotoxicity should be monitored with the use of valproate. Usual dose of valproate in younger patients is 250 mg three times per day. Dosage should be adjusted to keep serum concentration between 50 and 100 mg/L. Unfortunately, there are no studies in the literature to date reporting the effectiveness and the proper dosing of valproate in older adults.

REFERENCES

Ahles S, Gwirtzman H, Hilaris A, Sha P, Schwarcz G, et al: Comparative cardiac effects of maprotiline and doxepin in elderly depressed patients, *Journal of Clinical Psychiatry* 45:460-465, 1984.

Amsterdam J, Brunswick D, Mendels J: The clinical application of tricyclic antidepressant pharmacokinetics in plasma levels, *American Journal of Psychiatry* 137:653, 1980.

Ashford W, Ford CV: Use of monoamine oxidase inhibitors in elderly patients, *American Journal of Psychiatry* 136:1466-1467, 1979.

Branconnier RJ, Cole JO, Ghazviain S, Spera KF, Oxenkrug GF, et al: Clinical pharmacology of buproprion and imipramine in elderly depressives, *Journal of Clinical Psychiatry* 44:130-133, 1983.

Burgen ASU, Mitchell JF: *Gaddums' Pharmacology.* New York, Oxford University Press, 1978.

Burrows GD, Vorha J, Dumovic P, Maguire K, Scoggins BA, et al: Tricyclic antidepressant drugs in cardiac conduction, *Progress in Neuropsychopharmacology* 1:329-334, 1977.

Coppen A, et al: Prophylactic lithium in affective disorder, *Lancet* 2:275, 1971.

Coppen A, et al: Decreasing lithium dosage reduces morbidity and side-effects during prophylaxis. *Journal of Affective Disorders* 5:353-362, 1983.

Crook T: Central-nervous-system stimulants: a primer of use in geropsychiatric patients, *Journal of the American Geriatrics Society* 27:476-479, 1979.

Deptula D, Pomara N: Effects of antidepressants on human performance: a review, *Journal of Clinical Psychopharmacology* 10:105-111, 1990.

Dilsaver SC, Greden JF: Antidepressant withdrawal phenomenon, *Biological Psychiatry* 19:237-256, 1984.

Feighner JP, Cohn JB: Double-blind comparative trials of fluoxetine and doxepin in geriatric patients with major depressive disorders, *Journal of Clinical Psychiatry* 46:20-25, 1985.

Friedman AS, Granick S, Cohen HW, Cowitz B: Imipramine (tofanil) versus placebo in hospitalized psychotic depressives (a comparison of patients' selfratings, psychiatrists' ratings, and psychological test scores), *Journal of Psychiatric Research* 4:13-66, 1966.

Georgotas A, McCue RE, Cooper TB, Nagachandran N, Chang I: How effective and safe is continuation therapy in elderly depressed patients?—As factors affecting relapse rate, *Archives of General Psychiatry* 45:929-932, 1988.

Georgotas A, McCue RE, Cooper TB: A placebo-controlled comparison of nortriptyline and phenelzine in maintenance therapy of elderly depressed patients, *Archives of General Psychiatry* 46:783-786, 1989.

Gerner R, Esterbrook W, Steuer J, Jarvik L: Treatment of geriatric depression with trazodone, imipramine, and placebo: a double-blind study, *Journal of Clinical Psychiatry* 41:216-221, 1980.

Gershon SC, Plotkin DA, Jarvik LF: Antidepressant drug studies, 1964-1986: empirical evidence for aging patients, *Journal of Clinical Psychopharmacology* 8:311-322, 1988.

Glassman AH, Johnson LL, Giardina EV, Walsh T, Roose SP, et al: The use of imipramine in depressed patients with congestive heart failure, *Journal of the American Medical Association* 250:1997-2001, 1983.

Hayes PE, Kristoff CA: Adverse reactions to five new antidepressants, *Clinical Pharmacy* 5:471-480, 1986.

Hayes RL, Gerner RH, Fairbanks L, Moran R, Waltuch L: ECG findings in geriatric depressives given trazodone, placebo or imipramine, *Journal of Clinical Psychiatry* 44:180-183, 1983.

Helling DK, Lempke JH, Semla TP, Wallace RB, Lipson DP, et al: Medication use characteristics in the elderly: the Iowa 65+ rural health study, *Journal of the American Geriatrics Society* 35:4-12, 1987.

Heninger GR, Charney DS, Sternberg DE: Lithium carbonate augmentation of antidepressant treatment, *Archives of General Psychiatry* 40:1335-1339, 1983.

Jenike MA: The use of monoamine oxidase inhibitors in the treatment of elderly, depressed patients, *Journal of the American Geriatrics Society* 32:571-575, 1984.

Kane JM, Cole K, Sarantakos S, Howard A, Borenstein M: Safety and efficacy of buproprion in elderly patients: preliminary observations, *Journal of Clinical Psychiatry* 44:134-136, 1983.

Katon W, Raskind M: Treatment of depression in the medically-ill elderly with methylphenidate, *American Journal of Psychiatry* 137:963-967, 1980.

Klein HE, Muller N: Trazodone and endogenous depressed patients: a negative report and critical evaluation of the pertaining literature, *Progress in Neuro-psychopharmacology and Biological Psychiatry* 8:173-186, 1985.

Kramlinger KG, Post RM: The addition of lithium to carbomazepine: antidepressant efficacy in treatment-resistant depression, *Archives of General Psychiatry* 46:794-800, 1989.

Kushner SL: Lithium-antidepressant combinations in the treatment of depressed, physically ill geriatric patients, *American Journal of Psychiatry* 143:378-379, 1986.

Lundin DV: Medication-taking behavior of the elderly: a pilot study, *Drug Intelligence and Clinical Pharmacology* 12:518, 1978.

Miller F, Menninger J, Whitcup SM: Lithium-neuroleptic neurotoxicity in the elderly bipolar patient, *Journal of Clinical Psychopharmacology* 6:176-178, 1986.

Montleone P, Gnocchi G, Delrio G: Plasma and trazodone concentrations and clinical response in elderly depressed patients: a preliminary study, *Journal of Clinical Psychopharmacology* 9:284-287, 1989.

Nelson JC, Jatlow PI, Mazur EC: Desipramine plasma levels and response in elderly melancholic patients, *Journal of Clinical Psychopharmacology* 5:217-220, 1985.

O'Hanlan W: Driving skills and antidepressant therapy: an age comparison, *Proceedings of the Congress International Neuropsychopharmacology* (CINP), Munch, West Germany, 1988.

Physicians' Desk Reference (ed 44). Gradell, New Jersey, Medical Economics, 1990.

Pitts WM, Fann WE, Sajadi C, Snyder S: Alprazolam in older depressed inpatients, *Journal of Clinical Psychiatry* 44:213-215, 1983.

Pope HG, McElroy SL, Keck PE, Hudson JI: Valproate in the treatment of acute mania: a placebo-controlled study, *Archives of General Psychiatry* 48:62-68, 1991.

Post RM, Uhde TW, Roy-Byrne PP, Joffe RT: Correlates of antimanic response to carbomazepine, *Psychiatry Research* 21:71-83, 1987.

Prange AJ, Wilson IC, Knox A, McClane TK, Lipton MA: Enhancement of imipramine by thyroid-stimulating hormones: clinical and theoretical implications, *American Journal of Psychiatry* 127:191-199, 1971.

Quitkin F, Rifkin A, Klein DF: Monoamine oxidase inhibitors: a review of antidepressant effectiveness, *Archives of General Psychiatry* 36:749, 1979.

Robinson DS, Nies A, Davis JM, Bunney WE, Davis JM, et al: Aging: monoamines, and monoamine oxidase levels, *Lancet* 1:290-291, 1972.

Rodstein M, Oei LS: Cardiovascular side effects of long-term therapy with tricyclic antidepressants in the aged, *Journal of the American Geriatrics Society* 27:231-234, 1979.

Roose SP, Bone S, Haidorfer C, Dunner D, Fieve RR: Lithium treatment in older patients, *American Journal of Psychiatry* 136:843-844, 1979.

Roose SP, Glassman AH, Giardina EV, Johnson LL, Walsh BT et al: Nortriptyline in depressed patients with left ventricular impairment, *Journal of the American Medical Association* 256:3253-3257, 1986.

Rosenbaum A: Lithium use in geriatric patients, *Geriatric Medicine Today* 4:95-99, 1985.

Rowe JW, Andres R, Tobin JD, Norris AH, Shock NW: The effect of age on creatinine clearance in man: a cross-sectional and longitudinal study, *Journal of Gerontology* 31:155-163, 1976.

Salzman C: Caution urged in using monoamine oxidase inhibitors for the elderly (letter to the editor), *American Journal of Psychiatry* 143:118-119, 1986.

Schneider LS, Cooper TB, Staples FR, Sloane RB: Prediction of individual dosage of nortriptyline in depressed elderly outpatients, *Journal of Clinical Psychopharmacology* 7:311-314, 1987.

Schneider LS, Sloane RB, Staples FR, Bender M: Pre-treatment orthostatic hypotension as a predictor of response to nortriptyline in geriatric depression, *Journal of Clinical Psychopharmacology* 6:172-176, 1986.

Seppala T, Linnoila M: Effects of zimeldine and other antidepressants on skilled performance: a comprehensive review, *Acta Psychiatrica Scandinavica* 68:135-140, 1983.

Shulman KI, MacKenzie S, Hardy B: The clinical use of lithium carbonate in old age: a review, *Progress in Neuropsychopharmacology and Biological Psychiatry* 11:159-164, 1987.

Slater M, Milanes F, Talcott V, Okafor KC: Influence of age on lithium therapy, *Southern Medical Journal* 77:153-158, 1984.

Slotkin, TA, Whitmore WL, Dew KL, Kilts CD: Reduced inhibitory effects of imipramine on radiolabeled serotonin uptake into platelets in geriatric depression, *Biological Psychiatry* 25:687-691, 1989.

Spiker DG, Pugh DD: Combining tricyclic and monoamine oxidase inhibitors antidepressants, *Archives of General Psychiatry* 33:828, 1976.

Stein EM, Stein S, Linn MW: Geriatric sweet-tooth: a problem with tricyclics, *Journal of the American Geriatrics Society* 33:687-692, 1985.

vanMarwijk HWJ, Bekker FM, Nolan VA, Jansen PAF, vanNieuwkerk, et al: Lithium augmentation in geriatric depression, *Journal of Affective Disorders* 20:217-223, 1990.

Veith RC, Raskind MA, Caldwell JH, Barnes RF, Gumbrecht G, Ritchie JL: Cardiovascular effects of tricyclic antidepressants in depressed patients with chronic heart disease, *New England Journal of Medicine* 306:954-959, 1982.

Vestal RE, Cusak BJ: Pharmacology and aging, In Schneider E, Rowe JW: *Handbook of the Biology of Aging* (ed 3). New York, Academic Press, 1990, pp. 349-383.

Young RC, Alexopoulas G, Shamoian CA: *Depressive Disorders in the Aged . . . Sequella and Treatment Perspectives.* Scientific Exhibit, American Psychiatric Association (137th Annual Meeting). Los Angeles, California, May 5-11, 1984.

Young RC, Alexopoulas GS, Shindledecker R, Dahr AK, Kutt H: Plasma 10-hydroxinortriptyline and therapeutic response in geriatric depression, *Neuropsychopharmacology* 1:213-215, 1988.

20

Electroconvulsive Therapy

The initial therapies prescribed for treating depression in late life are usually antidepressant medications and psychotherapy. Clinicians are fortunate, however, to have adjunct therapies available that can complement or replace these interventions. Electroconvulsive therapy (ECT) is the most effective and one of the safest alternatives to traditional therapies for the severely depressed elderly.

ECT has been of great value in treating late life depression and is firmly established for severe depressive episodes. Convulsive therapies were introduced by von Meduna (1938) and were based on a series of observations in mental hospitals. Patients who experienced a spontaneous convulsion, usually associated with epilepsy, often experienced simultaneous remission of their symptoms. Von Meduna also observed that epilepsy and schizophrenia rarely occurred in the same patients. Camphor was the first seizure-inducing pharmacologic agent prescribed and was followed by the use of pentylenetetrazol (Metrazol). Cerletti and Bini (1938) substituted electrically induced seizures for pharmacologic convulsive therapies by developing a simple apparatus that used an alternating current whose source was an electric outlet. The technique has been greatly improved over the past 50 years.

In this chapter, after the case presentation, the indications, contraindications, and effectiveness of modern ECT in the elderly are reviewed. Then techniques of ECT are described with a special emphasis on modification of those techniques for the elderly. Adverse effects are discussed, with special attention directed to the cognitive deficits that are of great concern to patients receiving ECT. Finally, the long-term prognosis of older adults with severe depression who are treated with ECT is reviewed.

■ CASE PRESENTATION

A 71-year-old married man, a retired postal worker, was referred for inpatient therapy because of chronic and persistent complaints of pain, weight loss, and loss of interest in his usual activities. The patient reported no history of psychiatric disorder until 2 years before the referral at which time he withdrew progressively from his friends and family, complained of abdominal pains, and reported a 10-pound weight loss over 3 months.

His primary care physician referred him to a psychiatrist who admitted him to the hospital 18 months before the index admission. He was treated with imipramine and partially responded. On discharge, however, his symptoms soon returned and he was thereafter resistant to a variety of antidepressant medications. He was hospitalized on one other occasion, with little positive benefit. Throughout the 18 months between his first hospitalization and the index hospitalization, he was not so severely depressed that his family was concerned about suicide, but his preoccupation with physical problems, believing that he suffered from a cancer, was so much "unlike" the patient that the family sought additional help.

On index admission, the patient was found to be an alert, oriented, but disinterested and obviously depressed man whose depression manifested itself primarily through a flattened affect and somatic complaints. He reported no crying spells, no excessive guilt, and no suicidal ideation. A review of his history revealed that he had been treated with antidepressant therapy at adequate dosage with no effect. His medical condition was excellent for a 71 year old, and no evidence of physical difficulties could be identified. A computerized blood count was normal, electrolytes were normal, and his electrocardiogram (EKG) was normal. Given the chronicity of his depression and the significant change in his behavior over the prior 2 years, this patient was referred for ECT.

After appropriate workup, the patient received eight ECT treatments. He improved significantly, exhibited more interest in those around him, and even demonstrated a sense of humor after the fifth treatment. He also experienced significant memory loss (primarily an anterograde amnesia) during the ECT treatments.

The patient was discharged 2 days after the last ECT treatment and was begun on desipramine (50 mg po qhs). About 1 month after ECT, he reported that he was not sleeping as well as he had before the 2-year depressive episode but much better than he did during the episode. His wife complained that his memory was still somewhat impaired for recent events, although he had no difficulty in remembering remote events. She had difficulty in getting him to participate in activities outside the house. About 6 months after ECT, his sleep was greatly improved, his wife reported that his memory was virtually normal, and he was beginning to interact with family and old friends. About 1 year after ECT, his wife said that he was "totally back to normal." The patient was continued on desipramine because he experienced some sleep problems, especially on one occasion when the medication was withdrawn. The patient continued without a relapse of depression for 5 years, being evaluated by a psychiatrist at 6-month intervals. He enjoyed his retirement, maintained a sense of humor, and showed no evidence of any change in his mood during the 5-year follow-up.

■ INDICATIONS FOR ECT

Despite the negative reaction that often accompanies the mention of "shock" therapy, ECT has persisted as a treatment for severe depression since its introduction 50 years ago. This persistence is undoubtedly related to the obvious efficacy of the treatment for certain patients. From a summary of the literature, Weiner (1979) reported that ECT was considered the treatment of choice for certain conditions by more than

70% of psychiatrists. Since that time, the percentage has probably increased. Depression, especially depression with neurovegetative symptoms, such as sleep and appetite disturbance, psychomotor change, and mood-congruent psychotic symptoms, indicates a good prognosis from ECT in late life (Salzman, 1982; Weiner, 1982). Zorumski et al (1986) found ECT to be less effective in older adults with preexisting psychiatric disorders other than major depression, particularly if the preexisting condition was dementia or somatization disorder. Coryell et al (1985), however, found no evidence that ECT was less effective in the medically ill. Fraser and Glass (1980) also report that patients who experienced good outcomes from ECT in late life have higher scores on scales assessing guilt, agitation, overall severity of psychic anxiety, and impairment in work and outside interests. Mulsant et al (1991) found patients with psychotic depression in late life to improve more with ECT than patients with nonpsychotic depression. They also found that patients with organic mental disorders experienced the same improvement as other patients. Although ECT is an extremely effective treatment for depression in late life, it is not the first choice of treatment, even for severe depression.

Paul et al (1981) found ECT effective in about 80% of drug nonresponders overall. This appears to be the same for older persons as for persons earlier in the life cycle (Fraser and Glass, 1980; Kramer, 1987). Kendall (1981) notes that ECT is the first choice among treatments for the severely depressed who do not respond to medications, especially in individuals with life-threatening symptoms, such as refusal to eat or marked suicidal ideation. The Consensus Conference on ECT (1985) recommended that the immediate risk of suicide that cannot be managed otherwise is another indication for ECT.

ECT is also an effective treatment for mania in late life. Burke et al (1987) found that more than 90% of elderly manic patients show at least a partial improvement in manic symptoms after ECT. Although the issue has not been resolved in the literature, there is some suggestion that bilateral ECT may be more effective than unilateral ECT for treating manic episodes (Small, et al, 1988).

Magni et al (1988) studied 11 depressed patients who failed to respond to at least one course of antidepressant therapy and at least seven bilateral treatments with ECT, compared with 19 patients who did respond to ECT. The correlates of ECT nonresponse with onset of physical illness during the index episode, fewer life events preceeding the onset of the index episode, and a higher frequency of previous depressive episodes of long duration. There was some trend for the nonresponders to be older and bipolar, although the number of patients studied was far too small to generalize.

In a recent study by Benbow (1991), 205 practicing geriatric psychiatrists completed a questionnaire assessing their opinions about the use of ECT in late life. There is significant agreement regarding the indications for ECT in the elderly. They include the following: a depressive illness that fails to respond to tricyclic antidepressants (84%); a depressive illness in which the previous episode responded to ECT but not tricyclics (92%); a psychotic depressive illness (76%); and depressive illness with high risk for suicide (82%).

■ CONTRAINDICATIONS

There are no absolute contraindications to ECT. Three relative contraindications must be considered before administering ECT, however. The first is a central nervous system (CNS) lesion with evidence of increased intracranial pressure. Shapiro et al

(1957) suggest that a CNS lesion with increased intracranial pressure was an absolute contraindication. The seizure induced by ECT can produce a further increase in pressure, thus potentially leading to a life-threatening herniation of the brain stem. Coffey and Weiner (1990) suggest, however, that even an increase in intercranial pressure may be managed during ECT if the indications for the treatment are sufficient.

Cardiovascular complications are common side effects of ECT (Elliot et al, 1982; Zorumski et al). ECT is associated with profound changes in blood pressure and heart rate and can place significant strain on the cardiac reserve of patients with coronary artery disease, congestive heart failure, and hypertensive cardiovascular disease. Persons with a history of ventricular arrhythmias or those who have suffered a myocardial infarction are especially at risk. Steen et al (1978) found that patients with a recent myocardial infarction have a high risk of reinfarction associated with general anesthesia administered within 3 months of the first infarction. The same may be true for persons suffering a recent cerebrovascular accident.

The third relative contraindication is medication (Zorumski et al, 1988). Many drugs raise the seizure threshold, such as anticonvulsants, antiarrhythmic drugs, benzodiazepines, and sedative hypnotic agents (but these can be used during ECT if absolutely necessary). Some tricyclic antidepressants have neuron-membrane stabilizing properties and can interfere with the induction of seizures. Tricyclic antidepressants and other anticholinergic drugs also may augment the tendency of ECT to produce acute confusion and memory impairment. For this reason, peripheral-acting anticholinergics are now used for treatments before ECT, such as glycopyrrolate rather than atropine.

Other medications interfere with metabolism of succinylcholine and lead to a significant prolongation of the apnea after ECT (Packman et al, 1978). These include cholinesterase inhibitors (e.g., those found in some eyedrops prescribed for glaucoma), antibiotics, lithium carbonate, and the monoamine-oxidase inhibitors. The monoamine-oxidase inhibitors may also cause blood pressure changes. Lithium carbonate may also contribute to an increase in confusion and a spontaneous persistence of seizures during ECT.

■ EFFECTIVENESS OF ECT IN THE ELDERLY

Many investigators have documented the effectiveness of ECT in older adults. In 163 patients who were 65 years of age and older Godber et al (1987) found that 51% fully recovered and 23% were much improved after an average of 11 treatments. Those persons who improved were not necessarily individuals who spontaneously developed depressive episodes. In fact, 74% of those who improved had experienced precipitating events to the depressive illness, such as a physical illness and bereavement. In a study of 193 courses of ECT in 122 older patients, Benbow (1987) found that 80% were well or considerably improved at discharge. Most of these patients received between eight to ten treatments. At discharge, 52% were considered well and 28% much improved. Other investigators have generally agreed that approximately 80% of patients, regardless of age, respond positively to ECT. Fraser and Glass (1980) found a good response rate of over 90%, whereas Karlinsky et al (1984) found a good outcome in approximately 50%.

There is debate in the literature regarding the effect of age in response to ECT. Benbow (1989) suggests that older patients respond as well to ECT as younger patients.

Cattan et al (1990), in contrast, found a good outcome occurred significantly more often in persons 65 to 79 years of age (33%) than in persons 80+ years of age and older (13%). When both moderate and good outcomes were combined, however, there was no difference in response by age.

■ THE MEDICAL WORKUP FOR ECT

Once the clinician has determined that the older adult requires ECT, the treatment should be explained to the patient and his/her family. Many elders have exaggerated fears of ECT and are initially resistant. A careful and caring explanation, with emphasis on the safety and efficacy of treatment, usually alleviates patient and family fears. The family is often essential in encouraging the patient to agree to the treatment. Once the patient has agreed and has signed the release form, reasons for treating the patient should be documented in the chart. The nursing staff usually takes the patient to the treatment room before the treatment, explains the physical setting, and answers any questions about treatment.

The diagnostic workup for the patient who receives ECT is presented in Table 20-1. Other than the routine diagnostic procedures, special attention should be paid to the EKG, magnetic resonance imaging (MRI), or computerized tomography (CT) scans of the brain, and spinal x-ray films. MRI and CT scans can be helpful in identifying a cerebral neoplasm. The EKG alerts the clinician to an undocumented myocardial infarction, cardiac arrhythmia, or congestive heart failure. The identification of moderate-to-severe hypertension requires the stabilization of blood pressure before treatment is initiated.

Spinal x rays are important for documenting any evidence of compression fractures

TABLE 20-1. ECT Diagnostic Workup

Diagnostic Procedure	Notes
History	Previous history of ECT
	History of cardiovascular disease, neurologic disease
	Present drug use
	Family history of peculiar drug reactions or response to ECT
Physical examination	Evidence of cardiac arrhythmias, hypertension, neurologic signs of a brain tumor
Baseline mental status examination	Presence or absence of an organic brain syndrome, brief psychologic testing
Routine laboratory tests	Evidence of undetected medical illness
Complete blood cell count, urinalysis, chest x ray, blood chemistry studies	Routine medical screen
Special studies	
EKG	Evidence of cardiac arrhythmias or previous myocardial infarction
CT or MRI scan	Evidence of cerebral mass lesion
Spinal x rays	Evidence of compression fractures or degenerative spinal disease

or degenerative spinal disease. Although spinal disease does not preclude the use of ECT, the clinician should document any preexisting disease in case a compression fracture does occur during treatment. The use of a structured, brief cognitive rating scale is helpful before and during ECT. The test can be repeated after each treatment and after the treatments are completed. In most cases (as indicated later in this chapter), cognitive function actually improves as mood improves, given the cognitive dysfunction associated with the depressive disorder.

The patient should also be thoroughly evaluated by an anesthesiologist. ECT is commonly given in tertiary care facilities with a specialized team providing the treatments. The anesthesiologist is a key member of this team and should review medications and other medical problems that might complicate the successful treatment of the older adult.

■ TECHNIQUES OF ECT

Electroconvulsive treatments may be given at any time of the day but the preferred time is early morning, since patients will not worry or become obsessed about the treatments throughout the day, and breakfast can be served after the patient awakens from treatment. For the first treatment, it is helpful for the attending physician to accompany the patient to the treatment room and to be present during the treatment. In many teaching hospitals a specialist on the staff administers ECT and therefore the attending physician may not be present, thus heightening the patient's anxiety. If treatment is prescribed for the morning, no food should be given after midnight. The patient is instructed to empty his or her bladder and remove false teeth before treatment. About 30 minutes before treatment, an anticholinergic agent is given, usually glycopyrrolate (a peripheral-acting anticholinergic agent that does not increase problems with memory). Treatments are generally given three times per week.

Treatments now prescribed are increasingly unilateral, nondominant, and the stimulus is a pulse. Sinusoidal waves are associated with greater confusion than brief pulse stimulation (Daniel and Crovitz, 1983). A short-acting anesthetic (e.g., methohexital) is administered after the administration of a muscle relaxer (succinylcholine). Electrodes are placed over the frontotemporal and centroparietal areas and the stimulus is administered. Seizure activity is monitored by electroencephalographic tracings and cardiovascular response is monitored by continuous EKG and repeated measures of blood pressure. Most practitioners accept a seizure of 25 to 30 seconds as therapeutic. If a seizure does not occur after the initial stimulus, the patient can be restimulated 30 to 60 seconds afterwards with a higher energy stimulus. The seizure threshold is typically higher in males than in females and is higher in the elderly than younger persons (Coffey and Weiner, 1990).

Older persons are less likely to have a prolonged seizure requiring termination than younger persons. If a seizure is prolonged, it can be aborted by methohexital. Older persons are also more likely not to seizure with the first stimulus and therefore require higher electrical parameters (Hinkle et al, 1986). The seizure may be enhanced in duration by the use of caffeine in special cases (Coffey et al, 1987).

Considerable debate exists regarding the relative benefits of unilateral versus bilateral treatments. Small et al (1985) suggest that bilateral ECT may be more effective in the manic elderly than in unilateral patients. Fink (1985) notes that bilateral ECT is more often associated with memory impairment than unilateral treatment. That fewer cognitive difficulties are associated with unilateral treatments is now well-accepted (Abrams and Fink, 1985). In a study of 29 patients randomly assigned to unilateral versus bilateral ECT, Fraser and Glass (1980), found that all patients exhibited full recovery at 3 months and the number of treatments did not vary between unilateral and bilateral. Memory function was equally impaired in both groups, but after treatment recovery time was significantly longer in the bilateral group.

To ensure the maximum likelihood of successful treatment, all medications should be discontinued during treatment, if possible. As noted previously, lithium carbonate may prolong the half-life of succinylcholine and lead to acute neurologic toxicity and delirium. Benzodiazepines and sedative hypnotics increase the seizure threshold and monoamine-oxidase inhibitors can prolong the action of succinylcholine. The anticholinergic effects of the antidepressants may increase memory problems during therapy. There is no evidence that either the use of lithium or antidepressant therapy during the treatment improves the short- or long-term effects of ECT. If sleep problems are severe during the ECT treatments, then chlorylhydrate, a short-acting sedative hypnotic, is the preferred treatment (usually 500 mg at night). If agitation is a major problem during the course of treatment, haloperidol is the preferred treatment, as opposed to other antipsychotic agents or benzodiazepines.

After treatment, patients are typically placed on antidepressant medication for at least 6 months to prevent relapse. Patients who have not responded to tricyclic antidepressants (but who did not experience significant side effects from these medications) still benefit from antidepressant therapy after ECT. If the likelihood of relapse is high and the patient cannot tolerate antidepressant medication, then maintenance ECT may be indicated. Such treatments can be given as outpatient procedures and are usually given weekly for the first month after remission and then gradually decreased in frequency. Although outpatient ECT is expensive, it is a safe and frequently effective alternative for individuals at high risk for relapse (and subsequent hospitalization).

■ ADVERSE EFFECTS

Despite the relative safety of ECT, about one third of older persons who receive ECT experience at least one complication during the course of treatment. Burke et al (1987) found 50% of the complaints were falls, yet falls were no more frequent among inpatients undergoing ECT than other elderly inpatients on the ward at the same time. The major complications fell into the following three major groups: cardiovascular problems, severe confusion, and falls. These adverse effects were strongly related to age and health status. About 75% of individuals in two studies reviewed over 5 years had experienced complication during ECT. However, there was no relation between adverse effects and treatment outcome. Mulsant et al (1991), in a study of 40 patients 60+ years of age and older who received ECT, found that 7% developed significant medical complications, and 5% developed symptomatic vertebral compression fractures.

Cattan et al (1990) confirmed these findings, noting that, compared with the young-old (less than 80 years of age), the old-old (more than 80 years of age) given ECT were more likely to suffer cardiovascular complication and falls. Nevertheless, these investigators found ECT to be relatively safe regardless of age. The cardiovascular side effect (bradycardia, sinus arrhythmias, and atrial premature contractions) may occur immediately after the electrode stimulus and can be diminished by anticholinergics, such as glycopyrrolate or atropine. Most of these adverse effects are not serious. Alexopoulos et al (1984), in a retrospective chart review of 199 patients 65 years of age and older who received ECT, found that 10 suffered cardiovascular damage (three had myocardial infarctions and there was one death, with five individuals suffering some degree of heart failure). In addition, five subjects suffered aspiration pneumonia. Overall mortality from ECT ranges from 0.002% to 0.004% per treatment and 0.01% to 0.03% per patient (compared with mortality for anesthesia alone of 0.003% to 0.04% [Abrams and Fink, 1985]).

Although less severe, the more common side effects from ECT are headaches, nausea, and muscle pains (Coffey and Weiner, 1990). Headaches usually respond to mild analgesia. Although compression fractures can still occur, the use of muscle relaxants have greatly reduced their frequency.

There has been considerable interest in whether ECT may lead to permanent brain damage. Coffey et al (1988) found no short-term memory loss with ECT in nine patients, many of whom had changes on MRI scanning. There was no evidence that ECT produced long-term structural changes in the brain. Weiner (1981) found that EEG slowing occurs transiently after ECT, but that the EEG slowing returns to baseline by 1 month after ECT and is a function of the number of ECT treatments. EEG slowing is reduced by the use of unilateral electrode placement. In three patients with deep white matter hyperintensities and ventricular enlargement, Botteron et al (1991) found that these patients were less likely to respond to ECT (although the numbers are small) and that patients with caudate hyperintensities developed a prolonged interictal ECT-induced delirium. Delirium after ECT, however, is relatively rare.

There is some concern that individuals who receive ECT may be at greater risk for suicide. Rich et al (1984) could find no data to support the belief that suicide risk increases with improvement during ECT. The improvement in mood, for example, appears to predate the increase in energy and thus the risk for suicide may actually be decreased.

■ COGNITIVE EFFECTS

By far the most frequent adverse effects of ECT are interference with cognition. There is little evidence of permanent brain damage associated with ECT, although there have been case reports of neurologic deterioration closely after ECT (Weiner, 1981). These neurologic deficits usually derive from a cerebral vascular cause that may be fatal.

Memory loss (primarily retrograde and to some extent anterograde amnesia) is not specific to the seizure and is similar to changes in posttraumatic amnesia. A significant fraction of patients report memory difficulties months past treatment with ECT at the point at which objective measures of memory function reveal no cognitive abnormality (Squire and Chase, 1975; Small, 1974). Complaints usually persist of a spotty amnesia for past memories. The memory problem may be event-specific. On general testing, most investigators do not find significant memory loss 1 month after ECT (Cronholm and Molinda, 1964; Squire and Chase, 1975).

Frith et al (1983) studied 70 severely depressed patients randomly assigned to receive eight real or eight sham ECT treatments, and these patients were further subdivided on the basis of the degree of recovery from the depressive episode. In comparison with a nondepressed control group the depressed patients (both those who received ECT and those who did not) were impaired on a wide range of tests of memory and concentration. After treatment with ECT, performance on most tests had improved compared with those who received sham ECT. Real ECT increased impairment of concentration, short-term memory and learning, but significantly facilitated access to remote memories. At 6-month follow-up, all differences between the real and sham ECT had disappeared. There is some evidence that a subgroup of treatment-resistant patients (those who have a poor outcome after real ECT) were more likely to complain of memory problems 6 months later.

The clinical efficacy of ECT does not appear to be related to memory loss (Squire, 1984). In a comparison study of ECT and imipramine, Kelev et al (1989) found both ECT and imipramine treated patients showed a deficit in recent anterograde memory relative to pretreatment performance. ECT patients also had a significant impairment in retrograde remote memory (but not the imipramine-treated patients) 21 days after ECT treatments were completed (and at a comparative point for patients on imipramine).

There has been considerable interest as to whether ECT causes more memory problems in the old than in young. Fraser and Glass (1978) suggest that the elderly may be at greater risk for cognitive impairment from ECT secondary to diminished cognitive reserves. Rush, et al (1990), in a study of 12 elderly patients who were depressed and treated with ECT, found that one week after ECT there was a significant improvement in depression and ward behavior, but cognitive functioning was unchanged. They concluded that ECT was not associated with a functionally significant decrease in cognitive performance, however. Mulsant et al (1991), in a study of 40 patients 60 years of age and older given ECT, found that 31% were confused during ECT and that 10% reported persistent confusion at discharge from the hospital. Bachar et al (1990) found that older adults who respond to ECT actually reminisced more than they had before the ECT treatments (thus suggesting that remote memory is not significantly impaired and that older adults treated with ECT do recover their memory).

■ PROGNOSIS

Overall, ECT is an effective treatment for older adults, even elderly persons who do not respond to other psychologic and pharmacologic therapies. Nevertheless, the relapse rate from ECT can be relatively high. Godber et al (1987), in a study of 163 patients treated with ECT (all 65 years of age and older) and followed for 3 years (an average number of treatments of 11), found that, after the original course of ECT, 51% were fully recovered and 23% were somewhat improved. Two thirds experienced one or more relapses within 3 years, but one half of those who experienced a relapse regained a full remission. Benbow (1987) found that older patients improved with ECT and, when relapses occurred, they usually responded well to antidepressant therapy and therefore experienced a good long-term prognosis. Strain et al (1968) found a 34% to 37% relapse rate 1 year after ECT in 96 depressives (regardless of age). Mulsant et al (1991), in a study of 40 older patients who received ECT, found that all patients experienced a decrease in depressive symptoms and two thirds experienced a complete or partial remission from the depressive symptoms at discharge.

A number of investigators have examined predictors of recovery and relapse with ECT. Fink et al (1986), in a study of six patients whose dexamethasone-suppression test (DST) normalized after ECT, found that all remained well at 9-month follow-up. In a projective study after this initial finding, these investigators found that the risk of relapse was higher for patients with an abnormal DST at termination of ECT. Yet there was no relationship between the initial DST score change and DST with clinical outcome at discharge. In 50 hospitalized patients, Papakostas et al (1981) found no relationship between DST results and improvement or rehospitalization overall. Coffey et al (1988), in nine patients who had MRI scanning performed before and after ECT, found ECT produced no acute effects in brain structure (i.e., cortical atrophy). Brain abnormalities before ECT were common and did not predict outcome with ECT.

Other investigators have explored the relationship between ECT recovery, age, and cognition. Wessner and Winokur (1989) compared patients 40 years of age and older with persons less than 40. They found that ECT reduced the rate of chronicity of depressive illness in older patients but was associated with increased chronicity (i.e., relapse) after treatment in younger persons. Liang et al (1988), in two patients with mixed depression and dementia, found behavioral and mood improvement after treatment with ECT, but there was no improvement in cognition. These data parallel data regarding the efficacy of antidepressant therapy in improving mood in mixed depression and dementia but not improving cognition.

Other investigators have found that the risk of relapse can be mitigated by the use of maintenance medication. Perry and Tsuang (1979) found ECT followed by either lithium carbonate or tricyclic antidepressants to be more effective for preventing relapse from unipolar depression than ECT alone. Seager and Byrd (1962) found that, at 6 months, 17% of their subjects had experienced a relapse who were placed on imipramine after ECT versus 69% of the subjects who were placed on placebo after ECT.

REFERENCES

Abrams R, Fink M: The present status of unilateral ECT: some recommendations, *Journal of Affective Disorders* 7:245-247, 1985.

Alexopoulos GS, Shamoian CJ, Lucas J, et al: Medical problems in geriatric psychiatric patients and younger controls during electroconvulsive therapy, *Journal of the American Geriatrics Society* 32:651-654, 1984.

Bachar E, Dasberg H, Shapira B, Lerer B: Reminiscing in depressed, aging patients: effects of ECT and antidepressants, *International Journal of Geriatric Psychiatry* 5:251-256, 1990.

Benbow SM: Old-age psychiatrists' views of the use of ECT, *International Journal of Geriatric Psychiatry* 6:317-322, 1991.

Benbow SM: The role of electroconvulsive therapy in the treatment of depressive illness in old age, *British Journal of Psychiatry* 155:147-152, 1989.

Benbow SM: The use of electroconvulsive therapy in old-age psychiatry, *International Journal of Geriatric Psychiatry* 2:25-30, 1987.

Botteron K, Figiel GS, Zorumski CF: Electroconvulsive therapy in patients with late-onset psychoses and structural brain changes, *Journal of Geriatric Psychiatry and Neurology* 4:44-47, 1991.

Burke WJ, Rubin EH, Zorumski CF, Wetzel RD: The safety of ECT in geriatric psychiatry, *Journal of the American Geriatrics Society* 35:516-521, 1987.

Cattan RA, Barry PP, Mead G, Reefe WE, Gay A, et al: Electroconvulsive therapy in octogenarians, *Journal of the American Geriatrics Society* 38:753-758, 1990.

Cerletti V, Bini L: L'elettroshock, *Archivo Generale di Neurologia, Psichiatriaca e Psichoanalisi* 19:226, 1938.

Coffey CE, Figiel GS, Djang WT, Sullivan DC, Herfkens RJ, et al: Effects of ECT on brain structure: a pilot perspective magnetic resonance imaging study, *American Journal of Psychiatry* 145:701-706, 1988.

Coffey CE, Figiel GS, Djang WT, Cress M, Saunders WB, et al: Leukoencephalopathy in elderly depressed patients referred for ECT, *Biological Psychiatry* 24:143-161, 1988.

Coffey CE, Hinkle PE, Weiner RD, et al: Electroconvulsive therapy of depressin in patients with white matter hyperintensity, *Biological Psychiatry* 22:629-636, 1987.

Coffey CE, Weiner RD: Electroconvulsive therapy: an update, *Hospital and Community Psychiatry* 41:515-521, 1990.

Coryell W, Pohl B, Zimmerman M: Outcome following electroconvulsive therapy: a comparison of primary and secondary depression, *Convulsive Therapy* 1:10-14, 1985.

Cronholm B, Molander L: Memory disturbances after electroconvulsive therapy, V: conditions one month after a series of treatments, *ACTA Psychiatrica Scandinavia* 40:212-216, 1964.

Daniel F, Crovitz HF: Acute memory impairment following electroconvulsive therapy, I: Effects of electrostimulus waveform and number of treatments, *Acta Psychiatrica Scandinavica* 67:1-7, 1983.

Elliot TL, Linz DH, Kane JA: Electroconvulsive therapy: pretreatment medical evaluation, *Archives of Internal Medicine* 142:979-981, 1982.

Fink M: Reducing memory loss in electroconvulsive therapy, *Convulsive Therapy* 1:77-80, 1985.

Fink M, Gujavarty K, Greenberg GL: Serial dexamethasone suppression tests in ECT, *Clinical Neuropharmacology* 9(suppl 4):444-446, 1986.

Fraser RM, Glass IB: Recovery from ECT in elderly patients, *British Journal of Psychiatry* 133:524-528, 1978.

Fraser RM, Glass IB: Unilateral and bilateral ECT in elderly patients, *Acta Psychiatrica Scandinavica* 62:13-31, 1980.

Frith CD, Stevens M, Johnstone EC, Deakin JFW, Lawler P, et al: Effects of ECT and depression on various aspects of memory, *British Journal of Psychiatry* 142:610-617, 1983.

Godber C, Rosenvinge H, Wilkinson D, Smithes J: Depression in old age: prognosis after ECT, *International Journal of Geriatric Psychiatry* 2:19-24, 1987.

Hinkle P, Coffey CE, Weiner R, Moore J: *ECT Seizure Duration Varies with Age.* Paper presented at the Annual Meeting of the American Geriatrics Society, 1986.

Karlinsky H, Shulman KT: The clinical use of electroconvulsive therapy in old age, *Journal of the American Geriatric Society* 32:183-186, 1984.

Kelev A, Ben-Tsivi E, Shapira B, Drexler H, Carasso R, et al: Distinct memory impairment following electroconvulsive therapy and imipramine, *Psychological Medicine* 19:111-119, 1989.

Kendall RE: The present status of electroconvulsive therapy, *British Journal of Psychiatry* 139:265-283, 1981.

Kramer BA: Electroconvulsive therapy use in geriatric depression, *Journal of Nervous and Mental Diseases* 175:233-235, 1987.

Liang RA, Lam RW, Ancill RJ: ECT and the treatment of mixed depression and dementia, *British Journal of Psychiatry* 152:281-284, 1988.

Magni G, Fishman M, Helms E: Correlates of ECT-resistant depression in the elderly, *Journal of Clinical Psychiatry* 49:405-407, 1988.

Mulsant BH, Rosen J, Thornton JE, Zubenko GS: A prospective naturalistic study of electroconvulsive therapy in late-life depression, *Journal of Geriatric Psychiatry and Neurology* 4:3-13, 1991.

Packman PM, Meyer DA, Verdun RM: Hazards of succinyl administration during electrotherapy, *Archives of General Psychiatry* 35:1137-1141, 1978.

Papakostas Y, Fink M, Lee J, Irwin P, Johnson L: Neuroendocrine measures in psychiatric patients: course and outcome with ECT, *Psychiatry Research* 4:55-64, 1981.

Paul SM, Extein I, Calil HM, Potter WZ, Chodoff P, et al: Use of ECT with treatment-resistant depressed patients at the National Institute of Mental Health, *American Journal of Psychiatry* 138:486-490, 1981.

Perry P, Tsuang MT: Treatment of unipolar depression following electroconvulsive therapy, *Journal of Affective Disorders* 1:123-129, 1979.

Rich CL, Spiker DG, Jewell SW, et al: The efficacy of ECT, I: response rate in depressive episodes, *Psychiatry Research* 11:167-176, 1984.

Rush MJ, Ackerman SH, Burton SH, Shindledecker RD: Cognitive effects of ECT in the elderly: preliminary findings, *International Journal of Geriatric Psychiatry* 5:115-118, 1990.

Salzman C: Electroconvulsive therapy in the elderly patient, *Psychiatric Clinics of North America* 5:191-197, 1982.

Seager CB, Bird L: Imipramine with electrical treatment in depression—a controlled trial, *Journal of Mental Science* 108:704-707, 1962.

Shapiro MF, Goldberg HH: Electroconvulsive therapy in patients with a structural disease of the central nervous system, *American Journal of Medical Science* 233:286-295, 1957.

Small GL, Small IF, Milstein V, Kellams JJ, Klapper MH: Manic symptoms: an indication for bilateral ECT, *Biological Psychiatry* 20:125-134, 1985.

Small IF: Inhalant convulsive therapy. In Find M, Kity S, McGaugh J, Williams TA (eds): *Psychobiology of Convulsive Therapy.* Washington, DC, Winston, 1974, pp. 65-77.

Small JG, Klapper MH, Kellams JJ, Miller MJ, Milstein V, et al: Electroconvulsive treatment compared with lithium in the management of manic states, *Archives of General Psychiatry* 45:727-732, 1988.

Squire LR: ECT and memory dysfunction. In Lerer B, Weiner RD, Belmaker RH (eds): *ECT: Basic Mechanisms.* London, John Libbey, 1984.

Squire LR, Chase PM: Memory functions six to nine months after electroconvulsive therapy, *Archives of General Psychiatry* 32:1157-1164, 1975.

Steen PA, Tinker JH, Tarhin S: Myocardal reinfarction after anesthesia in surgery, *Journal of the American Medical Association* 239:2566-2570, 1978.

Strain JJ, Brunschwig L, Duffy JP, et al: Comparison of therapeutic effects and memory changes with bilateral and unilateral ECT, *American Journal of Psychiatry* 125:294-304, 1968.

von Meduna LJ: General discussion of cardizol therapy, *American Journal of Psychiatry* 94:40 (suppl), 1938.

Weiner RD: Electroconvulsive therapy: do persistent CNS changes occur? *Journal of Psychiatric Treatment and Evaluation* 3:309-313, 1981.

Weiner RD: The psychiatric use of electrically-induced seizures, *American Journal of Psychiatry* 136:1507, 1979.

Weiner RD: The role of electroconvulsive therapy in the treatment of depression in the elderly, *Journal of the American Geriatrics Society* 30:710-712, 1982.

Wessner RB, Winokur G: The influence of age on the natural history of unipolar depression when treated with electroconvulsive therapy, *European Archives of Psychiatry and Neurological Sciences* 238:149-154, 1989.

Zorumski CF, Rubin EH, Burke WJ: Electroconvulsive therapy for the elderly: a review, *Hospital and Community Psychiatry* 39:643-647, 1988.

Index